Baillière's
CLINICAL OBSTETRICS AND GYNAECOLOGY
INTERNATIONAL PRACTICE AND RESEARCH

Baillière's
CLINICAL OBSTETRICS AND GYNAECOLOGY
INTERNATIONAL PRACTICE AND RESEARCH

Volume 6/Number 4
December 1992

Prostaglandins

M. G. ELDER MD, FRCS, FRCOG
Guest Editor

Baillière Tindall
London Philadelphia Sydney Tokyo Toronto

This book is printed on acid-free paper.

Baillière Tindall 24–28 Oval Road,
W.B. Saunders London NW1 7DX

The Curtis Center, Independence Square West,
Philadelphia, PA 19106–3399, USA

55 Horner Avenue
Toronto, Ontario M8Z 4X6, Canada

Harcourt Brace Jovanovich Group (Australia) Pty Ltd,
30–52 Smidmore Street, Marrickville, NSW 2204, Australia

Harcourt Brace Jovanovich Japan, Inc,
Ichibancho Central Building,
22-1 Ichibancho, Chiyoda-ku, Tokyo 102, Japan

ISSN 0950–3552

ISBN 0–7020–1694–2 (single copy)

Baillière's Clinical Obstetrics and Gynaecology is published four times each year by Baillière Tindall. Prices for Volume 6 (1992) are:

TERRITORY	ANNUAL SUBSCRIPTION	SINGLE ISSUE
Europe including UK	£65.00 post free	£27.50 post free
All other countries	Consult your local Harcourt Brace Jovanovich Office	

The editor of this publication is Catriona Byres, Baillière Tindall, 24–28 Oval Road, London NW1 7DX.

Baillière's Clinical Obstetrics and Gynaecology was published from 1983 to 1986 as *Clinics in Obstetrics and Gynaecology*.

Typeset by Phoenix Photosetting, Chatham.
Printed and bound in Great Britain by Mackays of Chatham PLC, Chatham, Kent.

Contributors to this issue

ASIF S. AHMED PhD, BSc(Hons), Wellcome Research Fellow, Department of Obstetrics and Gynaecology, The Rosie Maternity Hospital, University of Cambridge, Robinson Way, Cambridge CB2 2SW, UK.

HENK A. BREMER MD, Research Fellow in Perinatal Medicine, Institute of Obstetrics and Gynaecology, School of Medicine and Health Sciences, Erasmus University, P.O. Box 1738, 3000 DR Rotterdam, The Netherlands.

MARC BYGDEMAN MD, PhD, Professor, Department of Obstetrics and Gynaecology, Karolinska Hospital; Chief Medical Officer, Karolinska Hospital, S-10401 Stockholm, Sweden.

ANDREW A. CALDER MD(Glas), FRCP(Glas), FRCOG, Head of Department of Obstetrics and Gynaecology, Centre for Reproductive Biology, University of Edinburgh; Honorary Consultant in Obstetrics and Gynaecology, Simpson Memorial Maternity Pavilion and Royal Infirmary of Edinburgh, Edinburgh, UK.

GAUTAM CHAUDHURI MD, PhD, Department of Pharmacology, UCLA School of Medicine, 10833 Le Conte Avenue, Room 22-188, Los Angeles, California 90025, USA.

CHRISTIAN H. EGARTER MD, Associate Professor, Department of Obstetrics and Gynaecology, Krankenhaus Vöcklabruck, Hatschekstraße 24, A-4840 Vöcklabruck, Austria.

M. G. ELDER MD, FRCS, FRCOG, Professor, Institute of Obstetrics and Gynaecology, Royal Postgraduate Medical School, Hammersmith Hospital, Du Cane Road, London W12 0HS, UK.

IAN S. FRASER MD, BSc(Hons), FRCOG, FRACOG, CREI, Associate Professor of Obstetrics and Gynaecology, University of Sydney, NSW 2006, Australia; Visiting Medical Officer, King George V Memorial and Royal Prince Alfred Hospitals, Camperdown, Sydney, Australia.

TIMOTHY J. GELETY MD, Department of Obstetrics and Gynaecology, UCLA School of Medicine, 10833 Le Conte Avenue, Room 22-188, Los Angeles, California 90025, USA.

IAN A. GREER MD, MRCP, MRCOG, Muirhead Professor of Obstetrics and Gynaecology, University of Glasgow; Honorary Consultant, Obstetrics and Gynaecology, Glasgow Royal Infirmary and Royal Maternity Hospital, Glasgow, UK.

PETER HUSSLEIN MD, Associate Professor, Department of Obstetrics and Gynaecology, 1st University of Vienna, Spitalgasse 23, A-1090 Wien, Austria.

MARC J. N. C. KEIRSE MD, Professor, Department of Obstetrics, Gynaecology and Reproduction, Leiden University Hospital, PO Box 9600, NL-2300 RC Leiden, The Netherlands.

MURRAY D. MITCHELL D.Phil, Professor, Department of Obstetrics and Gynaecology; Director, Division of Reproductive Sciences, University of Utah School of Medicine, Salt Lake City, Utah 84132, USA.

STEPHEN K. SMITH Professor of Obstetrics and Gynaecology, Department of Obstetrics and Gynaecology, The Rosie Maternity Hospital, University of Cambridge, Robinson Way, Cambridge CB2 2SW, UK.

LASSE VIINIKKA MD, Senior Lecturer in Clinical Chemistry, Head of Laboratory Services, Children's Hospital, University of Helsinki, SF-00290 Helsinki, Finland.

HENK C. S. WALLENBURG MD, PhD, FRCOG, Professor and Director of Obstetrics, Institute of Obstetrics and Gynaecology, School of Medicine and Health Sciences, Erasmus University, P.O. Box 1738, 3000 DR Rotterdam, The Netherlands.

OLAVI YLIKORKALA Professor and Chairman, Department of Obstetrics and Gynaecology, University of Helsinki, Haartmaninkatu 2, 00290 Helsinki, Finland.

Table of contents

PREVIOUS ISSUES

FORTHCOMING ISSUE

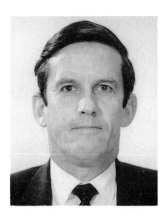

Foreword

Prostaglandins have been prominent in obstetrics and gynaecology for the last two decades, both as therapeutic tools and because of our increasing knowledge of their role in reproduction. They were first used clinically for induction of labour in the early 1970s and since then, obstetricians in many European countries have become used to their benefits. They are now widely used for cervical ripening, induction of labour, induction of second trimester abortions and increasingly so for first trimester abortions. What has taken longer to realize is their importance in a variety of aspects of reproductive physiology.

Arachidonic acid is metabolized via cyclo-oxygenase, lipoxygenase and epoxygenase enzyme pathways. The prostaglandins that we are familiar with are cyclo-oxygenase products and it is these that we appreciate as important second messengers. The roles of the lipoxygenase and epoxygenase products, of which there are many, are still unclear. Much research needs to be done to evaluate which compounds are important in reproduction and what their roles are. In five to ten years time there may well be a volume similar to this one addressing these aspects.

At present, however, the purpose of this volume is to examine systematically the biochemical role of the cyclo-oxygenase products and the processes in which they are involved in the reproductive organs. An understanding of this is crucial to providing a platform of knowledge on which to base improvements in treatment. The knowledge that prostaglandins cause uterine contractions and hence pain, and that women with primary dysmenorrhoea released excessive amounts of prostaglandins from the endometrium at the time of menstruation led to the use of non-steroidal anti-inflammatory drugs, which inhibit cyclo-oxygenase and so prostaglandin production, as effective treatments for dysmenorrhoea. However, much more needs to be known before manipulation of the many complex reproductive processes can take place logically.

While our knowledge of the role of prostaglandins in intracellular biochemistry has been advancing in the last five to ten years, there have been fewer advances on the purely clinical front. The development of new vehicles for the release of prostaglandins and of prostaglandin analogues are the most important recent advancements. This volume should bring doctors up to date with recent clinical advances and give them an insight into the scientific developments that are taking place. It should also provide a useful reference volume for the scientist wishing to be up to date with recent developments in the field. The contributors are all internationally well known and bring a very considerable experience to bear on the content of the chapters which they have written. I am grateful to them all for their contributions and as a consequence, this volume is as comprehensive and as up to date as any in the field of prostaglandins in reproduction.

M. G. ELDER

1

Biochemistry of the prostaglandins

MURRAY D. MITCHELL

INTRODUCTION

In 1935 von Euler first proposed the name 'prostaglandin' for one of the active principles in extracts that he was studying (von Euler, 1935). Information on these substances remained limited for over 30 years. From the 1960s onwards, however, a veritable explosion of interest and publications has occurred. This chapter provides a general overview of prostaglandin structure and nomenclature, biosynthesis and its inhibition and, finally, metabolism. Since these basic characteristics have not changed substantially with time, the background information will be provided with emphasis on the original descriptions and how the facts were deduced. Those who desire more detailed information on specific characteristics are directed to several excellent recent reviews (Smith, 1986, 1989; Eling et al, 1990; Vane and Botting, 1990; Holtzman, 1991; Smith et al, 1991).

PROSTAGLANDIN STRUCTURE AND NOMENCLATURE

The absolute configuration of the prostaglandins was defined by Nugteren et al (1966a) and is the basis for the extended modern nomenclature. 'Prostaglandin' is a generic term for a closely related family of C_{20} carboxylic acids. They are most easily envisaged as derivatives of the hypothetical prostanoic acid (Figure 1). As with all fatty acids, the C_{20} skeleton is numbered consecutively from the terminal carboxyl function, although when necessary it may be numbered from the terminal methyl group by addition of the prefix ω, such that $C-20 \equiv \omega-1$. The aliphatic side-chains project from the

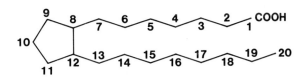

Figure 1. Hypothetical prostanoic acid skeleton.

ISBN 0–7020–1694–2

cyclopentane ring in a *trans* configuration with the chain containing the carboxyl function being assigned the α configuration to define its position in relation to the average plane of the ring. The α orientation thus refers to substituents nominally below the plane of the ring and the β orientation to substituents above the plane of the ring.

Prostaglandins may be divided into the A, B, C, D, E, F or J series, according to the substituents in the cyclopentane ring (Figure 2). The key endoperoxide intermediates in prostaglandin biosynthesis (see later) were named prostaglandin G (PGG) or PGH (Figure 3). Prostacyclin, which is PGI_2, and thromboxane A_2 both have unusual ring structures that do not fit easily into this simplified scheme (Figure 4). PGA, PGB and PGC may be derived from PGE by dehydration and isomerism. The hydroxyl group at C-11 is in the α configuration in PGE, and indeed in general for prostaglandin F, which also has an α-orientated hydroxyl function at C-9. It should

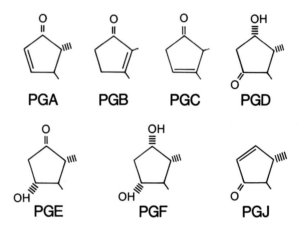

Figure 2. Structures of cyclopentane rings of common prostaglandins.

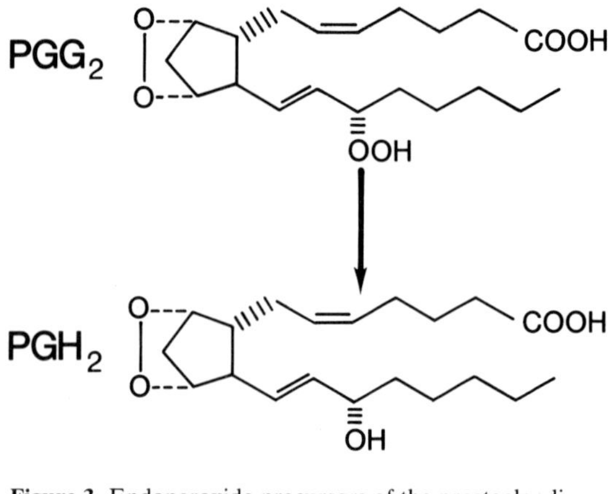

Figure 3. Endoperoxide precursors of the prostaglandins.

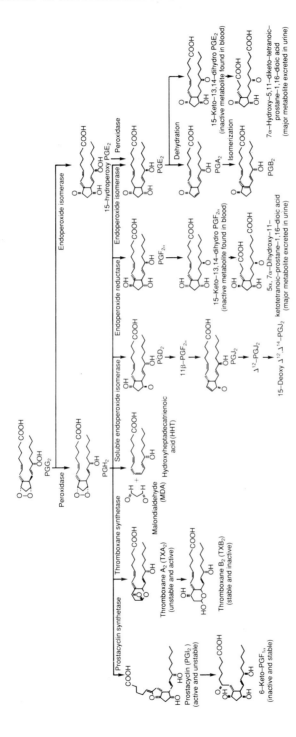

Figure 4. Structures and pathways in prostaglandin biosynthesis and metabolism.

be noted, however, that 9α,11β-PGF$_2$ can be formed by the action of PGF synthetase from bovine lung on PGD$_2$ (Watanabe et al, 1989). PGD has a ketone function at C-11 with an α-orientated hydroxyl group at C-9. PGJ also has a ketone function at C-11 with a double bond between C-9 and C-10. The hydroxyl function at C-15 is in the α configuration for all naturally occurring prostaglandins from mammalian sources: the only functions found

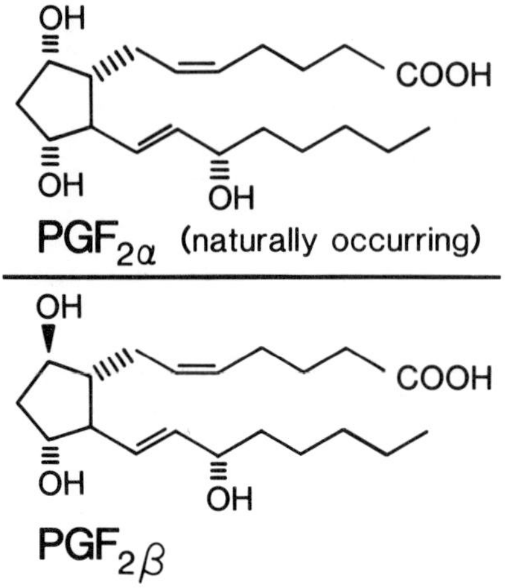

Figure 5. Structures of the α and β isomers of PGF$_2$.

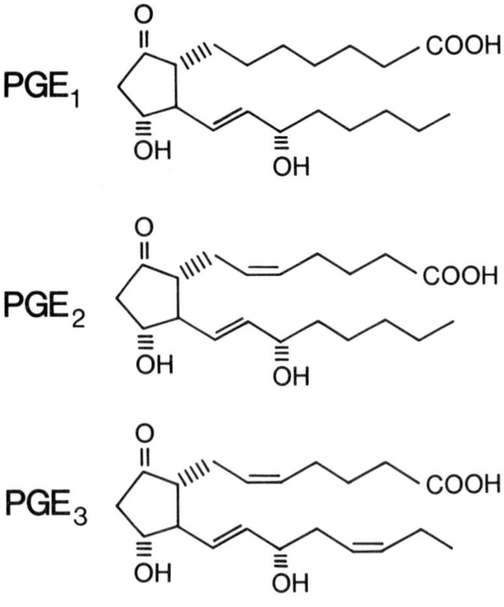

Figure 6. Structural characteristics that determine different numerical subscripts.

naturally in the β configuration are the hydroxyl group at C-19 in certain prostaglandins and the hydroxyl at C-11 in $9\alpha,11\beta$-PGF$_2$. In most naturally occurring mammalian prostaglandins the absolute stereochemical configurations at the asymmetric centres at C-9, 11, 15 and 19, respectively, are S, R, S, R (as defined by Cahn, 1964). The α subscript in PGF$_{2\alpha}$ (for example) actually denotes the configuration of the hydroxyl group at C-9 (Figure 5) and is thus absent when naming prostaglandins with a ketone group at this position. The numerical subscripts (1–3) in prostaglandin nomenclature refer to the number of double bonds in the side-chains of the molecule (Figure 6). In most naturally occurring prostaglandins their configurations are always 13,14-*trans*, 5,6-*cis* and 17,18-*cis*. The structures of both the intermediates in prostaglandin biosynthesis and the products of their enzymatic degradation will be described in the following sections.

PROSTAGLANDIN BIOSYNTHESIS

Substrates

The initial steps in the elucidation of the fatty acid precursors for prostaglandin biosynthesis came in 1964 when the conversion of arachidonic acid into PGE$_2$ by homogenates of sheep vesicular gland was reported (Bergstrom et al, 1964a; van Dorp et al, 1964a). The transformation of *all-cis*-8,11,14-eicosatrienoic acid and *all-cis*-5,8, 11,14,17-eicosapentaenoic acid into PGE$_1$ and PGE$_3$, respectively, were demonstrated in the same year (Bergstrom et al, 1964b; van Dorp et al, 1964b). Subsequently, PGF$_{1\alpha}$, as well as a number of monohydroxy acids, were isolated following incubation of *all-cis*-8,11,14-eicosatrienoic acid with preparations of sheep vesicular gland (Kupiecki, 1965; Hamberg and Samuelsson, 1966a; Nugteren et al, 1966a).

The findings that both PGE$_2$ and PGF$_{2\alpha}$ were formed by incubation of arachidonic acid with homogenates of guinea-pig lung (Angaard and Samuelsson, 1965) and rabbit kidney medulla (Hamberg, 1969) were the first indications that trienoic, tetraenoic and pentaenoic fatty acids serve as common precursors for prostaglandins containing, respectively, one, two or three double bonds in the side-chains (Figure 7). It was soon established that PGD was formed from the same set of precursors, although it was originally named *iso*-PGE (Nugteren et al, 1966a) and 11-dehydro-PGF$_{2\alpha}$ (Granstrom et al, 1968). Later studies also established that prostacyclin (Moncada et al, 1976) and thromboxane A$_2$ (Hamberg et al, 1975) were also derived from the same precursors.

Early studies had shown that prostaglandin synthetase could utilize *all-cis*-10,13,16-docosatrienoic acid and *all-cis*-7,10,13-nonadecatrienoic acid as substrates for conversion principally to ω-dihomo-PGE$_1$ and ω-nor-PGE$_1$, respectively (Bergstrom et al, 1964b; van Dorp et al, 1964b). A series of elegant studies by van Dorp's group further delineated the substrate specificity of prostaglandin synthetase. Initially they tested the conversion to prostaglandins of certain analogues and homologues of known prostaglandin precursors (Strujik et al, 1967). Both C$_{18}$ and C$_{22}$ homologues of

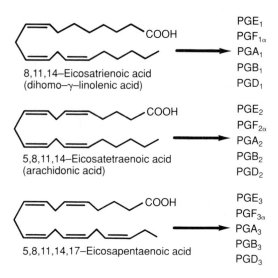

Figure 7. Fatty acid precursors of prostaglandins.

tetraenoic acids of the ω-6 type (in poor yield) and C_{19}–C_{21} trienoic acids of the ω-6 type (in good yield) were converted to prostaglandins. The C_{20} trienoic acids of the ω-5, -8 and -9 type did not serve as substrates, although a small conversion was found from the ω-7 isomer. This indicated that the position of the double bonds relative to the methyl end of the fatty acid was critical in determining its properties as a substrate for prostaglandin synthetase. The biological activity of the prostaglandins formed was in all cases low. Using additional synthetic analogues of prostaglandin precursors it was later demonstrated that fatty acids 21:4 ω-7, 19:4 ω-5, 21:3 ω-7 and 19:3 ω-5 (but not 18:3 ω-4 or 22:3 ω-7) could be converted into prostaglandin-like materials (Beerthuis et al, 1968).* These prostaglandin derivatives were biologically active, and indeed an interesting correlation was found in that only fatty acids that yielded biologically active prostaglandins showed high essential fatty acid activity. It is interesting to note that these studies were forming the early basis for the use of fish oils and fatty acid dietary supplements as potentially beneficial treatments for the prevention or amelioration of cardiovascular disease.

This work was extended by studying the conversion of substituted *all-cis*-8,11,14-eicosatrienoic acids into prostaglandins by incubation with a particulate fraction of sheep vesicular glands (van Dorp and Christ, 1975). Substitutions were made at the C-2, C-3, C-4, C-5, C-18 and C-19 positions. Prostaglandin derivatives were obtained in the majority of cases, although conversions were always lower than with the unsubstituted acid (20:3). The biological activities of the substituted prostaglandins formed were, in

---

* This nomenclature, e.g. 20:4 ω-6, defines a fatty acid with 20 carbon atoms and four double bonds in which the last double bond is six carbon atoms from the terminal methyl group.

general, less than those of PGE_1 although, interestingly, 19-methyl-PGE_1 was 1.6 times as potent as PGE_1 in smooth muscle-stimulating activity.

Originally it had been suggested that prostaglandins were bound in an esterified form to phospholipids (Eliasson, 1959). Eliasson had found that the addition of lecithinase A to homogenates of sheep vesicular glands would increase the formation of prostaglandins (Eliasson, 1958). Early theories on the mechanism of action of venoms and phospholipases on prostaglandin production were reviewed by Vogt (1967). Prostaglandins are not esterified to phospholipids, however (Lands and Samuelsson, 1968; Vonkeman and van Dorp, 1968), and the effects of lecithinase and phospholipase A_2 on prostaglandin formation are, in fact, due to the liberation of fatty acid precursors. This is a prerequisite for prostaglandin synthesis to occur, as it was shown that if the precursor fatty acids were esterified to phospholipids no synthesis occurred. Further evidence of the necessity of a free carboxyl group was provided by Struijk et al (1967), who demonstrated that *all-cis*-8,11,14-eicosatrienol and *all-cis*-5,8,11,14-eicosatetraenol, as well as the methyl esters of 20:3 ω-6 and 20:4 ω-6 fatty acids were not substrates for prostaglandin synthetase.

These findings, in conjunction with the fact that the capacity of prostaglandin-synthesizing enzymes in vesicular glands greatly exceeds the amount of non-esterified fatty acids available, led to the suggestion that the liberation of free fatty acids from their phospholipid stores may be a rate-limiting step in prostaglandin biosynthesis (Kunze and Vogt, 1971). The control and location of free fatty acid concentrations is highly complex, with high rates of fluxes between both plasma and cells and between different intracellular sites being a characteristic feature (Nikkila, 1971). Nowadays, considerable emphasis is placed on this release of substrate via the action of phospholipase C and the subsequent actions of diacylglycerol and mono-acylglycerol lipases. A simplified description of the sites of action of various phospholipases is given in Figure 8.

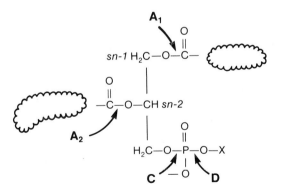

Figure 8. The structure of a generalized glycerophospholipid. The various alcohols that may be found in phosphomonoester linkage are depicted as X. The sites of hydrolysis catalysed by the various phospholipases are indicated by A_1, A_2, C and D. A saturated fatty acid is typically esterified at the *sn*-1 position and a polyunsaturated fatty acid commonly esterified at the *sn*-2 position. The fatty acids are represented by the rings.

Occurrence

Although sheep seminal vesicles provided the main source of prostaglandin synthetase in early studies, it was known that other tissues could synthesize prostaglandins, e.g. guinea-pig lung (Anggard and Samuelsson, 1965). Thereafter, data accumulated on tissues from which prostaglandins are released following the application of a suitable stimulus (Ramwell and Shaw, 1970; Horton et al, 1971; Piper and Vane, 1971). In a study of prostaglandin synthetase activity in various organs of sheep, guinea-pigs and rats, this enzyme system was found to be widespread in occurrence but generally low in activity (Nugteren et al, 1966a). Although exceptions exist, these findings remain surprisingly consistent many years later.

Christ and van Dorp (1972) then systematically investigated the activity of prostaglandin synthetase in a wide variety of tissues. Apart from vesicular glands, which possessed extremely high activities (about 75% conversion of substrate), mammalian tissues fell into three broad categories: those such as lung and kidney (medulla) in which approximately 10% conversion occurred; those such as gastrointestinal tract in which only 3% occurred; and those such as spleen and kidney cortex in which conversion was 1% or less. The synthetase was found in other vertebrate tissues (carp gills and frog lung) and in tissues from members of other *phyla*. These authors, however, stressed the importance of distinguishing between low enzymatic conversion (less than 2%) and auto-oxidation of the substrate. This latter problem still plagues research into prostaglandin biosynthesis in many organ, tissue and cell culture systems.

Mechanism

The biosynthetic pathway for prostaglandin production has mainly been studied using preparations of ovine seminal vesicles, as they are a rich and convenient source of prostaglandin synthetase. There is, however, no reason at present to suspect that prostaglandin synthesis catalysed by enzymes from other mammalian sources proceeds by a different pathway. The genetic conservation of cyclooxygenase at the molecular level (Bailey and Verma, 1990; Bennett and Moore, 1991) may be considered as consistent with this view. Interestingly, however, more than one form of cyclooxygenase has been proven to exist (Rosen et al, 1989; Kujuba et al, 1991; O'Banion et al, 1991; Xie et al, 1991). Thus, the potential for new mechanistic findings certainly exists.

Initial studies showed that prostaglandin synthetase activity is located mainly in the high-speed particulate fraction of cells but requires the supernatant fraction (as well as molecular oxygen) for appreciable activity to occur. The high-speed supernatant is needed to furnish a thermostable reducing cofactor, which may be replaced by glutathione or tetrahydrofolate, but not NADH or NADPH (Samuelsson, 1967; van Dorp, 1967). Additional reducing equivalents are required for PGF formation but glutathione cannot fulfil this requirement (van Dorp, 1967). Although Cu^{2+}, dithiol, dihydrolipoamide and L-adrenaline can stimulate $PGF_{2\alpha}$

formation from arachidonic acid, the identity of the reducing cofactor that operates under physiological conditions is still unknown. A comprehensive view of the activities involved in prostaglandin synthetase i.e. prostaglandin endoperoxide synthase (also known as fatty acid cyclooxygenase), peroxidase and various isomerases is outside the scope of this chapter but may be found in more specialized reviews (Holtzman, 1991; Smith et al, 1991).

Prostaglandin biosynthesis occurs via a series of enzymatic conversions, following what is assumed to be a free radical mechanism in the initial stages (Nugteren and Hazelhof, 1973). The mechanisms involved have been investigated both by isolation of natural intermediates and by the introduction of isotopically labelled precursors in which the subsequent fate of the 'label' has been monitored.

The initial step in the mechanism appears to be the stereospecific elimination of the 13L hydrogen, as demonstrated by the substitution of tritium for hydrogen at C-13 and the subsequently observed kinetic isotope effects (Hamberg and Samuelsson, 1967). This is followed by the addition of an oxygen molecule at C-11 and the isomerization of the Δ^{11}-cis double bond to a Δ^{12}-trans double bond. The resultant 11-peroxy fatty acid was the first postulated intermediate in prostaglandin synthesis (Nugteren et al, 1966a; Hamberg and Samuelsson, 1967). In the subsequent concerted reaction the oxygen radical attacks at C-9, ring closure occurs between C-8 and C-12, the Δ^{12}-trans double bond isomerizes into the Δ^{13}-trans position and there is addition of molecular oxygen at C-15. The endoperoxide thus formed is considered to be the common intermediate in prostaglandin biosynthesis and was isolated with either a hydroperoxy or hydroxyl group at C-15 (Hamberg and Samuelsson, 1973; Nugteren and Hazelhof, 1973; Hamberg et al, 1974). The presence of this intermediate had previously been postulated by Gryglewski and Vane (1972), following the discovery of a biologically active principle which had been named 'rabbit aorta contracting substance' (RACS). Van Dorp's group had named these compounds 15-hydroperoxy-PGF and PGR, whereas Samuelsson's group had given them their new accepted terms of PGG and PGH, respectively.

The final step in the reaction pathway involves either enzymatic conversion of the endoperoxide via isomerases or its reductive cleavage, although breakdown to 12-hydroxy-8,10-heptadecadienoic acid and malonaldehyde can occur (Hamberg and Samuelsson, 1966a, 1967; Nugteren et al, 1966a). Elimination of hydrogen at C-9 of the intermediate endoperoxide is the rate-limiting step in the formation of PGE_2 from the endoperoxide (Samuelsson, 1973). Nugteren and Hazelhof (1973) prepared both the prostaglandin endoperoxides and 15-hydroperoxy-PGE_1 and described the subsequent conversion to prostaglandins. A 15-hydroperoxyprostaglandin reductase was demonstrated, the bulk of which appeared to be in the $100\,000\,g$ supernatant of a homogenate of sheep vesicular glands. There were two distinct isomerases, requiring glutathione for activity: one was located in the particulate cell fraction and converted PGR to PGE, and the other was located in the high-speed supernatant and converted PGR to PGD. No evidence was found for an enzyme to convert PGE to PGF (such an enzyme is

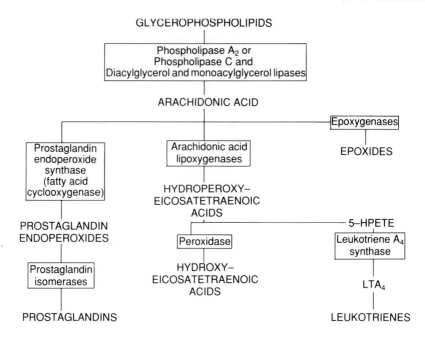

Figure 9. A simplified schematic representation of the enzymatic pathways of arachidonic acid metabolism.

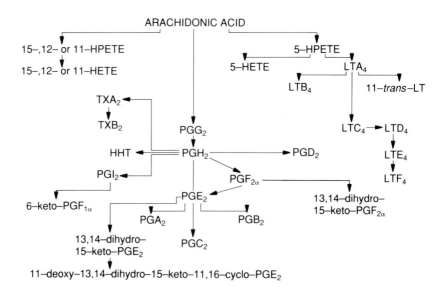

Figure 10. A simplified outline of the pathways of arachidonic acid metabolism.

now known to exist); increased PGF formation was, in fact, only found in tissues with no active isomerizing enzymes or under the influence of reducing substances not normally encountered in biological material. Although it has taken many years, a PGF synthetase has clearly been demonstrated (e.g. see Watanabe et al, 1989). Enzymes for the conversion of endoperoxides to PGI_2 and thromboxane A_2 have of course also been found. Other pathways for arachidonic acid metabolism have been described in the past few decades, e.g. lipoxygenase and epoxygenase. Simplified descriptions of these pathways and their products are presented in Figures 9 and 10.

Inhibition

Study of the biological activity of the prostaglandins under physiologically normal conditions is extremely difficult, due to the ubiquitous and labile nature of the prostaglandin-generating and -degrading systems. Such difficulties can, under certain circumstances, be reduced by the use of specific inhibitors of prostaglandin biosynthesis. These compounds may roughly be divided into three categories: (1) substrate analogues, (2) aspirin-like drugs and (3) various miscellaneous agents.

Substrate analogues and other fatty acids

Analogues of arachidonic acid and dihomo-γ-linolenic acid containing acetylenic or *trans* double bonds have been described which are potent inhibitors of prostaglandin synthetase (Ahern and Downing, 1970; Nugteren, 1970). The *trans* analogues of arachidonic acid and dihomo-γ-linolenic acid are competitive inhibitors (Nugteren, 1970) whereas 5,8,11,14-eicosatetraynoic acid exhibits a biphasic pattern of inhibition: a rapid concentration-dependent effect followed by a time-dependent destruction of the enzyme (Lands et al, 1972; Vanderhoek and Lands, 1973a). A similar biphasic pattern of inhibition has been noted for several naturally occurring fatty acids—oleic, linoleic and linolenic acids (Pace-Asciak and Wolfe, 1968)—although competitive inhibition has been described for decanoate (Wallach and Daniels, 1971). A competitive inhibitor of cyclooxygenase has been described in *all-cis*-5,8,11,14,17,20-docosahexaenoic acid (Marshall and Kulmacz, 1988).

A novel approach to synthetase inhibition was reported by Wlodawer et al (1971), who synthesized a series of compounds that were structurally related to the cyclic endoperoxide intermediate in prostaglandin synthesis. One of the bicyclo[2.2.1]heptene derivatives possessed the interesting property of inhibiting synthesis of PGE but not PGF. Certain prostaglandin-like compounds, such as 5- or 7-oxaprostaglandin derivatives, have antisynthetase activity (McDonald-Gibson et al, 1973). Inhibition is usually in a competitive manner, although some of the compounds were found to stimulate prostaglandin synthesis.

Aspirin-like drugs and other pharmacological agents

The term 'aspirin-like' refers to a group of compounds characterized by their antipyretic, analgesic and anti-inflammatory properties. Inhibition of prostaglandin synthesis is a fairly specific property of these compounds as many other pharmacologically active compounds are inactive in this respect (Gryglewski et al, 1972). In 1971 they were simultaneously shown to inhibit prostaglandin release from human platelets (Smith and Willis, 1971) and perfused dog spleen (Ferriera et al, 1971) and to inhibit prostaglandin synthesis in cell-free homogenates of guinea-pig lung (Vane, 1971).

Since then, much literature has accumulated on these compounds and their activities in inhibiting prostaglandin formation. From these accumulated data a general order of potency was put forward (Flower, 1974). In decreasing order of potency this was: meclofenamic acid > niflumic acid ≡ indomethacin > mefenamic acid > flufenamic acid > naproxen > phenylbutazone > aspirin or ibuprofen. Although minor variations were noted (Ham et al, 1972), this was, in general, an excellent guide to the potency of these compounds in inhibiting prostaglandin synthesis, despite the variables involved in measuring this parameter against synthetase systems from different tissues (Vane, 1972). Another list of kinetic data on these compounds came from Ku and Wasvary (1973), whose order of potency confirmed that of Flower. The wide range of newer drugs and differing test systems makes such comparisons nowadays extremely difficult and of limited usefulness. Most aspirin-like drugs were found to exhibit competitive, non-reversible inhibition of prostaglandin synthesis, only SU 21524 (a propionic acid derivative) and oxyphenylbutazone exhibited competitive reversible kinetics. It seems likely that these inhibitors combine irreversibly in a time-dependent fashion with the catalytic site of an enzyme before endoperoxide formation (Takeguchi and Sih, 1972; Flower, 1974). Presently, indomethacin, flurbiprofen and meclofenamate are thought to cause irreversible inactivation of cyclooxygenase in vitro but not in vivo. Non-steroidal anti-inflammatory agents such as flufenamate, ibuprofen, sulindac and naproxen are thought to be reversible competitive inhibitors of cyclooxygenase.

It is worthwhile to review briefly the reasons why aspirin is of so much benefit when used prophylactically to reduce the incidence and recurrence rate of pathologies such as myocardial infarction and stroke as well as being a possible prophylaxis against pregnancy-induced hypertension and intrauterine growth retardation. The net effect of low-dose aspirin is to increase the prostacyclin-to-thromboxane ratio of production. This is achieved by irreversible inactivation of cyclooxygenase in platelets (a key site of thromboxane production) which cannot synthesize new protein. Vascular endothelial cells (a key site of prostacyclin formation) are affected similarly but can generate fresh cyclooxygenase protein. Hence the relative shift to prostacyclin production.

Although synthetase inhibition is a fairly specific property of aspirin-like drugs, they do exert many other effects on a variety of enzymes and cellular systems (Smith and Dawkins, 1971; Shen, 1972; Paulus and Whitehouse, 1973). Taking indomethacin as one of the most widely used prostaglandin synthetase inhibitors, it has been shown to inhibit phosphodiesterase, oxidative phosphorylation, collagenase and enzyme release from lysosomes, as well as stabilizing proteins and erythrocyte membranes (Flower, 1974). Fortunately the concentrations of aspirin-like drugs required to inhibit prostaglandin synthesis are usually much lower than those required for their other pharmacological effects. It is perhaps best to refer to this class of compounds as preferential inhibitors of prostaglandin synthesis, rather than specific or selective inhibitors. The duration and onset of action of these drugs are variable (Hamberg, 1972; Horton et al, 1973; Vane and Botting, 1990), ranging from hours to days, and are dependent on individual clearance rates and the activity of metabolites as well as the kinetics of binding to the enzyme (Vane, 1972; Willis et al, 1972; Smith et al, 1991).

Miscellaneous agents

During investigations on the mechanism of prostaglandin synthesis it was found that some metal ions and antioxidants inhibited the conversion of eicosatrienoic acid into PGE_1 (Nugteren et al, 1966a). In the case of Cu^{2+}, it was subsequently found that there was a simultaneous increase in the production of PGF (Lee and Lands, 1972) which was enhanced by dithiol compounds. A wide range of antioxidants have been shown to have inhibitory actions, the majority exhibiting non-competitive inhibition without any time-dependent destruction of the enzyme (Vanderhoek and Lands, 1973b). A variety of other compounds were found to inhibit prostaglandin synthesis, including cyanide, some hydroxynaphthalene derivatives and rat liver GSH peroxidase (Flower, 1974). All these compounds have provided some information of prostaglandin synthesis in vitro, but their unusual and diverse nature renders them unlikely to be of great future use in elucidating the mechanism of prostaglandin synthesis in vivo.

PROSTAGLANDIN METABOLISM

Occurrence and mechanism

Homogenates of guinea-pig lung were originally found to convert PGE_1, into 13,14-dihydro-PGE_1, and 13,14-dihydro-15-keto-PGE_1 (Anggard and Samuelsson, 1964) whereas homogenates of swine lung produced 15-keto-PGE_1 (Anggard and Samuelsson, 1966). PGE_2 and PGE_3 were transformed in an analogous manner (Anggard and Samuelsson, 1965; Anggard et al, 1965). There was therefore an early indication of the species differences that exist for prostaglandin metabolism. Despite these differences which manifest themselves in the predominance of different metabolites and, occasionally, in the order of their formation, the basic steps in prostaglandin metabolism are similar and outlined in part in Figure 11. The major site of prostaglandin metabolism is the lung; almost all biologically active prostaglandins are metabolized during one passage through the lungs.

The enzymes involved in the initial steps of the metabolic pathway were found to be located in the particle-free fraction of cells (Anggard and

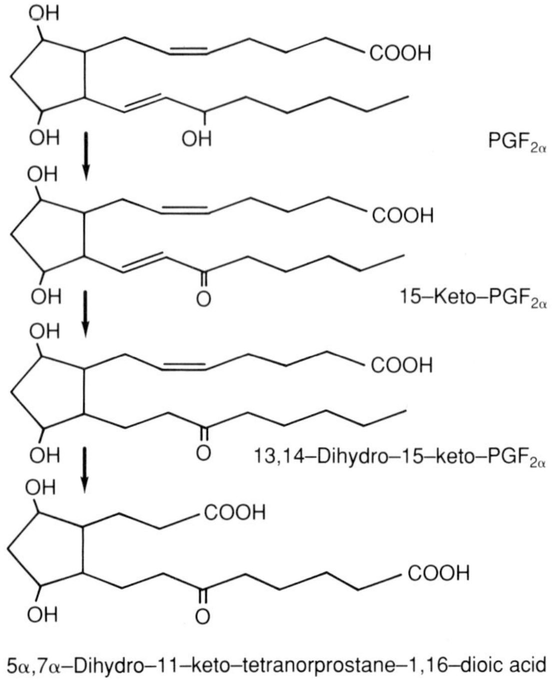

Figure 11. A simplified pathway for the metabolism of $PGF_{2\alpha}$.

Samuelsson, 1964). Their distribution throughout different swine tissues has been reported (Anggard et al, 1971). They were found to be widely distributed throughout the tissues studied. Dehydrogenase activity was greatest in lung, spleen and kidney with all other tissues showing far less activity, while reductase activity was greatest in spleen, kidney, liver, adrenal and small intestine. Data on the distribution of these enzymes in tissues from other species was more fragmentary in nature (Samuelsson et al, 1971) but has increased immensely in recent years.

It was demonstrated in early studies that 15-hydroxyprostaglandin dehydrogenase (PGDH) is both prostaglandin-specific (Anggard and Samuelsson, 1966) and specific with regard to configuration (15S) at C-15 (Nakano et al, 1969; Shio et al, 1970). Although prostaglandins of the B series are not substrates for this enzyme, the nature of the substituents in the cyclopentane ring did not seem to affect markedly the properties as a substrate whereas the length of the carboxyl side-chain was more important. Interestingly, however, PGD_2 is also a poor substrate for this enzyme. The enzyme requires NAD (Anggard and Samuelsson, 1966) and has been shown to be reversible (Yamasaki and Sasaki, 1975). Metabolism of prostaglandins, it should be noted, occurs firstly by uptake into pulmonary cells followed by the action of PGDH (and is completed by a series of β and ω oxidations in the liver and kidney). The uptake mechanism is of importance since prostacyclin, while a good substrate for PGDH action, is not a good substrate for the uptake mechanism and thus is incompletely cleared by the lungs.

The sequence of dehydrogenase and reductase actions was established by Hamberg and Samuelsson (1971a), who showed that the reduction of the Δ^{13} double bond must be preceded by the oxidation of the allylic alcohol group at C-15 (which results in activation of the double bond). Following the action of these enzymes, prostaglandin metabolism occurs via several pathways with marked interspecies differences (Samuelsson et al, 1971), although the basic reactions are ω-oxidation and a series of β oxidations. Evidence for dehydrogenase and reductase action preceding β oxidation originally came from the isolation and identification of plasma metabolites plus the fact that C_{18} and C_{16} metabolites are poor substrates for PGDH (Nakano et al, 1969). β oxidation eliminates two carbon atoms from the carboxyl side-chain and two steps of this reaction plus one of ω-oxidation results in the formation of $5\alpha,7\alpha$-dihydroxy-11-ketotetranorprostane-1,16-dioic and 7α-hydroxy-5,11-diketotetranorprostane-1,16-dioic acid, the major urinary metabolites of PGF and PGE, respectively, in man (Granstrom and Samuelsson, 1971a; Hamberg and Samuelsson, 1971b). PGE_1 and $PGF_{1\alpha}$ give rise to the same urinary metabolites of PGE_2 and $PGF_{2\alpha}$, respectively (Granstrom and Samuelsson, 1971b). Variations within the β and ω oxidation steps include C_{16} compounds, which are formed by one step of β-oxidation at each end of the molecule rather than two steps at the carboxyl end (Granstrom and Samuelsson, 1971b), and C_{14} metabolites, which are formed by two steps of β oxidation at the carboxyl end of the molecule and one at the methyl end of the molecule (Granstrom, 1973).

Studies on prostaglandins in human seminal fluid have shown high concentrations of ω-2 hydroxylated derivatives, i.e. 19-hydroxy-PGA_1, A_2, B_1 and B_2 (Hamberg and Samuelsson, 1966b). It is uncertain to what extent these may have been formed during work-up procedures, for 19-hydroxy-PGE has been identified as the major prostaglandin component of human semen (Taylor and Kelly, 1974). Whether these compounds should be regarded as metabolites or primary prostaglandins is also a matter for debate. Prostaglandin derivatives have been reported in which ω-1 has been hydroxylated (Granstrom and Samuelsson, 1971b; Hamberg and Wilson, 1973), and it is possible that the carboxyl function at ω-1 in other metabolites is derived from oxidation of a primary alcohol. Many urinary metabolites have been found to be unstable and may form lactones or dehydrate (Nugteren, 1975); several of them were isolated in their lactone form (Granstrom and Samuelsson, 1971b; Hamberg and Wilson, 1973).

Many other minor metabolic pathways have been described in various species but only two will be detailed here. One of the first prostaglandin metabolites to be identified was 13,14-dihydro-PGE_1 (Anggard and Samuelsson, 1964). This is derived from 13,14-dihydro-15-keto-PGE_1 via stereospecific reduction of the C-15 function by 15-ketoprostaglandin reductase, an enzyme which is not identical with PGDH (Anggard, 1971). The resulting derivatives are, however, still substrates for prostaglandin dehydrogenase (Anggard and Samuelsson, 1966; Nakano et al, 1969). This pathway was considered to be potentially of major physiological significance since 13,14-dihydro-$PGF_{2\alpha}$ was regarded as a potent stimulant of uterine activity and to circulate in human blood in about equal concentration with $PGF_{2\alpha}$ (Bygdeman et al, 1974).

Another pathway of interest that has been described in the guinea-pig is one in which reduction of the C-9 keto function of PGE_2 yields C_{16} urinary metabolites with both 5β-hydroxyl groups (Hamberg and Samuelsson, 1969) and 5α-hydroxyl groups (Hamberg and Israelsson, 1970). Similar enzymes have been described in other species (Hensby, 1974; Lee and Levine, 1974).

REFERENCES

Ahern DG & Downing DT (1970) Inhibition of prostaglandin biosynthesis by eicosa-5,8,11,14-tetraynoic acid. *Biochimica et Biophysica Acta* **210:** 456–461.

Anggard E (1971) Studies on the analysis and metabolism of the prostaglandins. *Annals of the New York Academy of Sciences* **180:** 200–217.

Anggard E & Samuelsson B (1964) Metabolism of prostaglandin E_1 in guinea pig lung: the structures of two metabolites. *Journal of Biological Chemistry* **239:** 4097–4102.

Anggard E & Samuelsson B (1965) Biosynthesis of prostaglandins from arachidonic acid in guinea-pig lung. *Journal of Biological Chemistry* **240:** 3518–3521.

Anggard E & Samuelsson B (1966) Purification and properties of a 15-hydroxy prostaglandin dehydrogenase from swine lung. *Arkiv für Kemi* **25:** 293–300.

Anggard E, Green K & Samuelsson B (1965) Synthesis of tritium labeled prostaglandin E_2 and studies on its metabolism in guinea pig lung. *Journal of Biological Chemistry* **240:** 1932–1940.

Anggard E, Larsson C & Samuelsson B (1971) The distribution of 15-hydroxy prostaglandin dehydrogenase and prostaglandin-Δ^{13}-reductase in tissues of the swine. *Acta Physiologica Scandinavica* **81:** 396–404.

Bailey JM & Verma M (1990) Identification of a highly conserved 3′ UTR in the translationally regulated mRNA for prostaglandin synthase. *Prostaglandins* **40:** 585–590.

Beerthuis RK, Nugteren DH, Pabon HJJ & van Dorp DA (1968) Biologically active prostaglandins from some new odd-numbered essential fatty acids. *Recueil des Travaux Chimiques des Pays-Bas* **87:** 461–480.

Bennett PR & Moore GE (1991) Genetic conservation of cyclo-oxygenase. *Prostaglandins* **41:** 135–142.

Bergstrom S, Danielsson H & Samuelsson B (1964a) The enzymatic formation of prostaglandin E_2 from arachidonic acid. *Biochimica et Biophysica Acta* **90:** 207–210.

Bergstrom S, Danielsson H, Klenberg D & Samuelsson B (1964b) The enzymatic conversion of essential fatty acids in to prostaglandins. *Journal of Biological Chemistry* **239:** PC4006–PC4008.

Bygdeman M, Green K, Toppozada M, Wiqvist N & Bergstrom S (1974) The influence of prostaglandin metabolites on the uterine response to $PGF_{2\alpha}$. A clinical and pharmacokinetic study. *Life Sciences* **14:** 521–531.

Cahn RS (1964) An introduction to the sequence rule: a system for the specification of absolute configuration. *Journal of Chemical Education* **41:** 116–125.

Christ EJ & van Dorp DA (1972) Comparative aspects of prostaglandin biosynthesis in animal tissues. *Biochimica et Biophysica Acta* **270:** 537–545.

Eliasson R (1958) Formation of prostaglandin in vitro. *Nature* **182:** 256–257.

Eliasson R (1959) Studies on prostaglandin: occurrence formation and biological actions. *Acta Physiologica Scandinavica* **46:** 1–73.

Eling TE, Thompson DC, Foureman GL, Curtis JR & Hughes MF (1990) Prostaglandin H synthase and xenobiotic oxidation. *Annual Review of Pharmacology and Toxicology* **30:** 1–45.

Ferreira SH, Moncada S & Vane JR (1971) Indomethacin and aspirin abolish prostaglandin release from the spleen. *Nature* **231:** 237–239.

Flower RJ (1974) Drugs which inhibit prostaglandin synthesis. *Pharmacology Review* **26:** 33–67.

Granstrom E (1973) Structure of C.14 metabolites of prostaglandin $F_{2\alpha}$. *Advances in Biosciences* **9:** 49–60.

Granstrom E & Samuelsson B (1971a) On the metabolism of prostaglandin $F_{2\alpha}$ in female subjects. *Journal of Biological Chemistry* **246:** 5254–5263.

Granstrom E & Samuelsson B (1971b) On the metabolism of prostaglandin $F_{2\alpha}$ in female subjects. II Structure of six metabolites. *Journal of Biological Chemistry* **246:** 7470–7485.

Granstrom E, Lands WEM & Samuelsson B (1968) Biosynthesis of 9α,15-dihydroxy-11-ketoprost-13-enoic acid. *Journal of Biological Chemistry* **243:** 4104–4108.

Gryglewski R & Vane JR (1972) The release of prostaglandins and rabbit aorta contracting substance (RACS) from rabbit spleen and its antagonism by anti-inflammatory drugs. *British Journal of Pharmacology* **45:** 37–47.

Gryglewski R, Flower RJ, Herbazynska-Cedro K & Vane JR (1972) Inhibition of prostaglandin synthetase by anti-inflammatory drugs. *Proceedings of the Fifth International Congress of Pharmacology*, San Francisco, p 90.

Ham EA, Cirillo VJ, Zanetti M, Shen TY & Juehl FA (1972) Studies on the mode of action of non-steroidal, anti-inflammatory agents. In Ramwell PW & Pharriss BB (eds) *Prostaglandins in Cellular Biology*, pp 345–352. New York: Plenum Press.

Hamberg M (1969) Biosynthesis of prostaglandins in the renal medulla of rabbit. *FEBS Letters* **5:** 127–130.

Hamberg M (1972) Inhibition of prostaglandin synthesis in man. *Biochemical and Biophysical Research Communications* **49:** 720–726.

Hamberg M & Israelsson U (1970) Metabolism of prostaglandin E_2 in guinea-pig liver. I Identification of seven metabolites. *Journal of Biological Chemistry* **245:** 5107–5114.

Hamberg M & Samuelsson B (1966a) Novel biological transformation of 8,11,14-eicosatrienoic acid. *Journal of the American Chemical Society* **88:** 2349–2350.

Hamberg M & Samuelsson B (1966b) Prostaglandins in human seminal plasma. *Journal of Biological Chemistry* **241:** 257–263.

Hamberg M & Samuelsson B (1967) On the mechanism of the biosynthesis of prostaglandins E_1 and $F_{1\alpha}$. *Journal of Biological Chemistry* **242:** 5336–5343.

Hamberg M & Samuelsson B (1969) The structure of a urinary metabolite of prostaglandin E_2 in the guinea-pig. *Biochemical and Biophysical Research Communications* **34:** 22–27.

Hamberg M & Samuelsson B (1971a) Metabolism of prostaglandin E_2 in guinea-pig liver. *Journal of Biological Chemistry* **246:** 1073–1077.

Hamberg M & Samuelsson B (1971b) On the metabolism of prostaglandins E_1 and E_2 in man. *Journal of Biological Chemistry* **246:** 6713–6721.

Hamberg M & Wilson M (1973) Structures of new metabolites of prostaglandin E_2 in man. *Advances in Biosciences* **9:** 39–48.

Hamberg M, Svensson J, Wakabayashi T & Samuelsson B (1974) Isolation and structure of two prostaglandin endoperoxides that cause platelet aggregation. *Proceedings of the National Academy of Sciences of the USA* **71:** 345–349.

Hamberg M, Svensson J & Samuelsson B (1975) Thromboxanes: a new group of biologically active compounds derived from prostaglandin endoperoxides. *Proceedings of the National Academy of Sciences of the USA* **72:** 2994–2998.

Hensby CN (1974) Reduction of prostaglandin E_2 to prostaglandin $F_{2\alpha}$ by an enzyme in sheep blood. *Biochimica et Biophysica Acta* **348:** 145–154.

Holtzman MJ (1991) Arachidonic acid metabolism. Implications of biological chemistry for lung function and disease. *American Review of Respiratory Diseases* **143:** 188–203.

Horton EW, Thompson C, Jones R & Poyser N (1971) Release of prostaglandins. *Annals of the New York Academy of Sciences* **180:** 351–362.

Horton EW, Jones RL & Marr GG (1973) Effects of aspirin on prostaglandin and fructose levels in human serum. *Journal of Reproduction and Fertility* **33:** 385–392.

Ku EC & Wasvary JM (1973) Inhibition of prostaglandin synthetase by SU 21524. *Federation Proceedings* **32:** 3302.

Kujubu DA, Fletcher BS, Varnum BC, Lim RW & Herschman HR (1991) TIS10, a phorbol ester tumor promoter-inducible mRNA from Swiss 3T3 cells, encodes a novel prostaglandin synthase-cyclooxygenase homologue. *Journal of Biological Chemistry* **266:** 12866–12872.

Kunze H & Vogt W (1971) Significance of phospholipase A for prostaglandin formation. *Annals of the New York Academy of Sciences* **180:** 123–125.

Kupiecki FP (1965) Conversion of homo-γ-linolenic acid to prostaglandin $F_{1\alpha}$ by ovine and bovine seminal vesicle extracts. *Life Sciences* **4:** 1811–1815.

Lands WEM & Samuelsson B (1968) Phospholipid precursors of prostaglandins. *Biochimica et Biophysica Acta* **164:** 426–429.

Lands WEM, Le Tellier PR, Rome LH & Vanderhoek JY (1972) Modes of inhibiting the prostaglandin synthetic capacity of sheep vesicular gland preparation. *Federation Proceedings* **31:** 476A.

Lee RE & Lands WEM (1972) Cofactors in the biosynthesis of prostaglandins $F_{1\alpha}$ and $F_{2\alpha}$. *Biochimica et Biophysica Acta* **260:** 203–211.

Lee SC & Levine L (1974) Prostaglandin metabolism. I Cytoplasmic reduced nicotinamide adenine dinucleotide phosphate-dependent and microsomal reduced nicotinamide adenine dinucleotide-dependent prostaglandin E 9-keto-reductase activities in monkey and pigeon tissues. *Journal of Biological Chemistry* **249:** 1369–1375.

McDonald-Gibson RG, Flack JD & Ramwell PW (1973) Inhibition of prostaglandin biosynthesis by 7-oxa and 5-oxa-prostaglandin analogues. *Biochemical Journal* **132:** 117–120.

Marshall PJ & Kulmacz RJ (1988) Prostaglandin H synthase: distinct binding sites for cyclooxygenase and peroxidase substrates. *Archives of Biochemistry and Biophysics* **226:** 162–170.

Moncada S, Gryglewski R, Bunting S & Vane JR (1976) An enzyme isolated from arteries transforms prostaglandin endoperoxides to an unstable substance that inhibits platelet aggregation. *Nature* **263:** 663–665.

Nakano J, Anggard E & Samuelsson B (1969) 15-hydroxy-prostanoate dehydrogenase. Prostaglandins as substrates and inhibitors. *European Journal of Biochemistry* **11:** 386–389.

Nikkila EA (1971) Transport of free fatty acids. *Progress in Biochemical Pharmacology* **6:** 102–129.

Nugteren DH (1970) Inhibition of prostaglandin biosynthesis by 8cis, 12trans, 14cis-eicosatrienoic acid. *Biochimica et Biophysica Acta* **210:** 171–176.

Nugteren DH (1975) The determination of prostaglandin metabolites in human urine. *Journal of Biological Chemistry* **250:** 2808–2812.

Nugteren DH & Nazelhof E (1973) Isolation and properties of intermediates in prostaglandin biosynthesis. *Biochimica et Biophysica Acta* **326:** 448–461.

Nugteren DH, Beerthuis RK & van Dorp DA (1966a) The enzymatic conversion of all-cis, 8,11,14-eicosatrienoic acid into prostaglandin E_1. *Recueil des Travaux Chimi ques des Pays-Bas* **85:** 405–419.

Nugteren DH, van Dorp DA, Bergstrom S, Hamberg M & Samuelsson B (1966b) Absolute configuration of the prostaglandins. *Nature* **212:** 38–39.

O'Banion KM, Sadowski HB, Winn V & Young DA (1991) A serum- and glucocorticoid-regulated 4-kilobase mRNA encodes a cyclooxygenase-related protein. *Journal of Biological Chemistry* **266:** 23261–23267.

Pace-Asciak C & Wolfe LS (1968) Inhibition of prostaglandin biosynthesis by oleic, linoleic and linolenic acids. *Biochimica et Biophysica Acta* **152:** 784–787.

Paulus HE & Whitehouse MW (1973) Non-steroid anti-inflammatory agents. *Annual Review of Pharmacology* **13:** 107–125.

Piper PJ & Vane JR (1971) The release of prostaglandins from lung and other tissues. *Annals of the New York Academy of Sciences* **180:** 363–385.

Ramwell PW & Shaw JE (1970) Biological significance of the prostaglandins. *Recent Progress in Hormone Research* **26:** 139–187.

Rosen GD, Birkenmeier TM, Raz A & Holtzman MJ (1989) Identification of a cyclooxygenase-related gene and its potential role in prostaglandin formation. *Biochemical and Biophysical Research Communications* **164:** 1358–1365.

Samuelsson B (1967) Biosynthesis and metabolism of prostaglandins. In Kraitchewsky R, Paoletti R & Steinberg D (eds) *Progress in Biochemical Pharmacology*, pp 59–70. New York: Karger.

Samuelsson B (1973) Biosynthesis and metabolism of prostaglandins. In *Seminaire—Les Prostaglandines*, pp 21–41. Paris: INSERM.

Samuelsson B, Granstrom E, Green K & Hamberg M (1971) Metabolism of prostaglandins. *Annals of the New York Academy of Sciences* **180**: 138–163.

Shen TY (1972) Perspectives in non-steroidal, anti-inflammatory agents. *Angewandte Chemie* **11**: 460–472.

Shio H, Ramwell PW, Andersen NH & Corey EJ (1970) Stereospecificity of the prostaglandin 15-dehydrogenase from swine lung. *Experientia* **26**: 355–357.

Smith JB & Willis AL (1971) Aspirin selectively inhibits prostaglandin production in human platelets. *Nature* **231**: 235–237.

Smith MJH & Dawkins PD (1971) Salicylate and enzymes. *Journal of Pharmacy & Pharmacology* **23**: 729–744.

Smith WL (1986) Prostaglandin synthesis and its compartmentation in vascular smooth muscle and endothelial cells. *Annual Reviews in Physiology* **48**: 251–262.

Smith WL (1989) The eicosanoids and their biochemical mechanisms of action. *Biochemical Journal* **259**: 315–324.

Smith WL, Marnett LJ & DeWitt DL (1991) Prostaglandin and thromboxane biosynthesis. *Pharmacologic Therapy* **49**: 153–179.

Struijk CB, Beerthuis RK & van Dorp DA (1967) Specificity in the enzymatic conversion of poly-unsaturated fatty acids into prostaglandins. In Bergstrom S & Samuelsson B (eds) *The Prostaglandins, Proceedings of the 2nd Nobel Symposium*, pp 51–56. Stockholm: Almqvist and Wiksell.

Takeguchi C & Sih CJ (1972) A rapid spectrophotometric assay for prostaglandin synthetase. Application to the study of non-steroidal, anti-inflammatory agents. *Prostaglandins* **2**: 169–184.

Taylor PL & Kelly RW (1974) 19-hydroxylated E prostaglandins as the major prostaglandins of human semen. *Nature* **250**: 665–667.

Vanderhoek JY & Lands WEM (1973a) Actylenic inhibitors of sheep vesicular gland oxygenase. *Biochimica et Biophysica Acta* **296**: 374–381.

Vanderhoek HY & Lands WEM (1973b) The inhibition of the fatty acid oxygenase of sheep vesicular gland by anti-oxidants. *Biochimica et Biophysica Acta* **296**: 382–385.

van Dorp DA (1967) Aspects of the biosynthesis of prostaglandins. In Editchewsky P, Paoletti R & Steinberg D (eds) *Progress in Biochemical Pharmacology*, pp 71–82. New York: Karger.

van Dorp DA & Christ EJ (1975) Specificity in the enzymic conversion of substituted cis-8, cis-11, cis-14-eicosatrienoic acids into prostaglandins. *Recueil des Travaux Chimi ques des Pays-Bas* **94**: 247–253.

van Dorp DA, Beerthuis RK, Nugteren DH & Vonkeman H (1964a) The biosynthesis of prostaglandins. *Biochimica et Biophysica Acta* **90**: 204–207.

van Dorp DA, Beerthuis RK, Nugteren DH & Vonkeman H (1964b) Enzymatic conversion of all-cis polyunsaturated fatty acids into prostaglandins. *Nature* **203**: 839–841.

Vane JR (1971) Inhibition of prostaglandin synthesis as a mechanism of action for aspirin-like drugs. *Nature* **231**: 232–235.

Vane JR (1972) Prostaglandins and the aspirin-like drugs. *Hospital Practice* **7**: 61–71.

Vane JR & Botting RM (1990) The mode of action of anti-inflammatory drugs. *Postgraduate Medical Journal* **66**: S2–17.

Vogt W (1967) Release of prostaglandins by venoms and endogenous mechanisms. In Leonardi A & Walsh J (eds) *International Symposium on Drugs of Animal Origin*, pp 29–33. Milan: Ferro Edizione.

von Euler US (1935) Uber die spezifische blutdrucksenkende Substanz des menschlichen Prostata und Samenblasensekretes. *Klinische Wochenschrift* **14**: 1182–1183.

Vonkeman H & van Dorp DA (1968) The action of prostaglandin synthetase on 2-arachidonyl-lecithin. *Biochimica et Biophysica Acta* **164**: 430–432.

Wallach DP & Daniels EG (1971) Properties of a novel preparation of prostaglandin synthetase from sheep seminal vesicles. *Biochimica et Biophysica Acta* **231**: 445–457.

Watanabe K, Fujii Y, Nakayama K, Ohkubo H, Kuramitsu S, Hayashi H, Kagamiyama H, Nakanishi S & Hayaishi O (1989) Cloning, nucleotide sequence and gene expression of bovine lung prostaglandin F synthetase. In Samuelsson B, Wong PYL & Sun FF (eds) *Advances in Prostaglandin, Thromboxane and Leukotriene Research*, vol. 19, pp 462–465. New York: Raven Press.

Willis AL, Davison P, Ramwell PW, Brocklehurst WE & Smith B (1972) Release and actions of prostaglandins in inflammation and fever. Inhibition by anti-inflammatory and anti-pyretic drugs. In Ramwell PW & Phariss B (eds) *Prostaglandins in Cellular Biology*, pp 227–259. New York: Plenum Press.

Wlodawer P, Samuelsson B, Albinoco SM & Corey EJ (1971) Selective inhibition of prostaglandin synthetase by a bicyclo (2:2.1) heptene derivative. *Journal of the American Chemical Society* **93:** 2815–2816.

Xie W, Chipman JG, Robertson DL, Erikson RL & Simmons DL (1991) Expression of a mitogen-responsive gene encoding prostaglandin synthase is regulated by mRNA splicing. *Proceedings of the National Academy of Sciences of the USA* **88:** 2692–2696.

Yamasaki M & Sasaki M (1975) Formation of prostaglandin E_1 from 15-keto-prostaglandin E_1 by guinea-pig lung 15-hydroxyprostaglandin dehydrogenase. *Biochemical and Biophysical Research Communications* **66:** 355–361.

2

Prostaglandins in the ovary and fallopian tube

TIMOTHY J. GELETY
GAUTAM CHAUDHURI

INTRODUCTION

Prostaglandins and leukotrienes (products of lipoxygenase metabolism of arachidonic acid) have been implicated in playing a role in virtually all aspects of reproductive physiology. A large body of contradictory data has been published regarding their various roles, which has led to a great deal of confusion regarding the physiological significance of these substances. It should be emphasized that, with respect to the prostaglandin literature, some of the confusion stems from the fact that many laboratories have used only radioimmunoassays to establish a physiological role, which may be inappropriate in some cases. There is a wide difference in cross-reactivity of the prostaglandin antibody with different prostaglandin metabolites, some of which may yet be uncharacterized. Therefore, it is important that in order to suggest a biological role of prostaglandins at a particular tissue site, whenever possible, one should demonstrate the presence of these substances with the use of a biological assay.

Another difficulty is the apparent marked interspecies differences observed in the physiological role of these bioactive substances, in particular with respect to the reproductive system. Significant advances in understanding the physiological roles for prostaglandins in the ovary has come from work involving the rat, rabbit, porcine and large ruminant models. However, there are numerous examples in which these findings are not applicable to human physiology.

In this chapter, the synthesis and distribution of prostaglandins and leukotrienes in the ovary and the fallopian tube will be reviewed. Prostaglandins are very rapidly metabolized by the lungs, and hence one has to consider the possibility that, with respect to the reproductive system, prostaglandins and leukotrienes may play an important role as 'local hormones' where they are produced locally, act locally, and are often metabolized locally. Prostaglandins appear to play a role in the modulation of action of other local hormones (epidermal growth factor (EGF), bovine insulin-like growth factor 1 (bIGF-1), norepinephrine), as well as other circulating hormones, including gonadotrophins and sex steroids. Prostaglandins and leukotrienes have been identified in ovarian tissue from all species studied. Prostaglandin synthesis has been demonstrated in the granulosa, thecal and

Baillière's Clinical Obstetrics and Gynaecology—
Vol. 6, No. 4, December 1992
ISBN 0–7020–1694–2

707

stromal compartments, and has also been identified in significant quantities in follicular fluid. Physiological roles which have been suggested for prostaglandins include the mechanism of ovulation, corpus luteum formation and function, and luteolysis. Prostaglandins have also been implicated in ovarian pathological states, including the ovarian hyperstimulation syndrome (OHSS). In addition, prostaglandins have been identified in varying amounts in the isthmic, infundibular and ampullary portions of the fallopian tube. The role of prostaglandins in tubal motility has been of great clinical interest with regard to fertility and ectopic gestations. More recently, prostaglandins have been used in the medical treatment of ectopic pregnancy, with promising results.

OVARY

Follicular compartment

Until recently, information regarding the biosynthetic potential of eicosanoids from the various compartments within the ovary (follicular, luteal and stromal) has been scant. Using a glutathione S-transferase (GST) coupled assay, the predominant prostaglandin synthesized in the ovine follicular compartment was demonstrated to be prostaglandin E_2 (PGE_2) (81%), followed by PGD_2 (17%) and then $PGF_{2\alpha}$ (2%) (Padmavathi et al, 1990). Follicular prostaglandins are known to increase dramatically in the hours after the preovulatory gonadotrophin rise in animals. In the rat and rabbit, accumulation of PGF in the follicle begins 2–3 h after endogenous luteinizing hormone (LH) surge, or following exogenous human chorionic gonadotrophin (hCG) administration, with peak levels observed about the time of ovulation (10–12 h) (LeMaire et al, 1979, 1980). PGF reaches a maximum level in the follicle by the time of ovulation and declines rapidly, whereas PGE continues to be produced for several hours after ovulation (Richman et al, 1974).

The gonadotrophin stimulation of follicular prostaglandin synthesis appears to be unique with respect to the usual pathways, which results in elevations of prostaglandins within seconds to minutes. Compounds that acutely increase prostaglandin synthesis primarily do so by increasing substrate availability (arachidonic acid) and by increasing phospholipase A_2 (Samuelsson et al, 1975), phospholipase C or diglyceride lipase activities (Bell et al, 1979). In studies on the rat ovary, stimulation with LH or hCG did not result in increased substrate availability (Clark et al, 1978a). However, an increase in the specific activity of prostaglandin synthetase was demonstrated in isolated granulosa cells treated with LH and hCG both in vitro and in vivo (Clark et al, 1978b, 1979). That this increase in enzyme activity might be due to an increase synthesis of enzyme protein was suggested by the demonstration of a reduction in ovarian prostaglandin accumulation by the use of protein and RNA synthesis inhibitors (Zor et al, 1977). More recently, the use of an enzyme immunoassay employing a monoclonal antibody for prostaglandin synthetase was employed to directly demonstrate a three-fold increase in prostaglandin synthetase with hCG in the rat (Huslig et al, 1987). Like LH, follicle-stimulating hormone (FSH) has been demonstrated to increase PGE_2 production in cultured rat granulosa cells (Wang et al, 1989). This increased production can be mimicked by cAMP, which has been suggested as the cellular mediator (Clark et al, 1978b).

PGE_2 synthesis in granulosa cells has been demonstrated to be associated with the phospholipid-sensitive calcium-dependent protein kinase, protein kinase C, in the rat and swine model (Kawai and Clark, 1985; Veldhuis and Demers, 1987). Activation of the protein kinase C effector pathway stimulates PGE_2 production in a dose- and time-dependent fashion and can be inhibited by indomethacin, an inhibitor of cyclooxygenase, or by the use of the protein synthesis inhibitor cycloheximide (Veldhuis and Demers, 1987). The mechanism of coupling between prostaglandin synthesis and the protein kinase C pathway is believed to involve calcium ions (Veldhuis and Demers, 1987). The precise physiological activators of protein kinase C are not clear. However, gonadotrophin-releasing hormone (GnRH) and $PGF_{2\alpha}$, have been shown to stimulate this pathway in rat granulosa cells (Kawai and Clark, 1986; Leung et al, 1986).

Protein kinase C, the calcium-activated phosphorylating enzyme system, has been demonstrated in the mammalian ovary. However, its role in ovarian cellular function is not entirely clear (Veldhuis and Demers, 1986). Protein kinase C stimulation has also been demonstrated to increase synthesis of Prostaglandin $F_{2\alpha}$ in porcine granulosa cells (Demers and Veldhuis, 1987) in a time- and dose-dependent manner. This increase could be inhibited by the cyclooxygenase inhibitor indomethacin and the protein synthesis inhibitor cycloheximide, which would suggest de novo synthesis of $PGF_{2\alpha}$ dependent on induction of enzyme synthesis (Demers and Veldhuis, 1987).

In addition to the gonadotrophins, LH and FSH, GnRH itself has been shown to increase PGE_2 synthesis in vitro in rat granulosa cells (Clark et al, 1980; Koos and Clark, 1982; Wang et al, 1989). Although GnRH has been demonstrated to simulate arachidonic acid release from granulosa cells (Minegishi and Leung, 1985), it appears that this effect is also linked to the activation of protein kinase C (Wang et al, 1989; Kawai and Clark, 1985). Wang and co-workers have suggested that the GnRH-induced activation of protein kinase C may involve two steps: the release of arachidonic acid from membrane phospholipid and the activation of cyclooxygenase, resulting in an increase in prostaglandin production (Wang et al, 1989). The mechanism of GnRH stimulation of prostaglandins appears to be different from that of the gonadotrophins (Clark, 1982). Treatment of rat granulosa cells in vitro with FSH and GnRH will increase PGE_2 ten-fold, and GnRH and FSH added concomitantly act synergistically to increase PGE_2 and $PGF_{2\alpha}$ formation (Wang et al, 1989). Activation of protein kinase C results in a dose-dependent inhibition of progesterone production by FSH by increasing FSH-stimulated production of PGE_2 (Wang et al, 1989).

Several other hormone/growth factors have been shown to influence prostaglandin synthesis in the ovarian granulosa, suggesting one of several mechanisms for activity of these paracrine ovarian hormones. These include

EGF (Berchuck et al, 1988), basic fibroblast growth factor (bFGF; LaPolt et al, 1990) and IGF-1 (McArdle and Holtorf, 1989). bFGF is an angiogenic factor which has been demonstrated in the granulosa cells (Neufeld et al, 1987). bFGF has been demonstrated to increase follicular PGE synthesis in a dose-dependent manner in the rat (LaPolt et al, 1990) and PGE_2 has been proposed as the mediator of bFGF oocyte maturation, which may also involve tissue mitogen activator (tPA), the expression of which can be stimulated in the granulosa cells by bFGF. In addition, PGE_1 and PGE_2 have been shown to increase granulosa cell plasminogen activator (PA) activity (Strickland and Beers, 1976), which has been proposed as yet another mediator of ovarian prostaglandin activity.

Prostacyclin (PGI_2) is produced from blood vessel microsomes of fresh vascular tissue by the action of prostacyclin synthetase on the prostaglandin endoperoxide PGH_2 (Bunting et al, 1976). Prostacyclin has been demonstrated in a wide variety of tissues, including decidua and myometrium of the pregnant rat (Williams et al, 1978), and the human chorion, amnion and decidua (Mitchell et al, 1978). Prostacyclin is chemically unstable with a half-life of 2–3 min and is rapidly metabolized to 6-keto-$PGF_{1\alpha}$. Early reports that prostacyclin was a major prostaglandin produced in rat ovarian homogenates may have reflected production predominantly by endothelial cells of the rich ovarian vasculature (Poyser and Scott, 1980). Prostacyclin has been demonstrated to stimulate cAMP production by rat granulosa in vitro (Goff et al, 1978). Recently, significant amounts of 6-keto-$PGF_{1\alpha}$ have been demonstrated by the technique of in vitro perfusion of human postmenopausal ovaries (Abrahamsson et al, 1990). Increased production of prostacyclin has been reported to be associated with benign ovarian cysts (Abrahamsson et al, 1990) and human ovarian cancer (Aitokallio-Tallberg et al, 1988). Evidence for prostacyclin production by human follicles has been reported by the identification of 6-keto-$PGF_{1\alpha}$ in the follicular fluid from hyperstimulated ovaries (Ylikorkala and Tenhuneu, 1984). 6-Keto-$PGF_{1\alpha}$ has also been characterized in preovulatory follicular fluid from women during spontaneous cycles. However, no increase in levels were noted with hCG administration or during ovulation (Priddy et al, 1989). 6-Keto-$PGF_{1\alpha}$ measurements have been used to demonstrate prostacyclin synthesis from rat granulosa cells in vitro (Koos and Clark, 1982). Prostacyclin synthesis in vitro can also be stimulated by LH and GnRH agonists (GnRHas), although in much smaller amounts when compared with PGE_2 synthesis (Koos and Clark, 1982).

The prostaglandin endoperoxides can also be transformed by the action of thromboxane synthetase to the unstable product thromboxane A_2 (TXA_2). The name 'thromboxane' was derived initially from the characterization of a vasoconstrictor substance in platelets (thrombocytes) which contained an oxane ring in its structure (Hamberg et al, 1975). TXA_2 has a chemical half-life of 30 seconds at body pH and temperature, and is inactivated to TXB_2. Piper and Vane (1969) originally described thromboxane, using bioassay, as rabbit aortic contracting substance (RCS). TXA_2 is primarily a product of platelets and is a strong contractor of large blood vessels and induces platelet aggregation. Other cells have been demonstrated to synthesize thromboxane, including polymorphonuclear leukocytes in human and rabbits (Higgs et al, 1976) and human umbilical artery (Tuvemo et al, 1981). TXB_2, the product of metabolism of the active TXA_2, has been characterized in follicular fluid from hyperstimulated human ovaries (Ylikorkala and Tenhuneu, 1984) and from spontaneous cycles (Priddy et al, 1989). The significance of the low levels of production of thromboxane in the ovary, however, is not clear.

In addition to arachidonic acid metabolism via the cyclooxygenase pathway, metabolism by lipoxygenase leading to the synthesis of leukotrienes has received increasing attention with respect to reproductive physiology. Arachidonic acid conversion by the enzyme lipoxygenase results in the formation of 5-hydroxyeicosatetraenoic acid (5-HETE). Subsequent metabolic products were named 'leukotrienes' by Samuelsson et al (1979), who characterized their synthesis from leukocytes which contain a conjugated triene in their structure. 5-HETE is converted by dehydrogenase to leukotriene A_4 (LTA_4). LTA_4 can be converted by hydroxylase to LTB_4, or by the enzyme glutathione S-transferase initially to LTC_4, which is converted to LTD_4, and then to LTE_4 and LTF_4. The peptitic LTB_4 has powerful chemotactic and chemokinetic properties with little direct smooth muscle stimulating activity (Ford-Hutchinson et al, 1980). The non-peptitic leukotrienes have direct smooth muscle stimulatory activity, and leukotrienes as a group may play an important role in the inflammatory process (Williams, 1983). Leukotrienes have been demonstrated in ovarian follicular fluid in humans in spontaneous ovulatory cycles with characterization of LTB_4, LTC_4, LTD_4 and LTE_4 (Priddy et al, 1989). In addition, the enzyme lipoxygenase has been characterized in human granulosa cells (Feldman et al, 1986). Subsequently, LTD_4 has been identified in human follicular fluid from hyperstimulated ovarian follicles (Heinonen et al, 1986).

In the rat, ovarian lipoxygenase activity has been shown to increase two- to five-fold in the periovulatory period and may be regulated by the preovulatory rise in gonadotrophins (Reich et al, 1983, 1985b). Furthermore, inhibition of lipoxygenase has been shown to inhibit ovulation in the rat (Reich et al, 1983). In rats treated with pregnant mare serum gonadotrophin (PMSG), LTB_4, LTC_4, LTD_4, and LTE_4 production was increased approximately two-fold after hCG, with peak production after 4 h and a significant decline in production observed prior to ovulation (Espey et al, 1989). The increase in leukotriene production observed for preovulation was much less than that observed with prostanoids. Small amounts of LTC_4 have been demonstrated to stimulate LH release from the rat anterior pituitary, suggesting a role as a mediator of positive feedback on the LH surge (Samuelsson et al, 1987). The functional role of ovarian leukotrienes, however, remains to be elucidated.

Ovulation

There now exists an increasing body of evidence implicating prostaglandins in the ovulatory process. In vivo studies in laboratory animals, including the rat, rabbit and rhesus monkey, suggest that the preovulatory increase of prostaglandin production by ovarian follicles plays a critical role in ovulation (LeMaire et al, 1973; Yang et al, 1974; Wallach et al, 1975; Armstrong, 1981; Dennefors et al, 1983). $PGF_{2\alpha}$ and PGI_2 appear to have a stimulatory role in ovulation, whereas PGE_2 has the opposite effect (Richman et al, 1974; Yoshimura et al, 1988). The evidence for the role of prostaglandins in this regard comes from work involving systemic administration of prostaglandin synthesis inhibitors, such as aspirin and indomethacin, which have been shown to inhibit ovulation in the rat (Armstrong and Grinwich, 1972; Tsafriri et al, 1973) and rabbit (O'Grady et al, 1972). In the rabbit, intrafollicular injection of either indomethacin or a specific antiserum to PGF prevents ovulation, which suggests a local ovarian site of action (Dennefors et al, 1983). Interestingly, in various species, including monkeys, inhibition of prostaglandin synthesis has been shown to prevent ovulation, but not luteinization (Armstrong and Grinwich, 1972; O'Grady et al, 1972; Tsafriri et al, 1973; Wallach et al, 1975). Wallach and co-workers demonstrated that the inhibitory action of prostaglandin synthetase inhibitors on ovulation in the rhesus monkey could be reversed with administration of $PGF_{2\alpha}$ (Wallach et al, 1975). Likewise, in the rat and rabbit models indomethacin has been shown to inhibit LH-induced follicular rupture without affecting steroidogenesis or oocyte maturation (Janson et al, 1988). In the rabbit, $PGF_{2\alpha}$ reverses the ovulatory blockade, and $PGF_{2\alpha}$ alone can induce follicular rupture with the release of immature follicles (Kitai et al, 1985b; Janson et al, 1988). Likewise, in this same species, PGI_2 alone has been shown to produce follicular rupture in the absence of gonadotrophins (Yoshimura et al, 1988).

Taken together it appears that prostaglandins mediate rupture of preovulatory follicles, and may not be involved in other LH-mediated ovulatory events, including oocyte maturation. Katz et al (1989) have demonstrated intact morphological and functional luteinization in the rabbit treated with indomethacin to block follicular rupture, using an in vitro perfused ovary system. Chaudhuri and Elder (1976), however, were unable to inhibit ovulation in women using high doses of aspirin and were also unable to demonstrate retained ova in the corpora lutea obtained from women treated with aspirin in that cycle. In the rabbit model, evaluation of the dose and type of prostaglandin synthesis inhibitors used suggests that ovarian prostaglandin levels must be inhibited by at least 80% in order to block ovulation (Espey et al, 1986, 1988, 1990). It is possible, therefore, that a more potent prostaglandin synthesis inhibitor may be able to inhibit ovulation; however, this remains to be demonstrated in the human.

The mechanism by which prostaglandins mediate follicular rupture in the process of ovulation is not clear. Stimulation of cAMP has been suggested to be mediated via prostaglandins (Kuehl et al, 1970; LeMaire and Marsh, 1975) and, in the rat, prostaglandin involvement in cAMP-induced ovulation independent of LH has been demonstrated (Brannstrom et al, 1987). Prostaglandins have also been proposed to have an action on the neuromuscular complex of the follicular wall, causing rupture by means of increased ovarian contractility; however, this remains controversial (Espey, 1978). Prostaglandins, in particular PGI_2, have been implicated in alterations of the follicular microvasculature, causing vasodilation and increased permeability of the perifollicular capillaries (Yoshimura et al, 1988). However, the finding of a lack of effect on the ultrastructure of the rabbit follicular wall and follicular microvasculature in the presence and absence of indomethacin does not support this as a mechanism for follicular rupture (Espey et al, 1981). Prostaglandins may stimulate proteolytic activity in the follicular wall, particularly collagenase (Reich et al, 1985a; Murdoch et al, 1986; Miyazaki et al, 1991). However, the preovulatory increase in collagenase activity has been shown to be independent of prostaglandin production in the rat (Curry et al, 1986). It has been proposed by Miyazaki and co-workers (1991) that prostaglandins may increase collagenase activity via activation of PA and plasmin. This group has recently demonstrated that inhibition of PA and/or plasmin can block $PGF_{2\alpha}$-induced ovulation in a dose-dependent manner. This supports the concept of prostaglandin activation of proteolytic enzymes in the follicular wall leading to follicular rupture.

In addition to the prostaglandins, the leukotriene products of the lipoxygenase pathway of arachidonic acid metabolism have been implicated in the ovulatory process (Espey, 1980; Tanaka et al, 1989). Follicular rupture has been likened to an inflammatory process which may be mediated by the well-recognized effects of leukotrienes, including vasodilatation, increased vascular permeability, and activation and chemotaxis of leukocytes. Reich and colleagues suggested a role for leukotrienes in this process by demonstrating a preovulatory increase in lipoxygenase activity in the rat model (Reich et al, 1983, 1985b). Furthermore, intrabursal injections into the rat ovary of nordihydroguaiaretic acid (NDGA), an inhibitor of lipoxygenase, resulted in inhibition of ovulation without affecting ovulation from the contralateral ovary (Reich et al, 1983). However, Hellberg and co-workers (1990), using the in vitro perfused rat ovary model, found an increase in the number of LH-stimulated ovulations after treatment with the lipoxygenase inhibitors NDGA and caffeic acid. These findings may reflect a shunting of arachidonic acid substrate from the lipoxygenase to the cyclooxygenase pathway, which is supported by the findings of a net increase in prostaglandins with a subsequent increase in ovulatory rate. The possible contributions of leukotrienes in the ovulatory process therefore remain to be elucidated.

Luteal compartment

In contrast to the follicular compartment, quantitative evaluation of the biosynthetic potential of prostaglandins in the ovine model has shown the major prostaglandin in the corpus luteum to be $PGF_{2\alpha}$ (59%), followed by PGD_2 (21%) and PGE_2 (20%) (Padmavathi et al, 1990). There is good evidence that the primate corpus luteum produces PGE_2, $PGF_{2\alpha}$ and PGI_2 (Challis et al, 1976; Patwardhan and Lanthier, 1985). Human corpus luteum has been shown to produce $PGF_{2\alpha}$ and PGE_2 in vitro (Challis et al, 1976). In addition, receptors have been identified in the human corpus luteum for $PGF_{2\alpha}$ and PGE_2 (Hamberger et al, 1979). The concentration of PGE_2 in human corpus luteum is increased during the early luteal phase and decreased during the late luteal phase, whereas $PGF_{2\alpha}$ concentration increases during the mid- and late luteal phase (Patwardhan and Lanthier, 1985).

In the rabbit corpus luteum, increased activity of the enzyme PGE_2 9-ketoreductase has been demonstrated in the late luteal phase, which is responsible for the conversion of PGE_2 to $PGF_{2\alpha}$ (Vijayakumar and Walters, 1987). In the cycling human, the early luteal phase is characterized by elevated PGE_2 concentrations, corresponding to peak progesterone levels, while the late secretory phase is associated with lower progesterone levels and markedly increased $PGF_{2\alpha}$ (Tanaka et al, 1981). The enzyme prostaglandin 15-dehydrogenase (PG-15-HDH), which is responsible for the metabolism of PGE_2 and $PGF_{2\alpha}$ to 13,14-dihydroxyketo-PGE_2 and 13,14-dihydroxyketo-$PGF_{2\alpha}$, respectively, has been demonstrated in the rabbit corpus luteum as well (Vijayakumar and Walters, 1987). However, changes in PG-15-HDH enzyme activity do not appear to be important in the regulation of $PGE_2/PGF_{2\alpha}$ production (Schlegel et al, 1988).

Prostaglandin-endoperoxide synthetase (PGHS) activity has been demonstrated in human corpus luteum tissue homogenates (Challis et al, 1976). More recently, immunoperoxidase staining techniques have been used to localize PGHS in the rat (Curry et al, 1990) and in the human corpus luteum (Kauma et al, 1990). Human corpus luteum contains immunoreactive PGHS primarily localized in well-differentiated granulosa lutein cells, with maximal staining noted in the mid-luteal phase, while theca lutein cells had less and stromal cells had almost no staining. PGHS activity has been suggested to be localized to the smooth endoplasmic reticulum of the large granulosa lutein cells (Curry et al, 1990; Kauma et al, 1990).

Stromal compartment

The ovarian stromal production of eicosanoids has only recently been the subject of investigation. In normally cycling women, ovarian stromal tissue PGE_2 content was found to vary with the stage of the menstrual cycle and was significantly elevated during the late proliferative and early secretory phases (Vijayakumar and Walters, 1987). This increased stromal production of PGE_2 parallels the early luteal production. Whereas the ovarian stromal tissue $PGF_{2\alpha}$ content was highest during the late secretory and early proliferative phase (Vijayakumar and Walters, 1987), stromal $PGF_{2\alpha}$ production was highest and paralleled late luteal production of $PGF_{2\alpha}$. An increase in stromal PGE_2 and $PGF_{2\alpha}$ occurs in the preovulatory period, as seen in the follicular compartment. In the rabbit, ovarian stromal concentrations of PGE_2, $PGF_{2\alpha}$, the enzymes PGE_2 9-ketoreductase and PGE 15-HAH, and prostaglandin metabolites were found to be similar, but generally lower in concentration than in luteal tissue (Schlegel et al, 1988).

Luteal function

Most theories regarding the role of prostaglandins in corpus luteum function were based on in vivo experimentation with laboratory animals. There are marked species differences in the factors responsible for maintenance of the corpora lutea, making it difficult to extrapolate data based on experimental models to humans. It appears that prostaglandins either promote or suppress luteal function. Despite the fact that PGE_2 seems to mimic the effects of LH in inducing luteinization, $PGF_{2\alpha}$ has the opposite effect; as both of these prostaglandins have been demonstrated in follicular fluid, their importance to the luteinization process and maintenance of the corpus luteum remains unclear.

Many studies have examined the primary role of $PGF_{2\alpha}$ in luteal function. However, findings of large quantities of PGE_2 and 6-keto-$PGF_{1\alpha}$ as a marker of PGI_2 in rabbit and human ovaries have suggested a luteotrophic role for these prostaglandins in these species. In vivo studies on the action of prostaglandins on luteal function have employed indomethacin in doses sufficient to affect ovulation in rats (Armstong and Grinwich, 1972), rabbits (O'Grady et al, 1972) and monkeys (Wallach et al, 1975), and have failed to demonstrate inhibition of luteinization with subsequent corpus luteum formation.

Using an in vitro perfusion technique of the isolated rabbit ovary, indomethacin significantly decreases prostaglandin production, including $PGF_{2\alpha}$, without affecting progesterone secretion from the corpus luteum (Dharmarajan et al, 1989). Furthermore, $PGF_{2\alpha}$ infusion does not affect luteal progesterone secretion (Hahlin et al, 1988). In the rhesus monkey, intraluteal infusion of the prostaglandin synthesis inhibitor sodium meclofenamate can cause premature luteolysis not seen with systemic administration, suggesting an obligatory luteotrophic role for locally produced metabolities of arachidonic acid (Sargent et al, 1988).

It should be pointed out that early studies showing conflicting results on luteal function with systemic administration of $PGF_{2\alpha}$ were thought to be due to a technical problem of adequate prostaglandin delivery to the site of action. Systemic treatment with $PGF_{2\alpha}$ analogues (Wilks, 1980, 1983) or infusion of $PGF_{2\alpha}$ directly into the corpus luteum (Auletta et al, 1984) results in decreased production of progesterone and premature menses in primates. Intraluteal infusion of prostaglandin synthetase inhibitors in primates results in decreased progesterone production and shortening of the luteal phase, which suggests a luteotrophic role for local prostaglandins (Sargent et al, 1988).

Many prostaglandins have been found to either stimulate or inhibit cAMP and progesterone production when added to luteal tissue in vitro. In the rhesus monkey, PGE_1 and PGE_2 added to cultured granulosa cells results in luteinization and increased synthesis of progesterone, similar to the effect of stimulation with LH (Channing, 1972). The luteinization seen with PGE was felt to be coupled to an increase in intracellular cAMP content, with the finding that this action could be mimicked by exogenous cAMP (Channing, 1972). Human granulosa cells in culture were also found to be stimulated by PGE_2, leading to increased progesterone production (McNatty et al, 1975). However, $PGF_{2\alpha}$ was found to inhibit progesterone production normally seen in granulosa cells obtained from gonadotrophin-exposed follicles (McNatty et al, 1975). PGA_2 has also caused inhibition of gonadotrophin-stimulated adenocyclase activity in the primate corpus luteum (Molskness et al, 1987), whereas PGI_2 and PGD_2 have been reported to stimulate cAMP and progesterone production in the primate and human ovary (Hamberger et al, 1987; Molskness et al, 1987).

The relevance of these in vitro and in vivo studies to the roles of endogenous prostaglandins in the regulation of human/primate corpus luteum remains unclear. This is in contrast to the situation with non-primate species where the role for $PGF_{2\alpha}$ derived from the uterus as the luteolytic factor is well established (Horton and Poyser, 1976). In laboratory and farm animals, including the guinea-pig and the sheep, hysterectomy leads to persistence of the corpus luteum, and $PGF_{2\alpha}$ derived from the uterus has been identified as the luteolytic factor (Blatchley et al, 1972; McCracken et al, 1972). Species in which the uterus has been demonstrated to regulate the life span of the corpus luteum such as the cow (Feilds et al, 1983; Wathes et al, 1983), ewe (Flint and Sheldrick, 1983) and the sow have been found to have high ovarian oxytocin concentrations which reach maximal levels on approximately day 11 of the luteal cycle and fall with oestrus. During the follicular phase, the oxytocin messenger RNA (mRNA) content of the granulosa cells and the oxytocin of the follicle are very low. Ovarian oxytocin gene expression increases rapidly after ovulation, with corpus luteum oxytocin mRNA concentrations increasing 100-fold within 2–4 days of ovulation (Ivell et al, 1985). $PGF_{2\alpha}$ administration has been demonstrated to cause ovarian oxytocin release in these species (Flint and Sheldrick, 1983; Rodgers et al, 1983). In addition, oxytocin results in $PGF_{2\alpha}$ production from the uterine endometrium and decidua (Roberts et al, 1976). Furthermore, immunization against oxytocin in bovine or ovine species prevents luteolysis (Cooke and Homeida, 1985; Schams et al, 1983; Sheldrick et al, 1980), which can be overcome by administration of exogenous $PGF_{2\alpha}$. Therefore, the positive-feedback loop between the ovary and the uterus may involve mediation by both prostaglandins and oxytocin to ensure luteolysis in species dependent on the uterus for the determination of luteal life span (Fuchs, 1987).

It is clear, therefore, in many subprimate species, including the sheep, cow and guinea-pig, that $PGF_{2\alpha}$ is the physiological luteolytic factor. In these species, corpus luteum regression is dependent on uterine $PGF_{2\alpha}$ production and local utero-ovarian blood flow (Blatchley et al, 1972; McCracken et al, 1972). Hysterectomy results in prolonged luteal function and luteolysis and subsequent menses can be induced with the administration of $PGF_{2\alpha}$. In primates and humans, however, cyclic ovarian function is not altered by hysterectomy. There are, however, several lines of evidence to suggest that local ovarian production of $PGF_{2\alpha}$ may play a role in corpus luteum functioning in these species. $PGF_{2\alpha}$ production by the primate and human corpus luteum is well established, as are the changes in relative concentrations of $PGE_2/PGF_{2\alpha}$ in early, mid- and late corpora lutea phases (Patwardhan and Lanthier, 1985). The rate of production of PGE_2 and $PGF_{2\alpha}$ has been shown to vary with the age of the corpus luteum during the human menstrual cycle (Patwardhan and Lanthier, 1985). In addition, there is good evidence that the action of prostaglandins on luteal tissue is dependent on the age or developmental stage of the corpus luteum (Khan, 1979).

Experiments designed to elucidate the role of $PGF_{2\alpha}$ on human corpus luteum steroid hormone production in vivo are contradictory. A systemic infusion of $PGF_{2\alpha}$ results in little effect on peripheral progesterone concentration (Wentz and Jones, 1973), whereas vaginal $PGF_{2\alpha}$ during early and mid-luteal phases has been shown to decrease progesterone levels and shorten the interval to menstrual bleeding (Hamberger et al, 1980b). Experiments designed to evaluate a local ovarian action of prostaglandins include injecting $PGF_{2\alpha}$ directly into human corpora lutea, which results in a decrease in progesterone and precipitation of menstrual bleeding (Korda et al, 1975). Infusion of $PGF_{2\alpha}$ into the corpus luteum of monkeys has also been shown to result in a fall of progesterone and the onset of menstrual bleeding (Auletta et al, 1984). In a more recent controlled study, injection of $PGF_{2\alpha}$ into the corpora lutea of eight women resulted in an immediate fall in serum progesterone by more than 30% and a shortening of the luteal phase by 2–5 days (Bennegard et al, 1991). This luteolytic effect of $PGF_{2\alpha}$ was not mediated by a decrease in serum LH, which is consistent with an intraluteal site of action (Bennegard et al, 1991).

The possibility of luteolysis being initiated by a primary vascular mechanism has been examined in animal studies. It has been clearly demonstrated that luteolysis precedes the decrease in luteal blood flow (Janson et al, 1975; Damber et al, 1981). Furthermore, in humans, direct injection of $PGF_{2\alpha}$ into the corpus luteum results in functional luteolysis without demonstrable changes in ovarian arterial blood flow or oxygen saturation as measured in the ovarian vascular pedicle (Bennegard et al, 1991).

Therefore, in humans, primates and other species in which hysterectomy does not interfere with luteolysis, it appears that local production of intraovarian factors, including prostaglandins, may play a role in the regulation of the corpus luteum. Ovarian oxytocin expression in the primate and the human has been demonstrated (Khan-Dawood and Dawood, 1983; Khan-Dawood et al, 1984; Schaeffer et al, 1984), but in much lower concentrations than in species in which uterine factors regulate corpus luteum life span. It has been suggested that oxytocin–$PGF_{2\alpha}$ interaction may occur in the ovary itself (Fuchs, 1987), in that luteal phase ovarian oxytocin may act in a paracrine manner to stimulate $PGF_{2\alpha}$ production, which in turn may suppress luteal progesterone production. In support of this concept, oxytocin infusion into the corpus luteum of the rhesus monkey has been shown to shorten the corpus luteum life span and to suppress progesterone production (Schaeffer et al, 1984). In addition, intraluteal $PGF_{2\alpha}$ infusion has also been demonstrated to result in luteolysis in primates (Auletta et al, 1984a), an effect not seen with systemic administration (Auletta et al, 1984b).

In the bovine model, $PGF_{2\alpha}$ has been shown to have a synergistic effect with insulin and IGF-1 to increase progesterone and oxytocin release from the granulosa (McArdle, 1990). In the early phase bovine corpus luteum, IGF-1-stimulated oxytocin can be inhibited by $PGF_{2\alpha}$ (McArdle and Holtorf, 1989). These findings suggest a functional interaction between prostaglandins and IGF-1 that may influence the development and regulation of the corpus luteum (McArdle, 1990). Using a microdialysis system designed to examine the paracrine interaction of the human corpus luteum in vitro, $PGF_{2\alpha}$ infusion has been shown to stimulate oxytocin, oestrogen and progesterone release. Furthermore, $PGF_{2\alpha}$ and oxytocin have both discrete inhibitory effects on progesterone release and oestrogen-mediated stimulatory effects, which results in a net stimulation of progesterone secretion in the young corpus luteum (Maas et al, 1992).

The paracrine regulation of luteal function in humans and primates has also been suggested to involve the interaction of catecholamines with $PGF_{2\alpha}$. It has been demonstrated that $PGF_{2\alpha}$ counteracts the stimulatory effects of hCG in vitro on cAMP formation by the human corpus luteum of the mid-luteal phase (Hamberger et al, 1979). $PGF_{2\alpha}$ also inhibits gonadotrophin-stimulated progesterone synthesis (Dennefors et al, 1980). This antigonadotrophin action of $PGF_{2\alpha}$ observed in vitro in humans (Hamberger et al, 1979; Dennefors et al, 1980) as well as rats (Lahav et al, 1976) is present only at a critical age of the corpus luteum. For instance, in the newly formed PMSG-induced corpus luteum of the pseudopregnant rat, $PGF_{2\alpha}$ cannot counteract the stimulatory effect of gonadotrophins on cAMP formation (Khan, 1979). Likewise, in the newly formed human corpus luteum, $PGF_{2\alpha}$ does not interfere with the stimulatory effect of hCG on cAMP formation in vitro, but does exhibit antigonadrotrophin effect on cAMP formation in the 7–11-day-old corpus luteum (Hamberger et al, 1979). This difference in response may be associated with the presence of noradrenergic terminals in the corpus luteum localized mainly in the blood vessels (Hamberger et al, 1980a). In rats, newly formed corpora lutea are almost totally devoid of noradrenergic innervation, whereas, in the 5–8 day postovulation corpus luteum, noradrenaline-innervated blood vessels appear (Dennefors et al, 1983). It is at this time that the inhibitory effect of $PGF_{2\alpha}$ on gonadotrophin-induced cAMP is maximal. Similarly, in humans, the amount of exogenous noradrenaline seems to be important for the interaction between $PGF_{2\alpha}$ and hCG (Dennefors et al, 1983). Noradrenaline or $PGF_{2\alpha}$ are ineffective in suppressing progesterone or cAMP production in human early phase luteal cells in vitro, but have a strong inhibitory effect when given together (Polishuk and Schenker, 1969). Furthermore, when luteal cells obtained from 7–10-day-old corpus luteum were preincubated with reserpine to release tissue catecholamines stores, $PGF_{2\alpha}$ was unable to counteract the stimulatory effect of hCG on cAMP formation (Hamberger et al, 1980a). Therefore, the hypothesis was formulated that the newly formed corpus luteum might be protected against $PGF_{2\alpha}$-induced luteolysis by the low noradrenaline content (Hamberger et al, 1980a).

It appears, therefore, that the regulation and life span of the human corpus luteum may involve the local production of luteotrophic and luteo-lytic prostaglandins, as well as interaction with other paracrine regulatory factors. However, the exact mechanisms of formation, maintenance and luteolysis in the human and the role of prostaglandins, if any, has yet to be clearly demonstrated.

Prostaglandins and the Ovarian Hyperstimulation Syndrome

The Ovarian Hyperstimulation Syndrome (OHSS) may be a severe and potentially fatal complication in women undergoing ovulation induction with gonadotrophins, clomiphene citrate and GnRHas, both alone or in combination. The syndrome is characterized by massive ovarian enlargement and increased capillary permeability, resulting in transudation of protein-rich fluid (Polishuk and Schenker, 1969; Dennefors et al, 1983). In the rabbit, gonadotrophin administration alone can result in ovarian enlargement and ascites formation, in the absence of ovulation (Dennefors et al, 1983). In the human, however, OHSS is a postovulatory event and it is well recognized that development of the syndrome can be prevented by withholding the ovulatory dose of hCG (Pride et al, 1990). This would suggest that a supraphysiological preovulatory LH surge or continuous stimulation in the luteal phase might trigger release of a critical vasoactive substance, resulting in the clinical manifestations of cystic ovarian enlargement, ascites formation, pleural and pericardial effusion, oliguria and decreased effective intravascular volume, with resultant arterial hypotension. Given the increased prostaglandin synthesis observed following the mid-cycle gonadotrophin surge and that follicular biosynthesis is enhanced by LH, prostaglandins have received intensive investigation as the likely candidate for the initiating factor in the development of this syndrome.

That the inciting vasoactive agent responsible for OHSS is of ovarian orgin was suggested by Polishuk and Schenker (see Dennefors et al, 1983), who were able to induce the syndrome with administration of gonadotrophins to female rabbits who had undergone hysterectomy or extraperitonealization of the ovaries, but not in males. These same investigators demonstrated that the prostaglandin synthetase inhibitor indomethacin could prevent fluid shifts associated with ascites, pleural effusion and hypovolaemia, suggesting a role for prostaglandin production in the development of the syndrome (Bennegaard et al, 1984). Furthermore, Kaitai and co-workers (see Pride et al, 1986) have demonstrated that perfusion of the rabbit ovary with hCG or $PGF_{2\alpha}$ results in vasodilatation of the microvasculature of prevulatory follicles, in contrast to the general vasoconstriction action of $PGF_{2\alpha}$. In the hamster model, treatment with LH infusion results in an increase of PGF and a decrease in PGE associated with superovulation (Schenker and Polinshuk, 1976). Indomethacin suppresses ovarian prostaglandin levels, prevents superovulation and is associated with increased ovarian blood flow, suggesting that superovulation may be mediated by prostaglandins via this mechanism (Schenker and Polishuk, 1976). However, although Pride et al (1986) demonstrated that ovarian PGF production was significantly decreased by indomethacin in rabbits with gonadotrophin-induced OHSS, they could demonstrate no effect on ascites formation. Likewise, in women with the syndrome treated with indomethacin, there appears to be no effect on the clinical course or ascites formation (Borenstein et al, 1989).

The use of indomethacin in patients with ovarian hyperstimulation has also raised concerns with respect to potential teratogenic effects (Balasch et al, 1991) as well as potential adverse systemic effects, especially with respect to renal function. Recently, a case of acute renal failure has been reported in a patient with severe OHSS who was treated with indomethacin (Balasch et al, 1990). Balasch and co-workers have demonstrated increased renal clearance of the vasodilators PGE_2 and PGI_2 in severe OHSS, and have suggested an essential role for prostaglandins in maintaining renal perfusion (Balasch et al, 1990). On this basis, the routine use of systemic prostaglandin synthetase inhibitors should be avoided in these patients.

PROSTAGLANDINS AND THE FALLOPIAN TUBES

Ovum pick-up and its subsequent transport through the ampulla takes place within a few hours of follicular rupture (Croxatto et al, 1978a). Important factors for the transport of ova are thought to include ciliary activity as well as muscular contractions (Hafez, 1979). It appears that endogenous oestrogens stimulate tubal contractility in humans, whereas progesterone is inhibitory (Lindblom et al, 1980).

On the basis of studies performed in rabbits, it was proposed that prostaglandins may play a role in oviductal motility. $PGF_{2\alpha}$, when administered subcutaneously to rabbits soon after ovulation, accelerates ovum transport (Chang and Hunt, 1972). Subsequently, Ellinger and Kirton (1971) observed in this same species that both PGE_2 and $PGF_{2\alpha}$ accelerated the transport of ova by 40 h and appreciably reduced the implantation rate if administered 13 h after ovulation. Furthermore, under oestrogen dominance as seen in rabbits, increased formation of $PGF_{2\alpha}$ (Spilman, 1974b; Saksena and Harper, 1975) and increased sensitivity of the musculature to $PGF_{2\alpha}$ stimulates tubal contractility (Coutinho and Maia, 1971). It is interesting to note, however, that administration of indomethacin to rabbits before and after ovulation does not affect ovum transport, thereby bringing into question the role of endogenous prostaglandins in the spontaneous oviductal motility in this species (El-Banna et al, 1976; Hodgson, 1976).

Early studies on the influence of various prostaglandins on human tubal motility yielded conflicting results (Sandberg et al, 1963, 1964, 1965), which may reflect differential responses in varying segments and smooth muscle layers of the fallopian tube. $PGF_{2\alpha}$ has been demonstrated to stimulate tubal motility in both the rhesus monkey (Spilman, 1974a) and human (Coutinho and Maia, 1971). In vitro studies evaluating the response of individual smooth muscle layers in the human suggest that $PGF_{2\alpha}$ and PGI_2 have a stimulatory effect in all layers, while PGE_2 has differential effects, with an overall inhibition of spontaneous contractions (Hahlin et al, 1987; Lindblom et al, 1978; Wilhelmsson et al, 1979).

Prostaglandins were isolated from extracts of human fallopian tube in 1969 by Zeller and Wiechell, who demonstrated the presence of PGE_1 and $PGF_{2\alpha}$ in the ampullary portion of the tube, but not in the isthmus. Subsequently, Ogra and co-workers (1974) measured $PGF_{2\alpha}$ in human tubal fluid using radioimmunoassay and suggested that prostaglandin synthesis was localized to the oviductal mucosa, primarily of the ampullary region, with the use of indirect immunofluorescence staining. Vastick-Fernandez and colleagues (1975), however, reported PGF_1 in the greatest quantity in the ampullary region and $PGF_{2\alpha}$ in the isthmic region from tubal segment extracts and suggested a role for $PGF_{2\alpha}$ in the spontaneous motility of the human fallopian tube.

However, despite the similarities with respect to prostaglandin effects on tubal motility, ovum transport in women shows marked differences when compared with the rabbit model, which has been studied most widely in this context. The duration of ovum transport in humans is approximately 80 hours, and retention at the ampullary–isthmic junction is not so distinct as in the rabbit (Croxatto et al, 1978a). More importantly, in a clinical trial designed to evaluate a possible contraceptive effect Croxatto and colleagues, using the PGF analogue $15(S)$-15-methyl-$PGF_{2\alpha}$ administered intravenously to women, were able to demonstrate an increase in tubal contractility. However, timed recovery of ova from tubal segments showed no evidence of accelerated ovum transport (Croxatto et al, 1978b).

Whether endogenous prostaglandins are responsible for the spontaneous motility of the human fallopian tube remains controversial. Elder et al (1977) have shown that prostaglandins released in vitro from the fallopian tube are a result and not a cause of spontaneous motility. Indomethacin was able to inhibit synthesis and prostaglandin release in vitro without affecting spontaneous motility. Similarly, papaverine, a smooth muscle relaxant, was able to block spontaneous motility and prostaglandin release. It was therefore concluded that prostaglandin was released as a result of tissue distortion resulting from the spontaneous motility rather than being responsible for the spontaneous motility. On this basis, it was concluded that it would be safe to use non-steroidal anti-inflammatory drugs during the menstrual cycle without increasing the risk of tubal pregnancy (Elder et al, 1977). It should be noted, however, that Lindblom et al (1983) were in fact able to inhibit the contractions of the fallopian tube with indomethacin, suggesting that prostaglandins may be involved in the spontaneous motility of the human fallopian tube.

PROSTAGLANDINS IN THE TREATMENT OF ECTOPIC PREGNANCY

The observation that early elective pregnancy termination using systemic prostaglandin analogues is associated with a very low rate of ectopic pregnancy (Borten and Friedman, 1985) has led to the investigation of a possible role for prostaglandins in the medical treatment of this disorder. In vitro studies of portions of fallopian tube and corpus luteum from surgical specimens of ectopic pregnancies have demonstrated an increase in tubal muscular contraction and tubal artery constriction with application of $PGF_{2\alpha}$, but not with PGE_2 (Hahlin et al, 1987). $PGF_{2\alpha}$ also decreased hCG-induced increases in progesterone production from the corpus luteum, suggesting a role for $PGF_{2\alpha}$ in the treatment of ectopic pregnancy (Hahlin et al, 1987). This same group of investigators went on to demonstrate that laparoscopic local injection of $PGF_{2\alpha}$ (0.5–1.5 mg) into an unruptured ectopic pregnancy and into the ovary containing the corpus luteum was highly successful in terminating the pregnancy (Lindblom et al, 1987). In a subsequent report, 18 cases of ectopic pregnancy treated with intratubal and intraovarian injection using higher doses (2.0 mg) of $PGF_{2\alpha}$ in addition to systemic PGE_2 were complicated by two episodes of cardiac arrhythmia and one episode of hypertension and massive pulmonary oedema (Egarter and Husslein, 1988). Further experience using $PGF_{2\alpha}$ and its 15-methyl derivative by intratubal and ovarian injection in 26 patients has resulted in a success rate of 92% without significant side-effects with a total subsequent fertility rate of 90% (Lindblom et al, 1991). It has been suggested that this form of treatment may represent an attractive alternative to surgical therapy in properly selected patients with an early intact ectopic gestation. However, the exact mechanism of action remains unclear.

SUMMARY

More than 20 years following the recognition of a possible role for eicosanoids in ovarian function a physiological role for prostaglandins and/or leukotrienes in human ovulation, corpus luteum function and tubal motility remains to be demonstrated. With respect to ovarian function, the well-characterized preovulatory rise in eicosanoid production in animal species and humans, in conjunction with the large body of experimental evidence employing inhibitors of prostaglandin synthesis and replacement of individual prostaglandins, has provided strong evidence for a role in follicular rupture independent of other LH-mediated ovulatory events. The possible mechanism of prostaglandin-induced follicle rupture may involve stimulation of proteolytic activity via substances such as plasmin and PA; however, this is controversial. A role for prostaglandins in ovarian luteal function is well established in laboratory animals and large ruminant species, where $PGF_{2\alpha}$ derived from the uterus has been demonstrated to be the luteolytic factor. In humans, luteal function may be influenced by local intraovarian eicosanoid production, which has been suggested to involve the paracrine interaction of local ovarian hormones such as oxytocin, noradrenaline, insulin and IGFs, to name but a few. Several lines of evidence have also implicated prostaglandins as an aetiological factor in ovarian pathological states such as seen in the OHSS. However, the bulk of clinical experimental evidence to date has failed to support this contention.

Prostaglandin production has likewise been well characterized in the fallopian tube in both humans and animal species. Whereas a role for prostaglandins in tubal transport has been demonstrated with animal species such as the rabbit, several studies have failed to define a similar function in humans. More recently, direct injections of prostaglandin analogues into the fallopian tube and the corpus luteum have been shown to be efficacious as a treatment for ectopic pregnancy. Whether the primary mechanism of action involves effects on tubal musculature or corpus luteum function, or is simply a local vascular effect, remains to be demonstrated. Therefore, although the physiological role for eicosanoids in ovarian and tubal function remains unclear, particularly in the human, an increasing body of recent evidence has suggested an important paracrine function for this class of cellular mediators whose interaction with other more recently characterized local ovarian factors has only begun to be recognized.

REFERENCES

Abrahamsson G, Janson PO & Kullander S (1990) An in vitro perfusion method for metabolic studies on human postmenopausal ovaries. *Acta Obstetrica et Gynecologica Scandinavica* **69:** 527.

Aitokallio-Tallberg A, Viinikka L & Ylikorkala O (1988) Ovarian cancer produces excessive amounts of prostacyclin and thromboxane (abstract). *1st European Congress of Prostaglandins in Reproduction* Vienna, Austria.

Armstrong DT (1981) Prostaglandins and follicular functions. *Journal of Reproduction and Fertility* **62:** 283.

Armstrong DT & Grinwich DL (1972) Blockade of spontaneous and LH-induced ovulation in rats by indomethacin, an inhibitor of prostaglandin biosynthesis. *Prostaglandins* **1:** 21.

Auletta FJ, Paradis DK, Wesley M & Duby RT (1984a) Oxytocin is luteolytic in the rhesus monkey. *Journal of Reproduction and Fertility* **72:** 401.

Auletta FJ, Kamps DL, Pories S, Bissett J & Gibson M (1984b). An intra-corpus luteal site for the luteolytic actions of $PGF_{2\alpha}$ in the rhesus monkey. *Prostaglandins* **27:** 285.

Balasch J, Carmona F, Llach J et al (1990) Acute prerenal failure and liver dysfunction in a patient with severe ovarian hyperstimulation syndrome. *Human Reproduction* **5:** 348.

Balasch J, Arroyo V, Carmona F et al (1991) Severe ovarian hyperstimulation syndrome: role of peripheral vasodilation. *Fertility and Sterility* **56:** 1077.

Bell RL, Kennerly DA, Stanford N & Majerus PW (1979) Diglyceride lipase: a pathway for arachidonate release from human platelets. *Proceedings of the National Academy of Sciences of the USA* **76:** 3238.

Bennegaard B, Bennefors B & Hamberger L (1984) Interaction betweeen catecholamines and prostaglandin F2alpha in human luteolysis. *Acta Endocrinologica (Copenhagen)* **106:** 532.

Bennegard B, Hahlin M, Wennberg E & Noren H (1991) Local luteolytic effect of prostaglandin $F_{2\alpha}$ in the human corpus luteum. *Fertility and Sterility* **56:** 1070.

Berchuck A, MacDonald PC, Milewich L & Casey ML (1988) Epidermal growth factor, vanadate, and 12-O-tetradecanoylphorbol-13-acetate inhibit growth and stimulate prostaglandin E2 production in A431 cells. *Molecular and Cellular Endocrinology* **57:** 87.

Blatchley FR, Donovan BT, Horton EW & Poyser NL (1972) The release of prostaglandins and progestin into the utero-ovarian venous blood of guinea pigs during the oestrous cycle and following oestrogen treatment. *Journal of Physiology (London)* **223:** 69.

Borenstein R, Elhalah U, Lunenfeld R et al (1989) Severe ovarian hyperstimulation syndrome: a reevaluated therapeutic approach. *Fertility and Sterility* **51:** 791.

Borten S & Friedman EA (1985) Ectopic pregnancy among early abortion patients: does prostaglandin reduce the incidence? *Prostaglandins* **30:** 891.

Brannian JD & Terranova PF (1991) Involvement of prostaglandins in LH-induced super-ovulation in the cyclic hamster. *Prostaglandins* **41:** 128.

Brannstrom M, Koos RD, LeMaire WJ & Janson PO (1987) Cyclic AMP induced ovulation in the perfused rat ovary and its mediation by prostaglandins. *Biology of Reproduction* **37:** 1047.

Bunting S, Gryglewski R, Moncada S & Vane JR (1976) Arterial walls generate from prosta-glandin endoperoxide a substance (prostaglandin X) which relaxes strips of mesenteric and coeliac arteries and inhibits platelet aggregation. *Prostaglandins* **12:** 897.

Challis JRG, Calder AA, Diley S et al (1976) Production of prostaglandins E and $F_{2\alpha}$ by corpora lutea, corpora albicantes and stroma from the human ovary. *Journal of Endocrinology* **68:** 401.

Chang MD & Hunt DM (1972) Effect of prostaglandin $E_{2\alpha}$ on the early pregnancy of rabbits. *Nature* **236:** 120.

Channing CP (1972) Stimulatory effects of prostaglandins upon luteinization of rhesus monkey grandulosa cell cultures. *Prostaglandins* **2:** 331.

Chaudhuri G & Elder M (1976) Lack of evidence for inhibition of ovulation by aspirin in women. *Prostaglandins* **11:** 727.

Clark MR (1982) Stimulation of progesterone and prostaglandin E accumulation by luteinizing hormone-releasing hormone (LHRH) and LHRH analogs in rat granulosa cells. *Endocrinology* **110:** 146.

Clark MR, Marsh JM & LeMaire WJ (1978a) Mechanism of luteinizing hormone regulation of prostaglandin synthesis in rat granulosa cells. *Journal of Biological Chemistry* **253:** 7757.

Clark MR, Triebwasser WF, Marsh JM & LeMarie WJ (1978b) Prostaglandins in ovulation. *Ann. Bio. Anim. Biochem. Biophys.* **18(2B):** 427.

Clark MR, Chainy GBN, Marsh JM & LeMaire WJ (1979) Stimulation of prostaglandin synthetase activity in rat granulosa cells by gonadotropin in vivo. *Prostaglandins* **17:** 967.

Clark MR, Thibier C, Marsh JM & LeMaire WJ (1980) Stimulation of releasing hormone (LHRH) and LHRH analogs in rat granulosa cells. *Endocrinology* **7:** 17.

Cooke RG & Homeida AM (1985) Suppression of PGF2alpha release and delay of the luteolysis after active immunization against oxytocin in the goat. *Journal of Reproduction and Fertility* **75:** 63.

Coutinho EM & Maia HS (1971) The contractile response of the human uterus, fallopian tubes and ovary to prostaglandins in vivo. *Fertility and Sterility* **22:** 539.

Croxatto HB, Ortiz ME, Diaz S et al (1978a) Studies on the duration of egg transport by the human oviduct. *American Journal of Obstetrics and Gynecology* **132:** 629.

Croxatto HB, Oriz ME, Guiloff E et al (1978b) Effect of 15(S)-15-methyl prostaglandin $F_{2\alpha}$ on human oviductal motility and ovum transports. *Fertility and Sterility* **30:** 408.

Curry TE Jr, Clark MR, Dean DD, Woessner JF Jr & LeMaire WJ (1986) The preovulatory increase in ovarian collagenase activity in the rat is independent of prostaglandin production. *Endocrinology* **118:** 1823.

Curry TE Jr, Bryant C, Haddix AC & Clark MR (1990) Ovarian prostaglandin endoperoxide synthase: cellular localization during the rat estrous cycle. *Biology of Reproduction* **42:** 307.

Damber JE, Janson PO, Axen C, Selstam G & Cederblad A (1981) Luteal blood flow and plasma steroids in rats with corpora lutea of different ages. *Acta Endocrinologica (Copenhagen)* **98:** 99.

Demers LM & Veldhuis JD (1987) A stimulatory role for the protein kinase C pathway in ovarian prostaglandin synthesis: studies with cultured swine grandulosa cells. *Advances in Prostaglandin, Thromboxane, and Leukotriene Research* **17:** 1117.

Dennefors B, Hamberger L & Sjogren A (1980) Acute antigonadotropic action of prostaglandin in $F_{2\alpha}$ in the human corpus luteum. *Acta Obstetrica et Gynecologica Scandinavica* **93** (supplement): 79.

Dennefors B, Hamberger L, Hillensjo T et al (1983) Aspects concerning the role of prostaglandins in ovarian function. *Acta Obstetrica et Gynecologica Scandinavica* **113** (supplement): 31.

Dharmarajan AM, Sueoka K, Miyazaki T et al (1989) Prostaglandins and progesterone secretion in the in vitro perfused pseudopregnant rabbit ovary. *Endocrinology* **124:** 1198.

Egarter C & Husslein P (1988) Prostaglandins in the treatment of tubal pregnancy. *Eicosanoids and Fatty Acids* **5:** 44.

El-Banna AA, Sacher B & Schilling E (1976) Effect of indomethacin on egg transport and pregnancy in the rabbit. *Journal of Reproduction and Fertility* **46:** 375.

Elder MG, Myatt L & Chaudhuri G (1977) The role of prostaglandins in the spontaneous motility of the fallopian tube. *Fertility and Sterility* **28:** 86.

Ellinger JV & Kirton KT (1971) Ovum transport in rabbits injected with prostaglandin E_1 and $F_{2\alpha}$. *Biology of Reproduction* **11:** 93.

Espey LL (1978) Ovarian contractility and its relationship to ovulation. A review. *Biology of Reproduction* **19:** 540.

Espey LL (1980) Ovulation as an inflammatory response—a hypothesis. *Biology of Reproduction* **22:** 73.

Espey LL, Coons PJ, Marsh M & LeMaire WJ (1981) Effect of indomethacin on preovulatory changes in the ultrastructure of rabbit graafian follicles. *Endocrinology* **108:** 1040.

Espey LL, Norris C & Saphire D (1986) Effect of time and dose of indomethacin on follicular prostaglandins and ovulation in the rabbit. *Endocrinology* **119:** 746.

Espey LL, Kohda H, Mori T & Okamura H (1988) Rat ovarian prostaglandin levels and ovulation as indicators of the strength of non-steroidal anti-inflammatory drugs. *Prostaglandins* **36:** 875.

Espey LL, Tanaka N & Okamura H (1989) Increase in ovarian leukotrienes during hormonally induced ovulation in the rat. *American Journal of Physiology* **256:** E753.

Espey LL, Adams RF, Tanaka N & Okamura H (1990) Effects of epostane on ovarian levels of progesterone, 17β-estradiol, prostaglandin E_2, and prostaglandin $F_{2\alpha}$ during ovulation in the gonadotropin-primed immature rat. *Endocrinology* **127:** 259.

Feilds PA, Eldridge RK, Fuchs AR, Roberts R & Fields MJ (1983) Human placental and bovine corpora luteal oxytocin. *Endocrinology* **112:** 1544.

Feldman E, Haberman S, Abisogun AO et al (1986) Arachidonic acid metabolism in human granulosa cells: evidence for cyclooxygenase and lipoxygenase activity in vitro. *Human Reproduction* **1:** 353.

Flint APF & Sheldrick EL (1983) Evidence for a systemic role for ovarian oxytocin in luteal regression in sheep. *Journal of Reproduction and Fertility* **67:** 215.

Ford-Hutchinson AW, Bray MA, Doig MV et al (1980) Leukotriene B, a potent chemokinetic and aggregating substance released from polymorphonuclear leukocytes. *Nature* **286:** 264.

Fuchs AR (1987) Prostaglandins F2alpha and oxytocin interactions in ovarian and uterine function. *Journal of Steroid Biochemistry* **27(4):** 1073.

Goff AK, Zamecnik J, Ali M & Armstrong DT (1978) Prostaglandin I_2 stimulation of granulosa cell cyclic AMP production. *Prostaglandins* **15:** 875.

Hafez ESE (1979) Function of the fallopian tube in human reproduction. *Clinical Obstetrics and Gynecology* **22:** 61.

Hahlin M, Bokstrom H & Lindblom B (1987) Ectopic pregnancy: in vitro effects of prostaglandins on the oviduct and corpus luteum. *Fertility and Sterility* **47:** 935.

Hahlin M, Dennefors B, Johanson C & Hamberger L (1988) Luteotropic effects of prostaglandin E_2 on the human corpus luteum of the menstrual cycle and early pregnancy. *Journal of Clinical Endocrinology and Metabolism* **6:** 909.

Hamberger L, Nillson L, Dennefors B et al (1979) Cyclic AMP formation of isolated human corpora lutea in response to HCG. Interference by $PGF_{2\alpha}$. *Prostaglandins* **17:** 615.

Hamberger L, Dennefors B, Hamberger B et al (1980a) Is vascular innervation a prerequisite for PG induced luteolysis in the human corpus luteum? *Advances in Prostaglandin and Thromboxane Research* **8:** 1365.

Hamberger L, Kallfelt B, Forshell S & Dukes M (1980b) A luteolytic effect of a prostaglandin $F_{2\alpha}$ analogue in non-pregnant women. *Contraception* **22:** 383.

Hamberger L, Hahlin M & Lindblom B (1987) The role of prostaglandins and catecholamines for human corpus luteum function. In Stouffer R, Brenner R & Phoenix C (eds) *The Primate Ovary*, p 191. New York: Plenum Press.

Heinonen PK, Punnonen R, Ashorn R et al (1986) Prostaglandins, thromboxane and leukotriene in human follicular fluid. *Journal of Reproduction and Fertility* **4:** 253.

Hellburg P, Holmes PV, Brannstrom M et al (1990) Inhibitors of lipoxygenase increase the ovulation rate in the in vitro perfused luteinizing hormone-stimulated rabbit ovary. *Acta Physiologica Scandinavica* **138:** 557.

Higgs GA, Bunting S, Moncada S & Vane JR (1976) Polymorph nuclear leukocytes produce thromboxane A_2-like activity during phagocytosis. *Prostaglandins* **12:** 749.

Hodgson BJ (1976) Effects of indomethacin and ICI 46,474 administered during ovum transport on fertility in rabbits. *Biology of Reproduction* **14:** 451.

Horton EW & Poyser NL (1976) Uterine luteolytic hormone: a physiological role for prostaglandin $F_{2\alpha}$. *Physiology Reviews* **56:** 595.

Huslig RL, Malik A & Clark MA (1987) Human chorionic gonadotropin stimulation of immunoreactive prostaglandin synthase in the rat ovary. *Molecular and Cellular Endocrinology* **50:** 237.

Ivell R, Brackett KH, Fields M & Richter D (1985) Ovulation triggers oxytocin gene expression in the bovine ovary. *FEBS Letters* **190:** 263.

Janson PO, Albrecht I & Ahren K (1975) Effects of prostaglandin $F_{2\alpha}$ on ovarian blood flow and vascular resistance in the pseudopregnant rabbit. *Acta Endocrinologica (Copenhagen)* **79:** 337.

Janson PO, Brannstrom M, Holmes PV & Sogn J (1988) Studies of the mechanism of ovulation using the model of the isolated ovary. *Annals of the New York Academy of Sciences* **541:** 22.

Katz E, Dharmarajan AM, Sueoka K et al (1989) Effects of systemic administration of indomethacin on ovulation, luteinization, and steroidogenesis in the rabbit ovary. *American Journal of Obstetrics and Gynecology* **161**: 1361.

Kauma SW, Curry TE Jr, Powell DE & Clark MR (1990) Localization of prostaglandin endoperoxide synthase in the human corpus luteum. *Human Reproduction* **5**: 800.

Kawai Y & Clark MR (1985) Phorbol ester regulation of rat granulosa cell prostaglandin and progesterone accumulation. *Endocrinology* **116**: 2320.

Kawai Y & Clark MR (1986) Mechanisms of action of gonadotropin releasing hormone on rat granulosa cells. *Endocrinology Research* **12**: 195.

Khan MI (1979) *Functional control of the corpus luteum: studies on the mechanism of luteolysis in the rat and human.* Thesis, Goteborg.

Khan-Dawood FS & Dawood MY (1983) Human ovaries contain immunoreactive oxytocin. *Journal of Clinical Endocrinology and Metabolism* **57**: 1129.

Khan-Dawood FS, Marut EL & Dawood MY (1984) Oxytocin in the corpus luteum of the cynomolgus monkey (*Macaca fascicularis*). *Endocrinology* **115**: 570.

Kitai H, Kobayashi Y, Santulli R, Wright KH & Wallach EE (1985a) The relationship between prostaglandins and histamine in the ovulatory process as determined with the in vitro perfused rabbit ovary. *Fertility and Sterility* **43**: 646.

Kitai H, Yoshimura Y, Wright KH, Santulli R & Walach EE (1985b) 'Microvasculature' of preovulatory follicles: comparison of in situ in in vitro perfused rabbit ovaries following stimulation of ovulation. *American Journal of Obstetrics and Gynecology* **152**: 889.

Koos RD & Clark MR (1982) Production of 6-keto-prostaglandin $F_{1\alpha}$ by rat granulosa cells in vitro. *Endocrinology* **111**: 1513.

Korda AR, Donald A, Shutt ID et al (1975) Assessment of possible luteolytic effect of intraovarian injection of prostaglandin $F_{2\alpha}$ in the human. *Prostaglandins* **3**: 443.

Kuehl FA Jr, Humes JL, Tranoff J et al (1970) Prostaglandin receptor site: Evidence for an essential role in the action of luteinizing hormone. *Science* **169**: 883.

Lahav M, Freud A & Linder HR (1976) Abrogation by prostaglandin $F_{2\alpha}$ of LH stimulated cyclic AMP accumulation in isolated rat corpora lutea of pregnancy. *Biochemical and Biophysical Research Communications* **68**: 1294.

LaPolt PS, Yamato M, Veljkovic M et al (1990) Basic fibroblast growth factor induction of granulosa cell tissue-type plasminogen activator expression and oocyte maturation: potential role as a paracrine ovarian hormone. *Endocrinology* **127**: 2357.

LeMaire WJ & Marsh JM (1975) Interrelationships between prostaglandins, cyclic AMP, and steroids in ovulation. *Journal of Reproduction and Fertility* **22**(supplement): 53.

LeMaire WJ, Yang NST, Behrman HH & Marsh JM (1973) Preovulatory changes in the concentration of prostaglandins in rabbit graafian follicles. *Prostaglandins* **3**: 367.

LeMaire WJ, Clark MR & Marsh JM (1979) Biochemical mechanisms of ovulation. In Hafez ESE (ed.) *Human Ovulation: Mechanisms, Detection and Regulation*, p 159. Amsterdam: Elsevier/North Holland.

LeMaire WJ, Clark MR, Chainy GBN & Marsh JM (1980) The role of prostaglandins in the mechanism of ovulation. In Tozzini RI, Reeves G & Pineda RL (eds) *Endocrine Physiopathology of the Ovary*, p 207. Amsterdam: Elsevier/North Holland.

Leung PCK, Minegishi T, Ma F, Zhou F & Ho-Yuen B (1986) Induction of polyphosphoinositide breakdown in rat corpus luteum by prostaglandin $F_{2\alpha}$. *Endocrinology* **119**: 12. ·

Lindblom B, Hamberger L & Wiqvist N (1978) Differentiated contractile effects of prostaglandins E and F on the isolated circular and longitudinal smooth muscle of the human oviduct. *Fertility and Sterility* **30**: 553.

Lindblom B, Wilhelmsson M, Wikland M, Hamberger L & Wiquist N (1983) Prostaglandins and oviductal function. *Acta Obstetrica et Gynecologica Scandinavica* (supplement) **113**: 43.

Lindblom B, Kallfelt B, Hahlin M & Hamberger L (1987) Local prostaglandin $F_{2\alpha}$, injection for termination of ectopic pregnancy. *Lancet* **i**: 776.

Lindblom B, Hahlin M, Lundorff P & Thorburn J (1991) Treatment of tubal pregnancy by laparoscope-guided injection of prostaglandin $F_{2\alpha}$. *Fertility and Sterility* **54**: 404.

Lindblom B, Hamberger L & Ljung B (1980) Contractile patterns of isolated oviductal smooth muscle under different hormonal conditions. *Fertility and Sterility* **33**: 283.

Maas S, Jarry H, Teichmann A et al (1992) Paracrine actions of oxytocin, prostaglandins $F_{2\alpha}$, and estradiol within the human corpus luteum. *Journal of Clinical Endocrinology and Metabolism* **74**: 306.

McArdle CA (1990) Chronic regulation of ovarian oxytocin and progesterone release by prostaglandins: opposite effects in bovine granulosa and early luteal cells. *Journal of Endocrinology* **126:** 245.

McArdle CA & Holtorf AP (1989) Oxytocin and progesterone release from bovine corpus luteal cells in culture: Effects of insulin-like growth factor I, insulin, and prostaglandins. *Endocrinology* **124:** 1278.

McCracken JA, Carlson JC, Glew ME et al (1972) Prostaglandin $F_{2\alpha}$ identified as a luteolytic hormone in sheep. *Nature* **238:** 129.

McNatty KP, Henderson KM & Sawers RS (1975) Effects of prostaglandin F_2 and E_2 on the production of progesterone by human granulosa cells in tissue culture. *Journal of Endocrinology* **67:** 231.

Minegishi T & Leung PCK (1985) Luteinizing hormone-releasing hormone stimulated arachidonic acid release in rat grandulosa cells. *Endocrinology* **117:** 2001.

Mitchell MD, Bibby JC, Hicks BR & Turnbull AC (1978) Possible role of prostacyclin in human parturition. *Prostaglandins* **16:** 931.

Miyazaki T, Dharmarajan AM, Atlas SJ, Katz E & Wallach EE (1991) Do prostaglandins lead to ovulation in the rabbit by stimulation proteolytic activity? *Fertility and Sterility* **55:** 1183.

Molskness TA, VandeVoort CA & Stouffer RL (1987) Stimulatory and inhibitory effects of prostaglandins on the gonadotropin-sensitive adenylate cyclase in the monkey corpus luteum. *Prostaglandins* **34:** 279.

Murdoch WJ, Peterson TA, Van Kirk EA, Vincent DL & Inskeep EK (1986) Interactive roles of progesterone, prostaglandins, and collagenase in the ovulatory mechanism of the ewe. *Biology of Reproduction* **35:** 1187.

Neufeld G, Ferrara N, Mitchell R, Schweigerer L & Gospodarowicz D (1987) Grandulosa cells produce basic fibroblast growth factor. *Endocrinology* **121:** 597.

O'Grady JP, Caldwell BV, Auletta FJ & Speroff L (1972) The effects of an inhibitor of prostaglandin synthesis (indomethacin) on ovulation, pregnancy, and pseudopregnancy in the rabbit. *Prostaglandins* **1:** 97.

Ogra SS, Kirton KT, Tomasi TB Jr & Lippes J (1984) Prostaglandins in the human fallopian tube. *Fertility and Sterility* **25:** 250.

Padmavathi O, Pandu Ranga Reddy G, Ramesh Reddy G & Reddanna P (1990) Biosynthesis of prostaglandins in ovarian follicles and corpus luteum of sheep ovary. *Biochemistry International* **20:** 455.

Patwardhan VV & Lanthier A (1985) Luteal phase variations in endogenous concentrations of prostaglandins PGE and PGF and the capacity for their in vitro formation in the human corpus luteum. *Prostaglandins* **30:** 91.

Piper PJ & Vane JR (1969) Release of additional factors in anaphylaxis and its antagonism by anti-inflammatory drugs. *Nature* **223:** 29.

Polishuk WZ & Schenker JG (1969) Ovarian overstimulation syndrome. *Fertility and Sterility* **20:** 443.

Poyser NL & Scott FM (1980) Prostaglandin and thromboxane production by the rat uterus and ovary in vitro during the estrus cycle. *Journal of Reproduction and Fertility* **60:** 33.

Pride SM, Ho Yeun B & Moon YS (1984) Clinical, endocrinological and intraovarian prostaglandin-F response to H-1 receptor blockade in the ovarian hyperstimulation syndrome. *American Journal of Obstetrics and Gynecology* **148:** 670.

Priddy AR, Killick SR, Elstein M et al (1989) Ovarian follicular fluid eicosanoid concentration during the pre-ovulatory period in humans. *Prostaglandins* **38:** 197.

Pride SM, Ho Yuen B, Moon YS et al (1986) Relationship of GnRH, danazol and prostaglandin blockade to ovarian enlargement and ascites formation of the ovarian hyperstimulation syndrome in the rabbit. *American Journal of Obstetrics and Gynecology* **154:** 1155.

Pride SM, James C St J & Ho Yuen B (1990) The ovarian hyperstimulation syndrome. *Seminars in Reproduction and Endocrinology* **8:** 247.

Reich R, Kohen F, Naor Z & Tsafriri A (1983) Possible involvement of lipoxygenase products of arachidonic acid pathway in ovulation. *Prostaglandins* **26:** 1011.

Reich R, Tsafriri A & Mechanic GL (1985a) The involvement of collagenolysis in ovulation in the rat. *Endocrinology* **116:** 522.

Reich R, Kohen F, Slager R & Tsafriri A (1985b) Ovarian lipoxygenase activity and its regulation by gonadotropin in the rat. *Prostaglandins* **30:** 581.

Richman KA, Wright KH & Wallach EE (1974) Local ovarian effects of prostaglandin E_2 and

F_2 on human chorionic gonadotropin-induced ovulation in the rabbit. *Obstetrics and Gynecology* **43**: 203.

Roberts JS, McCrakcen JA, Gavagan JE & Soloff MS (1976) Oxytocin-stimulated release of PGF2alpha from ovine endometrium in vitro. *Endocrinology* **99**: 1107.

Rodgers RJ, O'Shea JD, Findlay JK, Flint APF & Sheldrick EL (1983) Large luteal cells the source of luteal oxytocin in the sheep. *Endocrinology* **113**: 2302.

Rollins T & Smith W (1980) Subcellular localization of prostaglandin forming cyclooxygenase in Swiss mouse 3T3 fibroblast by electron microscopic immunocytochemistry. *Journal of Biological Chemistry* **255**: 4872.

Saksena SK & Harper MJK (1975) Relationship between concentration of prostaglandin F (PGF) in the oviduct and egg transport in rabbits. *Biology of Reproduction* **13**: 68.

Samuelsson B, Granstrom E, Green K, Hamberg M & Hammarstrom S (1975) Prostaglandins. *Annual Review of Biochemistry* **44**: 669.

Samuelsson B, Borgeat P, Hammarstrom S & Murphy R (1979) Introduction of nomenclature, leukotrienes. *Prostaglandins* **17**: 785.

Samuelsson B, Dahlen SE, Lindgren JA, Rouzer CA & Serhan CN (1987) Leukotrienes and lipoxins: structures, biosynthesis, and biological effects. *Science* **237**: 1171.

Sandberg F, Ingelman-Sundberg A & Ryden G (1963) The effect of prostaglandin E_1 on the human uterus and the fallopian tubes in vitro. *Acta Obstetrica et Gynecologica Scandinavica* **42**: 269.

Sandberg F, Ingelmens-Sundberg A & Ryden G (1965) The effect of prostaglandin $F_{1\alpha}$, $F_{1\beta}$, $F_{2\beta}$ on the human uterus and the fallopian tubes in vitro. *Acta Obstetrica et Gynecologica Scandinavica* **44**: 585.

Sandberg F, Ingelman-Sundberg A & Ryden G (1964) The effect of prostaglandin E_2 and E_3 on the human uterus and fallopian tubes in vitro. *Acta Obstetrica et Gynecologica Scandinavica* **43**: 95.

Sargent EL, Baughman WL, Novy MJ & Stouffer RL (1988) Intraluteal infusion of a prostaglandin synthesis inhibitor, sodium meclofenamate, causes premature luteolysis in rhesus monkeys. *Endocrinology* **123**: 2261.

Schaeffer JM, Liu J, Hsueh AJW & Yen SSC (1984) Presence of oxytocin and arginine vasopressin in human ovary, oviduct and follicular fluid. *Journal of Clinical Endocrinology and Metabolism* **59**: 970.

Schams D, Prokopp S & Barth D (1983) The effect of active and passive immunization against oxytocin on ovarian cyclicity in ewes. *Acta Endocrinologica (Copenhagen)* **103**: 337.

Schenker JG & Polinshuk WZ (1976) The role of prostaglandins in ovarian hyperstimulation syndrome. *European Journal of Obstetrics, Gynecology and Reproductive Biology* **6**: 47.

Schlegel W, Kruger S, Daniels D et al (1988) Studies on prostaglandin metabolism in corpora lutea of rabbits during pregnancy and pseudopregnancy. *Journal of Reproduction and Fertility* **83**: 365.

Sheldrick EL, Mitchell MD & Flint APF (1980) Delayed luteal regression in ewes immunized against oxytocin. *Journal of Reproduction and Fertility* **59**: 37.

Spilman CH (1974a) Oviduct motility in the rhesus monkey: spontaneous activity and response to prostaglandins. *Fertility and Sterility* **25**: 935.

Spilman CH (1974b) Oviduct response to prostaglandins: Influence of estradiol and progesterone. *Prostaglandins* **7**: 465.

Strickland S & Beers WH (1976) Studies on the role of plasminogen activator in ovulation. *Journal of Biological Chemistry* **251**: 5694.

Tanaka N, Espey LL & Okamura H (1989) Increase in ovarian 15-hydroxyeicosatetraenoic acid during ovulation in the gonadotropin-primed immature rat. *Endocrinology* **125**: 1373.

Tanaka S, Shimoya Y, Azumaguchi A et al (1981) Studies on the prostaglandin E_2 receptor in human corpora lutea. *Nippon Sanka Fujinka Gakkai Zasshi* **33**: 1888.

Tsafriri A, Koch Y & Linder HR (1973) Ovulation rate and serum LH levels in rats treated with indomethacin or prostaglandin E_2. *Prostaglandins* **3**: 461.

Tuvemo T, Strandberg K, Hamberg M & Samuelsson B (1981) Maintenance of the tone of the human umbilical artery by prostaglandin and thromboxane formation. *Advances in Prostaglandin and Thromboxane Research* **1**: 425.

Vastick-Fernandez J, Gimeno MF, Lima F & Gimeno AL (1975) Spontaneous motility and distribution of prostaglandins in different segments of human fallopian tubes. *American Journal of Obstetrics and Gynecology* **122**: 663.

Veldhuis JD & Demers LM (1986) An inhibitory role for the protein kinase C pathway in ovarian steroidogenesis: studies in cultured swine grandulosa cells. *Biochemical Journal* **239:** 505.

Veldhuis JD & Demers LM (1987) Activation of protein kinase C is coupled to prostaglandin E_2 synthesis in swine grandulosa cells. *Prostaglandins* **33:** 819.

Vijayakumar R & Walters AW (1987) Ovarian stromal and luteal tissue prostaglandins, 17β-estradiol, and progesterone in relation to the phases of the menstrual cycle in women. *American Journal of Obstetrics and Gynecology* **156:** 947.

Wallach EE, Bronson R, Hamada Y et al (1975) Effectiveness of prostaglandin $E_{2\alpha}$ in restoration of HGM–HCG-induced ovulation in indomethacin treated rhesus monkeys. *Prostaglandins* **10:** 129.

Wang J, Lee V & Leung PC (1989) Differential role of protein kinase C in action of luteinizing hormone-releasing on the hormone production in rat ovarian cells. *American Journal of Obstetrics and Gynecology* **160:** 984.

Wathes DC, Swann RW, Birkett SD, Porter DJ & Pickering BT (1983) Characterization of oxytocin, vasopressin and neurophysin from the bovine corpus luteum. *Endocrinology* **113:** 693.

Wentz AC & Jones GS (1973) Transient luteolytic effect of prostaglandin $F_{2\alpha}$ in the human. *Obstetrics and Gynecology* **42:** 172.

Wilhelmsson L, Lindblom B & Wiqvist N (1979) The human uterotubal junction: contractile patterns of different smooth muscle layers and the influence of prostaglandin E_2, prostaglandin $F_{2\alpha}$, and prostaglandin I_2 in vitro. *Fertility and Sterility* **32:** 303.

Wilks JW (1980) Effects of (15S)-15-methyl PGF$_{2\alpha}$ methyl ester and estrogens upon the corpus luteum and conceptus of the rhesus monkey. *Prostaglandins* **20:** 807.

Wilks JW (1983) Pregnancy interception with a combination of prostaglandins: studies in monkeys. *Science* **221:** 1407.

Williams KI, Dembinska-Kiec A, Zmuda A & Gryglewski RJ (1978) Prostacyclin production by myometrial and decidual fractions of the pregnant rat uterus. *Prostaglandins* **15:** 343.

Williams TJ (1983) Interactions between prostaglandins, leukotrienes, and other mediators of inflammation. *British Medical Bulletin* **39:** 239.

Yang NST, Marsh JM & LeMaire WJ (1974) Post-ovulatory changes in the concentration of prostaglandins in rabbit graafian follicles. *Prostaglandins* **6:** 37.

Ylikorkala O & Tenhuneu A (1984) Follicular fluid prostaglandins in endometriosis and ovarian hyperstimulation. *Fertility and Sterility* **41:** 66.

Yoshimura Y, Dharmarajan AM, Gips S et al (1988) Effects of prostacyclin on ovulation and microvasculature of the in vitro perfused rabbit ovary. *American Journal of Obstetrics and Gynecology* **159:** 977.

Zetler G & Wiechell H (1969) Pharmakologisch Aktive lipide in extrakten aus tube und ovardes Menschen. Nauym Schneideberg. *Archiv der Pharmazie (Weinheim)* **165:** 101.

Zor U, Strulovici B, Nimrod A & Lindner HR (1977) Stimulation by cyclic nucleotides of prostaglandin E production in isolated graafian follicles. *Prostaglandins* **14:** 947.

3

The endometrium: prostaglandins and intracellular signalling at implantation

ASIF S. AHMED
STEPHEN K. SMITH

BACKGROUND

It is now almost 30 years since prostaglandins (PGs) were first found to be synthesized by human endometrium. In that time there has been considerable interest in the ability of endometrium to release these compounds which initially centred on the direct effects that PGs could exert on endometrial and myometrial function. This research was prompted by the possible role of disturbances of PG release by endometrium of women complaining of menstrual dysfunction, most particularly dysmenorrhoea. In addition, there was increasing interest in the use of non-steroidal anti-inflammatory drugs for the alleviation of menstrual problems. This interest has largely been successful in that primary dysmenorrhoea is now seen to be a disorder which in the main has a clearly defined aetiology and for which there is effective treatment available.

The function of the cyclical development of endometrium is, of course, to provide an environment for successful implantation of the primate embryo. Much of the initial interest in the role of PGs in the process of implantation was derived from animal studies, in which uterine PGs were found to be luteolytic. Changes in the release of PGs by endometrium influenced corpus luteal function. This release of PGs was found to be mediated by ovarian steroids and, in view of this interaction, interest changed to the role of PGs in the process of primate implantation. Whilst evidence in rodents pointed to an obligatory role of PGs in implantation, no such relationship has been shown for human pregnancy.

It is now clear that PGs are part of a complex intracellular signalling system which permits external ligands to transfer their signal to the nucleus by binding to cell surface receptors. In this respect, the study of PG synthesis has become exceedingly complicated, interacting as it does with a wide range of intracellular molecules and a wide range of ligands, most specifically locally derived growth factors. In addition, the complexity of the origin of the cells of the endometrium is increasingly appreciated and each of these groups of cells is capable of synthesizing PGs.

This chapter will address the known factors involved in the synthesis of PGs by human endometrium, and will speculate on their function at implantation.

PG BIOSYNTHESIS AND METABOLISM

PGs are synthesized from free intracellular arachidonic acid (AA) by the action of cyclo-oxygenase. $PGF_{2\alpha}$ is derived from PG endoperoxide by the action of $PGF_{2\alpha}$ reductase and from PGE_2 under the influence of 9-keto-reductase (Samuelsson et al, 1978). PGE_2 is derived from its precursor either by non-enzymatic degradation or by catalysis of PGE isomerase. Less than 5% of intracellular AA is present in the free form, most being bound to the membrane phospholipids. PGS are not stored in tissue but are derived from de novo synthesis. They are metabolized by PG dehydrogenase, itself expressed in human endometrium.

Previously, it was assumed that the rate-limiting step in the synthesis of PGs was the release of AA from the C-2 position of membrane phospholipids such as phosphatidylethanolamine and phosphatidylcholine Samuelsson et al, 1978). It is now clear that the generation of AA for eicosanoid synthesis within the cell can occur through a receptor-mediated GTP-binding protein-linked or calcium-dependent activation of phospholipases (Burgoyne and Morgan, 1990). These will be considered before establishing the relevant importance of each pathway to PGs and endometrial function.

PHOSPHODIESTERASES

Phospholipases A_2

The phospholipases A_2 (PLA_2) are a diverse family of enzymes which hydrolyse the sn-2 fatty acyl bond of phospholipids. Type I PLA_2s are found in elapid snakes but are also present in human pancreas and lung. Type II PLA_2s are present in viperid and crotalid snake venom and a 124 amino acid peptide has been found in human rheumatoid arthritic synovial fluid (Seilhamer et al, 1989a), platelets (Kramer et al, 1989) and placental membranes (Lai and Wada, 1988). It is likely that there are multiple forms of PLA_2 probably arising from alternate slicing (Seilhamer et al, 1989b). There is as yet little evidence to suggest that PLA_2 is linked to ligand receptor activation—which is the case for other phospholipases—making it difficult to determine specific effects for agents like growth factors. It is clear that PLA_2 activity is enhanced by elevated intracellular calcium, ($[Ca^{2+}]_i$), changes which probably arise secondary to activation of the other phospholipases to be discussed below. It is possible that PLA_2 exists free in the cytoplasm but becomes activated by being incorporated into the cell membrane. Human endometrium has PLA_2 activity (Bonney, 1985) and, in the rat, stimulation of this activity is suppressed by progesterone (Pakrasi et al, 1983). A cDNA probe identifies a PLA_2 in amnion of pregnant women (Aitken et al, 1990), but has not yet been reported in human endometrium.

Phospholipases C

Ca^{2+}-mobilizing agonists are believed to initiate intracellular signalling by receptor-mediated hydrolysis of a quantitatively minor membrane phospholipid, phosphatidylinositol 4,5-bisphosphate (PIns 4,5-P_2) by a phosphoinositide-specific phospholipase C (PI-PLC) (Berridge and Irvine, 1989). This hydrolysis generates two second messengers, inositol 1,4,5-trisphosphate (Ins 1,4,5-P_3) and sn-1,2-diacylglycerol (DAG). Ins 1,4,5-P_3 stimulates the release of calcium from endoplasmic reticulum, thus raising $[Ca^{2+}]_i$, whilst DAG is the main physiological activator of phosphatidylserine-dependent protein kinase C (PKC) (Berridge and Irvine, 1989). PKC phosphorylates cellular proteins and thereby controls a host of cellular processes (Nishizuka, 1989) (Figure 1).

Isoenzymes

The past 5 years has seen a remarkable increase in the identification of multiple forms of PLC not only with respect to their substrate but also the molecular heterogeneity within substrate groups. Several PI-PLC isozymes have been identified (Rhee et al, 1989). The three of particular interest are PI-PLCβ, γ and δ which were initially identified in rat and bovine brain but which are now known to be expressed in humans. The molecular masses measured by sodium dodecyl sulphate–polyacrylamide gel electrophoresis of the three peptides are 150–154 kDa for PLCβ, 145–148 kDa for PLCγ and 85–88 kDa for PLCδ. A fourth PI-PLCα has been identified in guinea-pig uterus with a molecular mass of 62–68 kDa (Bennett and Crooke, 1987) and is expressed in human endometrium, amnion, chorion and placenta (Jones and Smith, 1991). However, PI-PLC activity of the cloned product was not demonstrated by these investigators. Furthermore, a recent study suggests that cDNA of PI-PLCα may encode for a microsomal protein of unknown function (Martin et al, 1991).

The three initial PI-PLCs share two regions of sequence identity, but function differently. PI-PLCβ appears linked to a G protein whilst PI-PLCγ is activated following phosphorylation of tyrosine kinase receptors such as epidermal growth factor (Koch et al, 1991). The role of PI-PLCα in endometrium is yet to be determined, and although PI-PLCδ is present in amnion its expression and activity in human endometrium is not clear. Endometrium does contain PLC activity but it is not known which isozymes are active in endometrium in health or disease.

PI-PLC activation by a number of agonists such as oxytocin in the ovine endometrium (Flint et al, 1986; Mirando et al, 1990), bombesin and bradykinin in human endometrial stromal cells (Endo et al, 1991), and in tissue explants of human endometrium by platelet-activating factor (PAF) (Ahmed and Smith, 1992) and endothelin-1 (Ahmed et al, 1992a) has been reported. The rapid formation of inositol phosphate has also been reported in cultured rabbit endometrial cells with 1 μM $PGF_{2\alpha}$ (Orlicky et al, 1986). However, $PGF_{2\alpha}$ failed to stimulate inositol phosphate formation in human endometrial stromal cells (Endo et al, 1991).

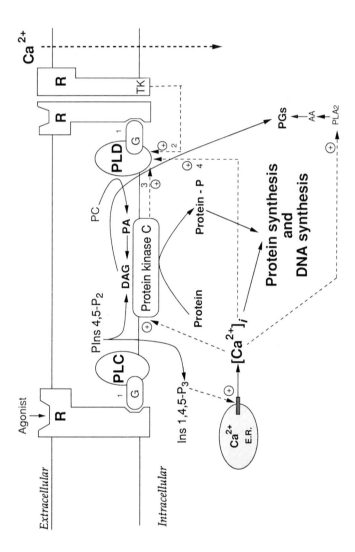

Figure 1. Model of agonist–receptor (R) signal transduction pathways in the endometrium. (1) Phospholipase C (PLC) and D (PLD) activation via a GTP-binding protein (G). (2) Phosphorylation by a receptor–tyrosine kinase (TK) complex of PLC and PLD, or a factor necessary for PLD activation. (3) PLD activation resulting in a protein kinase C-dependent manner via PLC activation, hydrolysis of phosphatidylinositol 4,5-bisphosphate (PIns 4,5-P_2) and activation of protein kinase C (PKC) by diacylglycerol (DAG) formation. (4) Ca^{2+}-dependent activation from PLC-dependent formation of inositol 1,4,5-trisphosphate (Ins 1,4,5-P_3) and intracellular Ca^{2+} ([Ca^{2+}]$_i$) mobilization from stores such as the endoplasmic reticulum (ER) or uptake. Phosphatidylcholine (PC) hydrolysis via PLD yields phosphatidic acid (PA) which is a putative second messenger. These signals, such as a rise in [Ca^{2+}]$_i$ and protein phosphorylation (protein-p) co-operate in initiating many of the early events associated with protein and DNA synthesis.

Transient phenomena and other phospholipid pools

In a wide variety of tissues and cells, agonist-stimulated PIns $4,5\text{-}P_2$ hydrolysis is a transient process which is rapidly desensitized (Cook and Wakelam, 1989), whilst accumulation of DAG mass is kinetically distinct from and exceeds the mass of inositol phosphates (Cook et al, 1990). Increasing evidence points to an important role for cellular phosphatidylcholine (PC) as the substrate for promoting sustained elevation of DAG levels which is needed for prolonging cellular activation (Billah and Anthes, 1990; Exton, 1990). PC is the principal phospholipid class in mammalian tissues and can account for up to 50% of the total cellular phospholipid content. PC hydrolysis can result in the direct formation of DAG and phosphocholine by PC-specific phospholipase C (PC-PLC) (Slivka et al, 1988) (Figure 2). In addition, hydrolysis of PC by the PC-PLA_2 produces lyso-PC and AA ($C_{20:4}$), an immediate precursor of eicosanoids. Lyso-PC may be re-esterified to PC or catabolized to glycerophosphocholine (GPC), which can be further degraded to glycerol 3-phosphate and choline. Glycerol 3-phosphate can be converted back to DAG via phosphatidic acid (PA) synthesis (Billah and Anthes, 1990). PC-PLC may be present in human endometrium (Ahmed et al, 1992b).

Phospholipase D

An additional alternative to the degradation of PC is via a novel mammalian phospholipase D (PLD), initially thought to be expressed only in plants.

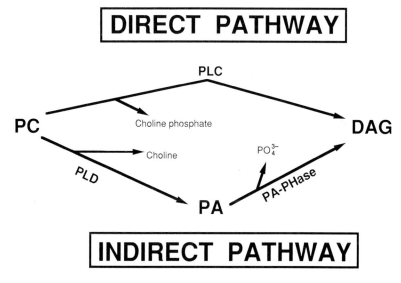

Figure 2. Direct and indirect pathways of phosphatidylcholine (PC) breakdown. The diacylglycerols (DAG) can be generated directly via PC-specific phospholipase C (PLC) or by the action of phospholipase D (PLD) to yield phosphatidic acid (PA), which is cleaved to DAG by PA phosphohydrolase (PA-PHase).

Mammalian PLD was first detected using a microsomal preparation from rat brain (Saito et al, 1975). PLD is now seen as being a crucial pathway in generating choline and PA, the latter compound being a potential second messenger, which can be further degraded by a PA phosphohydrolase to DAG (Bocckino et al, 1987; Billah et al, 1989) (Figure 2).

Transphosphatidylation

A unique feature of PLD is its ability to catalyse a transphosphatidylation reaction between the phosphatidyl moiety of labelled PC and primary alcohols such as butanol to produce phosphatidylalcohol (Dawson, 1967; Kobayashi and Kanfer, 1987). The phosphatidylalcohol product of this reaction is not a substrate for PA phosphohydrolase and thus accumulates in the cell providing a marker of PLD activity (Figure 3).

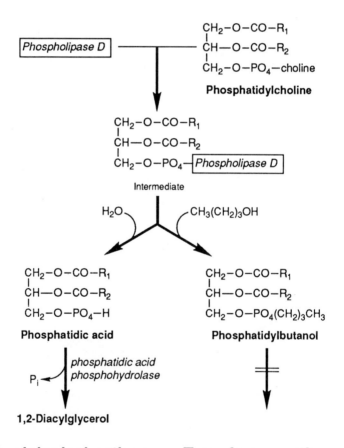

Physiological pathway   Transferase pathway

Figure 3. The hydrolytic and transferase activities of phospholipase D.

The method described by Randall and co-workers (Randall et al, 1990) which measures the PLD-catalysed transfer of high specific activity [^{3}H]butan-1-ol (25.8 Ci mmol^{-1}) to [^{3}H]phosphatidylbutanol ([^{3}H]PBut) has been used to measure PLD activity in endometrial tissue explants. Two distinct advantages of this technique over the conventional method of labelling cellular phospholipid pools are that the method does not require cellular phospholipids to be prelabelled and uses a much lower concentration of alcohol. Since this reaction is not catalysed by PLC, transphosphatidylation has been used to detect PLD activity in intact cells. Requirements of Ca^{2+}, fatty acids and detergents for PLD expression vary from cell to cell, suggesting that multiple PLD isoforms may exist (Billah and Anthes, 1990).

Receptor regulation

The regulatory mechanisms of PLD activation and its coupling to cellular function is illustrated in Figure 1. In the presence of 30 mM butanol, a number of agonist receptor systems such as endothelin-1-stimulated Rat-1 fibroblast (MacNulty et al, 1990) and bombesin-stimulated Swiss 3T3 fibroblasts (Cook et al, 1990) generated [^{3}H]PBut which was found to be kinetically downstream of Ins 1,4,5-P$_3$ formation. This favours a sequential pathway involving the activation of PKC, since PKC activators stimulate the accumulation of [^{3}H]PBut in the concentration range consistent with their activation of PKC. Down-regulation of PKC by chronic phorbol ester pretreatment prevents subsequent activation of PLD (MacNulty et al, 1990). Phorbol esters or DAG activate PKC by increasing its sensitivity to Ca^{2+}, thus a rise in cytosolic free Ca^{2+} following PIns 4,5-P$_2$ hydrolysis will activate PKC. A negative-feedback signal to limit the magnitude and duration of receptor signalling is provided by the ability of phorbol esters or DAG to attenuate receptor-coupled PI-PLC activity.

However, another possibility is a receptor-linked activation of PLD via a GTP-binding regulatory protein (Billah et al, 1989), as has been demonstrated in vasopressin-stimulated hepatocytes (Bocckino et al, 1987) and in chemotactic-peptide-stimulated HL-60 cells (Pai et al, 1988).

Functional significance

The steroid interaction and biological effect of this activity is still unclear, although increasing evidence suggests that this pathway may be important in chronic activation of cellular processes. PC hydrolysis provides an alternative pathway for the generation of second messengers derived from membrane phospholipids. The product of PLD-catalysed hydrolysis of PC, PA, provides a sustained source of DAG for the prolonged activation of PKC (Billah and Anthes, 1990), a family of enzymes central to the initiation of the growth process. However, Leach et al (1991) recently demonstrated that, in intact thrombin-stimulated IIC-9 fibroblasts, DAG derived from PC does not translocate the α isoform of PKC. However, PKC activity can be activated in vitro by PC-derived DAG extracted from the same cells. One possible explanation for this is that the PC-derived DAG may preferentially activate a Ca^{2+}-independent isoform of PKC (δ, ϵ or ζ).

The products of PC hydrolysis may also be involved in the regulation of transcription and other events related to cell growth and differentiation (Exton, 1990). A unique feature of PLD is that the enzyme or a factor crucial for PLD can be induced in virally transformed lymphocytes (Thompson et al, 1991) and in neutrophils primed by pretreatment with PAF or granulocyte-macrophage colony-stimulating factor (Bourgoin et al, 1990). The presence of PLD was recently demonstrated in secretory endometrium (Ahmed et al, 1992b) and, more recently, the same group showed that ovarian steroids induce PAF-stimulated PLD activity in HEC-1B cells, a transformed endometrial cell line (Ahmed et al, 1992c). These observations suggest that PLD may be particularly involved in cell transformation, implantation and in leukocyte response at inflammation sites.

Diacylglycerol also has functions other than the activation of PKC. One is to serve as a source of AA for eicosanoid production. AA is released not only by the direct action of PLA_2 but also indirectly, following the release of DAG from membrane-bound phospholipids, under the influence of a wide range of PLCs. DAG acts as a substrate for diacyl- and monoacylglycerol lipases which release AA for eicosanoid production (Exton, 1990). Other possible actions include the translocation of diacylglycerol kinase to membrane-bound compartments (Besterman et al, 1986) and the activation of PLA_2 (Kolesnick and Paley, 1987). In addition, PA and AA also function as mitogenic stimuli, possibly through an interaction with the p21[ras]-regulating protein GAP (Tsai et al, 1990). These findings strongly implicate the PC pathway in the regulation of mitogenesis.

LOCAL ENDOMETRIAL FACTORS AT IMPLANTATION

Prostaglandins

PGE_2 and $PGF_{2\alpha}$ are the principal PGs in the endometrium of non-pregnant women (Abel and Kelly, 1979). Immunohistochemical studies show that cyclo-oxygenase is found primarily in the glandular epithelium of the endometrium (Rees et al, 1982). The production of PGE_2 and $PGF_{2\alpha}$ is significantly greater in the glandular epithelium than in the stroma of the endometrium (Smith and Kelly, 1988). The endometrium is not only the site of PG synthesis, but also the site of action for PGs. Consistent with this idea is the demonstration of PGE_2 binding sites within the rat (Kennedy et al, 1983) and human (Hofmann et al, 1985) endometrium as well as endometrial epithelial cell uptake of PGs in the rabbit (Jones and Harper, 1983).

Ovarian steroids

The evidence of steroid regulation of PG synthesis has been available for 20 years but the interpretation of the data remains controversial. Initial studies measured endogenous levels of PGs in endometrium. They showed increased levels of $PGF_{2\alpha}$ and PGE_2 in the luteal phase of the cycle (Downie et al, 1974; Singh et al, 1975; Maathuis and Kelly, 1978). Further studies in vitro in both endometrial explants and separated cells confused this interpretation.

Animal studies

In non-primate species, the site of implantation is characterized by local oedema and an increased vascular permeability around the blastocyst, readily demonstrated by the extravasation of Evans blue dye (Psychoyos and Martel, 1985). Levels of PGE_2, $PGF_{2\alpha}$ and 6-keto-$PGF_{1\alpha}$ are elevated at the site of implantation (Kennedy and Zamecnik, 1978). PGE_2 increases local vascular permeability and stromal oedema (Kennedy, 1983). Indomethacin, an inhibitor of PG synthesis, alters the local increase in endometrial vascular permeability in rabbits (Hoffman et al, 1984), hamsters (Evans and Kennedy, 1978), mice (Lundkvist and Nilsson, 1980) and rats (Phillips and Poyser, 1981), and blocks or delays implantation in mice (Saksena et al, 1976), rabbits (Hoffman et al, 1978) and pigs (Kraeling et al, 1985). Blockage of implantation in indomethacin-treated mice (Lau et al, 1973) and rats (Garg and Chaudhury, 1983) can be reversed by injection of PGs. An increase in vascular permeability in the stroma at the site of impending blastocyst implantation occurring over the 24 hour period prior to attachment is an obligate accompaniment of normal implantation and decidualization. An exception to this is the sheep. The treatment of ewes from days 7 to 22 after mating with either indomethacin or acetylsalicylic acid at doses which significantly reduce endometrial PG levels had no apparent effect on the establishment of pregnancy (Lacroix and Kann, 1982).

Due to ethical constraints, such studies cannot be performed in women. There is, however, good morphological evidence obtained during early pregnancy in women to suggest that the site of implantation is characterized by an expansion of extracellular fluid volume and increased vascular permeability (Hertig, 1964). It would appear that many of the aspects of implantation are similar in both rodents and humans and it is likely that similar mechanisms may operate.

Leukotrienes

The products of the 5-lipoxygenase pathway of AA metabolism may be involved in endometrial function. Activation of this pathway at the time of implantation has been observed in the rat (Malathy et al, 1986) and mouse (Gupta et al, 1989) uterus. A selective leukotriene receptor antagonist, FPL 55712, prevents the decidual cell reaction in the rat, an action antagonized by the infusion of leukotriene C_4 (LTC_4) (Tawfik and Dey, 1988). It has been suggested that LTC_4 interacts with PGE_2 to enhance decidual cell reaction (Tawfik and Dey, 1988).

Studies with $[^3H]$-LTC_4 demonstrated that luminal epithelial cells of the human endometrium, stromal cells, and muscle cells of the myometrium as well as arteriolar smooth muscle cells contained numerous LTC_4 binding sites (Chegini and Rao, 1988). In contrast, glandular epithelium and vascular endothelium contained few or no LTC_4-binding sites (Chegini and Rao, 1988).

The importance of the pro-inflammatory peptidoleukotriene LTC_4 is not fully established in the endometrium. In other tissues, such as rat gastric mucosa, topical application of LTC_4 is known to cause intense vasoconstriction of submucosal venules, leading to reduced mucosal blood flow (Whittle et al, 1985) which is considered to be a major contributory factor in the pathogenesis of peptic ulceration (Ahmed et al, 1992d,e). Furthermore, LTC_4 provokes extensive plasma leakage in a number of vascular beds in the guinea pig (Hau et al, 1985). In the endometrium, the physiological significance of LTC_4 may be that it interacts with PGE_2 to modulate endometrial blood flow. The role of lipoxygenase pathways needs further investigation in this tissue.

Platelet-activating factor

Biosynthesis of PAF

PAF (1-O-alkyl-2-acetyl-sn-glycero-3-phosphocholine) is a family of acetylated glycerophospholipids strongly implicated in the events associated with early implantation. The biosynthesis of PAF involves the action of PLA_2 on alkylacylglycero-3-phosphocholine to release lyso-PAF, which is metabolized to PAF by acetyltransferase (Snyder, 1990). This is termed the remodelling pathway, although PAF can also be synthesized by a *de novo* route. In the remodelling pathway the subclass of membrane phospholipids that serves as the precursor of PAF is 1-alkyl-2-acyl-sn-glycero-3-phosphocholine. Of considerable importance is that the long-chain fatty acid at the sn-2 position of the alkylacylglycerophosphocholine consists mainly of arachidonic acid. Thus, formation of PAF via the remodelling route is always accompanied by the release of AA (Snyder, 1990). AA can then serve as a substrate for potent bioactive eicosanoid mediators as well as itself being an important second messenger, possibly through an interaction with the $p21^{ras}$-regulating protein GAP (Tsai et al, 1990).

PAF synthesis by the embryo

Rabbit embryos in culture produce maximal PAF at a time corresponding to the development of the morula (Angle et al, 1987). One of the first measurable maternal responses to conception is the development of a mild systemic transient thrombocytopenia in mice (O'Neil, 1985a) and women (O'Neil et al, 1985). Biochemical and pharmacological characterization of embryo culture media demonstrated that the embryo-derived factor capable of inducing systemic platelet depletion in mice (O'Neil, 1985b,c) and women (Roberts et al, 1987) was homologous to synthetic PAF (Collier et al, 1988).

PAF and the endometrium

PAF, like PGE_2, is a highly potent inducer of vascular permeability (Humphrey et al, 1984). PAF is produced not only by human embryos during early pregnancy (Roberts et al, 1987), but also by the stromal cells of human endometrium, where its levels are hormonally regulated and progesterone and PGE_2 augment these levels (Alecozay et al, 1991). Uterine PAF production is highest just prior to implantation and drops in areas of the uterus adjacent to the embryo at the time of implantation (Johnston et al, 1990). Further support for the role of PAF in implantation has come from a number of recent studies which indicate that cultures of embryos in media supplemented with PAF enhanced the oxidative metabolism of glucose and lactate in the polyploid pre-implantation human embryos (O'Neil et al, 1989; Ryan et al, 1990a) and increased the implantation potential of embryos cultured in vitro (Ryan et al, 1990b).

INTRACELLULAR REGULATION OF PG SYNTHESIS

Calcium-mobilizing agonists transmit their intracellular messages by binding to specific receptors on the cell surface. The ligand-bound receptors activate effector systems including PLA_2, PLC and PLD via a receptor-coupled G protein to generate second messengers (see Figure 1). The addition of PAF to enriched glandular fractions of human endometrium removed in the luteal phase of the menstrual cycle caused a dose-dependent increase in the synthesis of PGE_2 but not of $PGF_{2\alpha}$ (Smith and Kelly, 1988). The cellular mechanism whereby PAF enhances PG biosynthesis may play a pivotal role in local cellular events at the time of implantation in human endometrium.

Inositol phosphates as markers of PLC

In ex vivo experiments using human endometrial explants, PAF stimulated PIns $4,5$-P_2 hydrolysis by a PI-PLC mechanism, resulting in the generation of inositol phosphates in endometrium obtained from women during the secretory phase of the menstrual cycle (Figure 4). However, in the same system PAF did not significantly alter the inositol phosphate turnover in proliferative endometrium (Figure 5) (Ahmed and Smith, 1992), as was the case for PGE_2 synthesis (Smith and Kelly, 1988), thus implying that the PAF response may be under ovarian steroid regulation. It is interesting to note that PAF production in endometrium has been shown to be regulated by ovarian steroids (Alecozay et al, 1991). It is also possible that PAF did not increase inositol phosphate turnover in proliferative tissue due to a relatively small number of PAF receptors present on the endometrium at this time of the cycle.

PAF receptors in the endometrium

The pattern of distribution of PAF receptors as well as the presence of PAF receptors in the endometrium has not been fully elucidated. Although

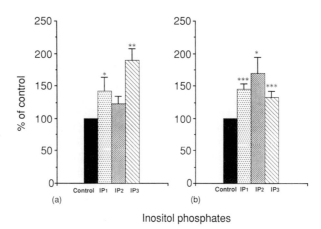

Figure 4. PAF-evoked inositol phosphate accumulation in human secretory endometrium ($n = 12$). After the addition of $1.8\,\mu M$ PAF, incubations were determined in the presence of $10\,mM$ LiCl, at (a) 1 minute and (b) 30 minutes. Results are presented as the mean ($\pm$ SEM) percentage of basal activity (solid columns), which is expressed as 100. IP_1 (dashed columns), IP_2 (crossed columns) and IP_3 (hatched columns) are inositol monophosphate, bisphosphate and trisphosphate fractions, respectively. Statistical analysis was performed using non-parametric Wilcoxon's signed rank. $*p < 0.05$, $**p < 0.002$, $***p < 0.003$, when compared with basal values of inositol phosphates.

autoradiography studies have shown binding sites for PAF in the rabbit endometrium (Kudolo et al, 1991), the presence of a specific PAF receptor or its location in specific cells of the endometrium has not been clearly determined. A recent study demonstrated the presence of PAF receptors in explants of human endometrium using a specific PAF receptor antagonist, WEB 2086. PAF-induced PIns $4,5$-P_2 hydrolysis was inhibited in a dose-dependent manner (Figure 6), suggesting the effect was mediated via a specific endometrial PAF receptor (Ahmed and Smith, 1992). The same group have also shown that the PAF receptors are located on the epithelial cells of HEC-1B cells (Ahmed et al, 1992c). These findings are further strengthened by experiments with [³H]WEB which indicate that its binding site on human platelets is identical to the specific [³H]PAF-binding sites (Ukena et al, 1988).

The cDNA for a PAF receptor has now been cloned from a human leukocyte cDNA library using a $0.8\,kb$ fragment of the guinea-pig lung PAF receptor cDNA (Nakamura et al, 1991). It will now be possible to clearly demonstrate the expression of PAF receptor throughout the menstrual cycle as well as to study the presence of PAF receptor mRNA in embryos and infertile women.

G protein coupling

PAF-mediated responses in endometrium are consistent with those in other tissues. PAF has been shown to stimulate accumulation of inositol phosphates

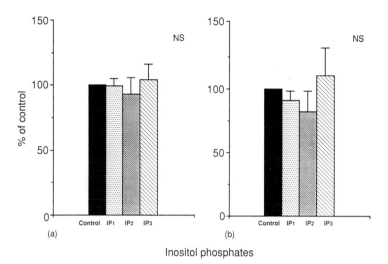

Figure 5. Effect of PAF on inositol phosphate accumulation in human proliferative endometrium. After the addition of 1.8 μM PAF, incubations were determined in the presence of 10 mM LiCl, at (a) 1 minute and (b) 30 minutes. Results are presented as the mean ($\pm$ SEM) percentage of basal activity (solid columns), which is expressed as 100. IP$_1$ (dashed columns), IP$_2$ (crossed columns) and IP$_3$ (hatched columns) are inositol monophosphate, bisphosphate and trisphosphate fractions, respectively. Statistical analysis using non-parametric Wilcoxon's signed rank test was performed ($n = 6$). $p <$ NS when compared with basal values of inositol phosphates.

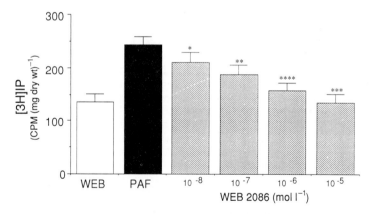

Figure 6. Effect of varying concentrations of WEB 2086 on total inositol phosphate accumulation by PAF in human endometrium. Endometrial explants were pre-incubated for 10 minutes with WEB 2086 and, in the presence of 10 mM LiCl, incubations were determined at 30 minutes after addition of 1.8 μM PAF. The open column represents the effect of WEB 2086 alone, and the effect of PAF on increasing concentration of WEB 2086 is shown by the hatched columns. Results are expressed as the mean ($\pm$ SEM) of six separate experiments. Statistical analysis was by the Student paired t test on log-normalized data. $^*p < 0.02$, $^{**}p < 0.004$, $^{***}p < 0.001$, and $^{****}p < 0.0005$ when compared with PAF-stimulated values of inositol phosphates in the absence of the antagonist (solid column).

in human platelets (Shukla, 1985), in bovine pulmonary artery endothelial cells (Kawaguchi et al, 1990), in rat and bovine cultures of anterior pituitary cells (Grandison, 1990) and in strips of rat (Varol et al, 1989) and human (Schrey et al, 1988) myometrium. These studies indicate that PAF binds to a specific membrane receptor and activates PI-PLC via a G protein, resulting in the hydrolysis of PIns $4,5$-P_2. In addition, it has been reported that PAF stimulated protein tyrosine phosphorylation and caused the rapid trans-location of tyrosine kinase from cytosol to membranes in rabbit platelets (Dhar and Shukla, 1991). It is not known whether the activation of PI-PLC by PAF occurs via a GTP-binding protein or through a tyrosine kinase pathway in endometrium. The PAF response seems to be through both these pathways in HEC-1B cells (A. Ahmed and S. K. Smith, unpublished work).

Ca^{2+} mobilization

PAF-induced PLC activation results in increased production of Ins $1,4,5$-P_3, which elevates $[Ca^{2+}]_i$ levels required for Ca^{2+}-dependent processes. Although the effect of PAF on $[Ca^{2+}]_i$ release in endometrial cells has not been reported, PAF was shown to induce $[Ca^{2+}]_i$ mobilization in a human endometrial cell line—HEC-1B (Figure 7) (Ahmed et al, 1992c). Ins $1,4,5$-P_3 releases Ca^{2+} from a non-mitochondrial pool which has character-istics to suggest that it is the endoplasmic reticulum, but only part of this pool seems to be Ins $1,4,5$-P_3-sensitive (Streb et al, 1984). Immunocytochemical studies using a specific antibody on Purkinje cells reveal that the Ins $1,4,5$-P_3 receptor is localized on the nuclear envelope and on parts of the endo-plasmic reticulum, near the nucleus (Ross et al, 1989). To release Ca^{2+}, Ins $1,4,5$-P_3 must bind to receptors that are linked to Ca^{2+} channels connected with the Ins $1,4,5$-P_3-sensitive Ca^{2+} pool. This Ins $1,4,5$-P_3-induced Ca^{2+} signal can drive a process of Ca^{2+}-induced Ca^{2+} release from the Ins $1,4,5$-P_3-insensitive pools to produce a spike which might be organized in the form of a wave, so spreading the signal throughout the cell (Berridge and Irvine, 1989). As Ins $1,4,5$-P_3 is a key regulator of the periodic release of internal calcium, it is reasonable to assume that activation of endometrial PIns $4,5$-P_2-specific phospholipase C by PAF may result in the elevation of $[Ca^{2+}]_i$.

PC hydrolysis in endometrium

PAF has been shown to stimulate the breakdown of PC by multiple phospholipase pathways in endometrial explants obtained from women during the secretory phase of the menstrual cycle (Ahmed et al, 1992b). These results provide further evidence to support the view that the signal transduction pathways in the human endometrium are complex and may be under ovarian steroid regulation.

The generation of [³H]choline in response to stimulation with PAF in [³H]choline-labelled endometrial explants precedes [³H]GPC and [³H]phosphocholine formation, suggesting PLD-catalysed PC breakdown (Figure 8). PAF-evoked [³H]PBut formation conclusively demonstrates

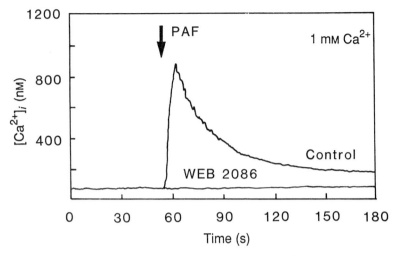

Figure 7. Effect of the PAF antagonist WEB 2086 on intracellular Ca^{2+} release in Hec-1B cells. Fura-2-loaded cells were stimulated with 10 nM PAF in the presence of 1 mM external Ca^{2+} after pre-incubation with 10 μM WEB 2086 for 2 minutes or the vehicle alone (control).

PLD activity in human secretory endometrium as the transphosphatidyla-tion reaction is unique to the activation of PLD (Figure 9). [³H]PBut formation in response to PAF was rapid, dose related and attenuated by the specific PAF receptor antagonist, indicating a receptor-mediated mechan-ism (Ahmed et al, 1992b). As the rise in intracellular [³H]choline and the rise in [³H]PBut formation were similar, it would suggest that the initial route of hydrolysis is likely to be PLD-catalysed PC breakdown. The product of this pathway, PA, provides a sustained source of DAG for the prolonged activation of PKC (Billah and Anthes, 1990). PAF-stimulated [³H]PBut accumulation was found to be kinetically downstream of inositol phosphate formation in human endometrium (Ahmed et al, 1991). This result is similar to that obtained in other systems and suggests that, in the endometrium, PI-PLC is activated before PLD.

Ahmed et al suggested that the slower rise in intracellular [³H]phospho-choline in response to PAF in [³H]choline-labelled endometrial explants (Figure 8(b)) may be due to the inactivation of PC-PLC, but could also be due to phosphorylation of liberated [³H]choline by choline kinase (Cook and Wakelam, 1989). It is difficult to predict which of these two sources of [³H]phosphocholine is the more likely, due to lack of selective choline kinase inhibitors.

A delayed increase in intracellular [³H]GPC is probably due to sequential activation of PLA_2 and lysophospholipase, the enzymes responsible for the sequential deacylation of PC (Billah and Anthes, 1990). Activation of PLA_2 activity after exposure to PAF represents a potential source of AA for PG synthesis from PC breakdown. In addition, lysophosphatidyl-choline generated by the activation of $PC-PLA_2$ could ensure local cell fusion and invasion of the endometrium at the implantation site (Morin et al, 1992).

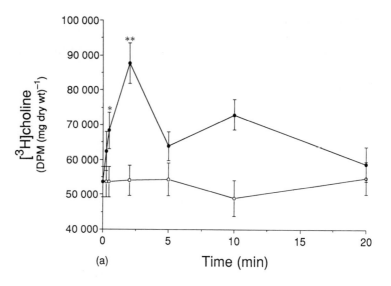

(a)

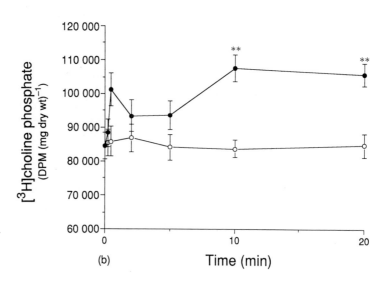

(b)

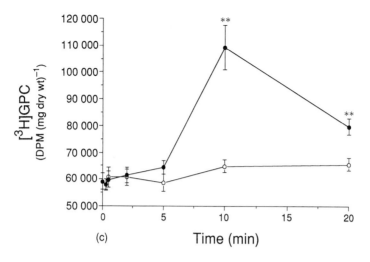

Figure 8. Time-course of PAF-evoked (A) [³H]choline ([³H]Cho) (B) [³H]choline phosphate ([³H]ChoP) and (C) [³H]glycerophosphocholine ([³H]GPC) formation. Endometrial explants were prelabelled with 5 μCi of [³H]choline ml⁻¹ for 24 hours and water-soluble choline metabolites separated by the method described by Cook and Wakelam (1989). The amount of intracellular [³H]choline, [³H]choline phosphate and [³H]GPC generated in response to 1.0 μM PAF were expressed as percentage of control values obtained at each time point. Results presented are the mean (± SEM) of four separate experiments, all of which were done in triplicate. Statistical analysis was performed using the Student paired t test on log-normalized data. $^*p<0.05$, $^{**}p<0.02$ and $^{***}p<0.01$.

Animal experimentation has shown that the levels of PGE_2, $PGF_{2\alpha}$ and 6-keto-$PGF_{1\alpha}$ are elevated at the site of implantation (Kennedy and Zamecnik, 1978). PAF-evoked PC degradation products such as PA and DAG may serve not only as potential second messengers during signal transduction, but could also provide an alternative and important pathway for the generation of PGs as well as serve as potent promoters of mitogenesis in human endometrium.

Apart from PAF and PKC activators, a number of endometrial growth factors such as bradykinin and basic fibroblast growth factor also activate PLD in human endometrium (Ahmed and Smith, unpublished data) and trophoblast cells from first trimester pregnancy exhibit epidermal growth factor-stimulated PLD activity (Figure 10). These studies suggest that the PLD pathway may play a central role in endometrial growth and differentiation at implantation.

CONCLUSIONS

An attempt has been made to explain the complex heterogeneity of intracellular signalling systems operating in the endometrium which are

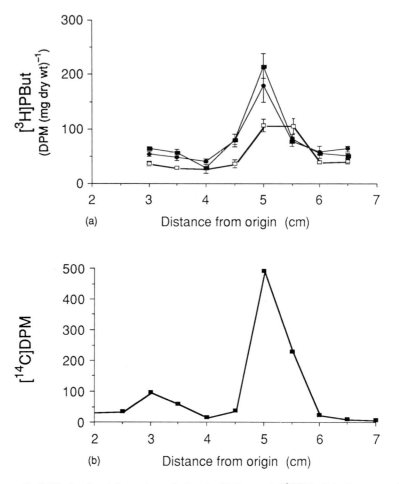

Figure 9. PAF-stimulated formation of phosphatidylbutanol ([³H]PBut) in human endometrium. (A) Tissue explants were pre-incubated with [³H]butan-1-ol for 90 minutes at 37°C
prior to the addition of buffer alone (open squares), 1.0 μM PAF for 2 minutes (solid circles) and
1.0 μM PAF for 5 minutes (solid squares). The [³H]PBut formed was separated by thin-layer
chromatography (TLC); 0.5 cm bands were scraped from the chromatogram and radioactivity
quantified by liquid scintillation spectrometry. Results are expressed as mean (± SEM) triplicate
determinations and are from one typical experiment where $n = 4$. (B) The TLC profile of a
[¹⁴C]PBut standard prepared by incubating 1-stearoyl-2-[¹⁴C]arachidonyl phosphatidylcholine
with cabbage phospholipase D in the presence of [³H]butan-1-ol.

involved in the regulation of PG synthesis and implantation, some of which
may be dependent on ovarian steroids. Considerable information points to a
significant role of PGs in implantation and a case has been made for the
involvement of local regulators of PG synthesis such as PAF in the processes
associated with implantation. The findings support the hypothesis that, at
the site of blastocyst implantation, the localized high concentration of PAF

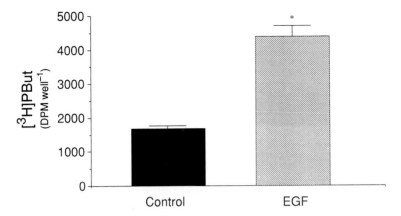

Figure 10. EGF-stimulated phosphatidylbutanol ([³H]PBut) accumulation in human trophoblasts. Trophoblast cells from the first trimester were prelabelled with 3 μCi/ml [³H]myristic acid at 37°C for 48 hours. Cells were stimulated with 50 nM EGF (hatched column) or the vehicle alone (solid column) in the presence of 30 mM butanol. Lipids were extracted and separated by TLC. The results presented are the mean (± SEM) of three separate experiments, all of which were done in triplicate. Statistical analysis was performed using the Student paired t test on log-normalized data. $**p < 0.02$.

released either by the embryo or from the stroma displaces the biologically inactive PAF precursor, lyso-PAF, from receptors on the endometrium; thus enabling PAF–receptor coupling to take place. The study provides evidence of endometrial PAF receptors and shows that the action of PAF is mediated via a specific receptor, which when coupled to the agonist activates endometrial PIns 4,5-P_2-specific PLC and PLD, resulting in the generation of second messengers likely to play a crucial role in cellular events involved in very early recognition of human pregnancy. Evidence to support the hypothesis that PG synthesis and PAF-mediated processess in the endometrium may be under ovarian steroid regulation has been presented. It is concluded that the ability of the endometrium to respond to PAF appears to be a feature of the preparation of this tissue for implantation in women.

Acknowledgements

This work was supported by grant 030060/1.5. from the Wellcome Trust.

REFERENCES

Abel MH & Kelly RW (1979) Differential production of prostaglandins within the human uterus. *Prostaglandins* **10:** 821–828.
Ahmed A & Smith SK (1992) Platelet-activating factor stimulates phospholipase C activity in human endometrium. *Journal of Cellular Physiology* **152:** 207–214.

Ahmed A, Ferriani RA & Smith SK (1991) Stimulation of the hydrolysis of phosphatidyl-inositol 4,5-bisphosphate and phosphatidylcholine by platelet-activating factor (PAF) in human endometrium. *Journal of Reproduction and Fertility, Abstract Series* **8**: abstract 105.

Ahmed A, Cameron IT, Ferriani RA & Smith SK (1992a) Activation of phospholipase A_2 and phospholipase C by endothelin-1 in human endometrium. *Journal of Endocrinology* **135**: 383–390.

Ahmed A, Ferriani RA, Plevin R & Smith SK (1992b) Platelet-activating factor mediated phosphatidylcholine hydrolysis by phospholipase D in human endometrium. *Biology of Reproduction* **47**: 59–65.

Ahmed A, Sage SO, Shoaibi MA, Ferriani RA & Smith SK (1992c) Ovarian steroids modulate stimulated phospholipase D but not phospholipase C by platelet-activating factor in the human endometrial cell line, HEC-1B. *Journal of Biological Chemistry* (in press).

Ahmed A, Hobsley M, Cairns CR, Salmon PR & Hoult JRS (1992d) Eicosanoid synthesis in duodenal ulcer disease: decrease in leukotriene C_4 by colloidal bismuth subcitrate. *Gut* **33**: 159–163.

Ahmed A, Holton J, Vaira D, Smith SK & Hoult JRS (1992e) Eicosanoid synthesis and *Helicobacter pylori* associated gastritis: increase in leukotriene C4 generation associated with *H. pylori* colonisation. *Prostaglandins* **44**: 75–86.

Aitken MA, Rice GE & Brennecke SP (1990) Gestational tissue phospholipase A_2 messenger RNA content and the onset of spontaneous labour in the human. *Journal of Reproduction, Fertility, and Development* **2**: 575–580.

Alecozay AA, Harper MJK, Schenken RS & Hanahan DJ (1991) Paracrine interaction between and prostaglandins in hormonally-treated human luteal phase endometrium in vitro. *Journal of Reproduction and Fertility* **91**: 301–312.

Angle MJ, Byrd W & Johnston JM (1987) Embryonic production of in culture. *Fertility and Sterility* **566 (supplement)**: 158.

Bennett CF & Crooke ST (1987) Purification and characterisation of a phosphoinositide-specific phospholipase C from guinea pig uterus. *Journal of Biological Chemistry* **262**: 13789–13797.

Berridge MJ & Irvine RF (1989) Inositol phosphates and cell signalling. *Nature* **341**: 197–205.

Besterman JM, Pollenz RS, Booker EL Jr & Cuatrecasas P (1986) Diacylglycerol-induced translocation of diacylglycerol kinase: use of affinity-purified enzyme in a reconstitution system. *Proceedings of the National Academy of Sciences of the USA* **83**: 9378–9382.

Billah MM & Anthes JC (1990) The regulation and cellular functions of phosphatidylcholine hydrolysis. *Biochemical Journal* **269**: 281–291.

Billah MM, Pai JK, Mullmann TJ, Egan RW & Siegel MI (1989) Regulation of phospholipase D in HL-60 granulocytes. *Journal of Biological Chemistry* **264**: 9069–9076.

Boeckino SB, Blackmore PF, Wilson PB & Exton JH (1987) Phosphatidate accumulation in hormone-treated hepatocytes via a phospholipase D mechanism. *Journal of Biological Chemistry* **262**: 15309–15315.

Bonney RC (1985) Measurement of phospholipase A_2 activity in human endometrium during the menstrual cycle. *Journal of Endocrinology* **107**: 183–189.

Bourgoin S, Plante E, Gaudry M et al (1990) Involvement of a phospholipase D in the mechanism of action of granulocyte-macrophage colony-stimulating factor (GM-CSF): priming of human neutrophils in vitro with GM-CSF is associated with accumulation of phosphatidic acid and diacylglycerol. *Journal of Experimental Medicine* **172**: 767–777.

Burgoyne RD & Morgan A (1990) The control of free arachidonic acid levels. *Trends in Biochemical Sciences* **15**: 365–366.

Chegini N & Rao CV (1988) The presence of leukotriene C_4 and prostacyclin binding sites in non-pregnant human uterine tissue. *Journal of Clinical Endocrinology and Metabolism* **66**: 76–87.

Collier M, O'Neil C, Ammit AJ & Saunders DM (1988) Biochemical and pharmacological characterization of human embryo-derived platelet-activating factor. *Human Reproduction* **3**: 993–998.

Cook SJ & Wakelam MJO (1989) Analysis of the water-soluble products of phosphatidyl-choline breakdown by ion-exchange chromatography. *Biochemical Journal* **263**: 581–587.

Cook SJ, Palmer S, Plevin P & Wakelam MJO (1990) Mass measurement of inositol 1,4,5-trisphosphate and sn-1,2-diacylglycerol in bombesin-stimulated Swiss 3T3 mouse fibroblasts. *Biochemical Journal* **265**: 617–620.

Dawson RMC (1967) The formation of phosphatidylglycerol and other phospholipids by the transferase activity of phospholipase D. *Biochemical Journal* **102**: 205–210.

Dhar A & Shukla SD (1991) Involvement of pp60$^{c\text{-src}}$ in platelet-activating factor-stimulated platelets. *Journal of Biological Chemistry* **266**: 18797–18801.

Downie J, Poyser N & Wunderlich M (1974) Levels of prostaglandins in human endometrium during the normal menstrual cycle. *Journal of Physiology* **236**: 465–472.

Endo T, Fukue H, Kanaya M et al (1991) Bombesin and bradykinin increase inositol phosphates and cytosolic free Ca^{2+}, and stimulate DNA synthesis in human endometrial stromal cells. *Journal of Endocrinology* **131**: 313–318.

Evans CA & Kennedy TG (1978) The importance of prostaglandin synthesis for the initiation of blastocyst implantation in the hamster. *Journal of Reproduction and Fertility* **54**: 255–261.

Exton JH (1990) Signaling through phosphatidylcholine breakdown. *Journal of Biological Chemistry* **265**: 1–4.

Flint APF, Leat WMF, Sheldrick EL & Stewart HJ (1986) Stimulation of phosphoinositide hydrolysis by oxytocin and the mechanism by which oxytocin controls prostaglandin synthesis in the ovine endometrium. *Biochemical Journal* **237**: 797–805.

Garg SK & Chaudhury RR (1983) Evidence for a possible role of prostaglandins in implantation in rats. *Archives Internationales de Pharmacodynamie et de Therapie* **262**: 299–305.

Grandison L (1990) Platelet-activating factor induces inositol phosphate accumulation in cultures of rat and bovine anterior pituitary cells. *Endocrinology* **127**: 1786–1791.

Gupta A, Huet YM & Dey SK (1989) Evidence for prostaglandins and leukotrienes as mediators of phase I of estrogen action in implantation in the mouse. *Endocrinology* **124**: 546–548.

Hertig AT (1964) Gestational hyperplasia of endometrium; a morphologic correlation of ova, endometrium, and corpora lutea during early pregnancy. *Laboratory Investigation* **13**: 1153–1191.

Hoffman LH, Di Pietro DL & McKenna TJ (1978) Effect of indomethacin on uterine capillary permeability and blastocyst development in rabbits. *Prostaglandins* **15**: 823–828.

Hoffman LH, Davenport GR & Brash AR (1984) Endometrial prostaglandins and phospholipase activity related to implantation in rabbits: effects of dexamethasone. *Biology of Reproduction* **38**: 544–555.

Hofmann GE, Rao ChV, De Leon FD, Toledo AA & Sanfilippo JS (1985) Human endometrial prostaglandin E2 binding sites and their profiles during the menstrual cycle and in pathologic states. *American Journal of Obstetrics and Gynecology* **151**: 369.

Hua, XY, Dahlen SE, Lundberg S, Hammarstrom S & Hedqvist P (1985) Leukotriene C_4, D_4 and E_4 cause widespread and extensive plasma extravasation in the guinea-pig. *Naunyn-Schmeideberg's Archive of Pharmacology* **330**: 136–141.

Humphrey DM, McManus LM, Hanahan DJ & Pinckard RN (1984) Morphologic basis of increased vascular permeability induced by acetyl glyceryl ether phosphorylcholine. *Laboratory Investigation* **50**: 16–25.

Johnston JM, Noriei M, Angle MJ & Hoffman DR (1990) Regulation of the arachidonic acid cascade and platelet-activating factor metabolism in reproductive tissues. In Mitchell MD (ed.) *Eicosanoids in Reproduction*, pp 5–37. Boston: CRC Press.

Jones DSC & Smith SK (1991) Cloning and sequencing of human uterine phospholipase C isozymes. In Bailey JM (ed.) *Prostaglandins, Leukotrienes, Lipoxins & PAF. XIth Washington International Spring Symposium*, p 88.

Jones MA & Harper MJK (1983) Prostaglandin accumulation by isolated uterine endometrial epithelial cells from six-day pregnant rabbits. *Biology of Reproduction* **29**: 1201–1209.

Kawaguchi H, Sawa H & Yasuda H (1990) Mechanism of increased angiotensin-converting enzyme activity stimulated by platelet-activating factor. *Biochemical Biophysical Acta* **1052**: 503–508.

Kennedy TG (1983) Embryonic signals and the initiation of blastocyst implantation. *Australian Journal of Biological Science* **36**: 531–543.

Kennedy TG & Zamecnik J (1978) The concentration of 6-keto-prostaglandin F1alpha is markedly elevated at the site of blastocyst implantation in the rat. *Prostaglandins* **61**: 599–605.

Kobayashi M & Kanfer JN (1987) Phosphatidylethanol formation via transphosphatidylation by rat brain synaptosomal phospholipase D. *Journal of Neurochemistry* **48:** 1597–1603.

Koch CA, Anderson D, Moran MF, Ellis C & Pawson T (1991) SH2 and SH3 domains: elements that control interactions of cytoplasmic signalling proteins. *Science* **252:** 668–674.

Kolesnick RN & Paley AE (1987) 1,2-Diacylglycerol and phorbol esters stimulate phosphatidylcholine metabolism in GH3 pituitary cells. Evidence for separate mechanisms of action. *Journal of Biological Chemistry* **262:** 9204–9210.

Kraeling RR, Rampacek GB & Fiorello NA (1985) Inhibition of pregnancy with indomethacin in mature gilts and prepubertal gilts induced to ovulate. *Biology of Reproduction* **32:** 105–110.

Kramer RM, Hession C, Johansen B et al (1989) Structure and properties of a human non-pancreatic phospholipase A_2. *Journal of Biological Chemistry* **264:** 5738–5775.

Kudolo GB, Kasamo N & Harper MJ (1991) Autoradiographic localization of platelet-activating factor (PAF) binding sites in the rabbit endometrium during the peri-implantation period. *Cell Tissue Research* **265:** 231–241.

Lacroix MC & Kann G (1982) Comparative studies of prostaglandin $F_{2\alpha}$ and E_2 in late cyclic and early pregnant sheep: in vitro synthesis by endometrium and conceptus—effects of in vivo indomethacin treatment on establishment of pregnancy. *Prostaglandins* **23:** 507–526.

Lai CY & Wada K (1988) Phospholipase A_2 from human synovial fluid: Purification and structural homology to the placental enzyme. *Biochemical and Biophysical Research Communications* **157:** 488–493.

Lau IF, Saksena SK & Chang MC (1973) Pregnancy blockade by indomethacin, an inhibitor of prostaglandin synthesis: its reversal by prostaglandins and progesterone in mice. *Prostaglandins* **4:** 795–803.

Leach KL, Ruff VA, Wright TM, Pessin MS & Raben DM (1991) Dissociation of protein kinase C activation and sn-1,2-diacylglycerol formation. Comparison of phosphatidyl-inositol- and phosphatidylcholine-derived diglycerides in alpha-thrombin-stimulated fibroblasts. *Journal of Biological Chemistry* **266:** 3215–3221.

Lundkvist O & Nilsson BO (1980) Ultrastructural changes of the trophoblast–epithelial complex in mice subject to implantation blocking treatment with indomethacin. *Biology and Reproduction* **22:** 719–726.

Maathuis JB & Kelly RW (1978) Concentrations of prostaglandins $F_{2\alpha}$ and E_2 in the endometrium throughout the human menstrual cycle, after the administration of clomiphene or an oestrogen-progestogen pill and in early pregnancy. *Journal of Endocrinology* **77:** 361–371.

MacNulty EE, Plevin R & Wakelam MJO (1990) Stimulation of the hydrolysis of phosphatidyl-inositol 4,5-bisphosphate and phosphatidylcholine by endothelin, a complete mitogen for rat-1 fibroblasts. *Biochemical Journal* **272:** 761–766.

Malathy PV, Cheng HC & Dey SK (1986) Production of leukotrienes and prostaglandins in the rat uterus during periimplantation period. *Prostaglandins* **32:** 605–614.

Martin JL, Pumford NR, La Rosa AC et al (1991) A metabolite of halothane covalently binds to an endoplasmic reticulum protein that is highly homologous to phosphatidylinositol-specific phospholipase C-α but has no activity. *Biochemical and Biophysical Research Communications* **178:** 679–685.

Mirando MA, Ott TL, Vallet JL, Davis M & Bazer FW (1990) Oxytocin-stimulated inositol phosphate turnover in endometrium of ewes is influenced by stage of the estrous cycle, pregnancy, and intrauterine infusion of ovine conceptus secretory proteins. *Biology of Reproduction* **42:** 98–105.

Morin C, Langlais J & Lambert RD (1992) *Possible implication of lysophosphatidyl-choline in cell fusion accompanying implantation in the rabbit.* Satellite Symposium of the Ninth International Congress of Endocrinology (Endocrinology of Embryo–Endometrial Interactions), Bordeaux, France. Abstract 19.

Nakamura N, Honda Z, Izumi T et al (1991) Molecular cloning and expression of platelet-activating factor receptor from human leukocytes. *Journal of Biological Chemistry* **266:** 20400–20405.

Nishizuka Y (1989) The molecular heterogeneity of protein kinase C and its implication for cellular regulation. *Nature* **334:** 661–665.

O'Neil C (1985a) Thrombocytopenia is an initial maternal response to fertilization in mice. *Journal of Reproduction and Fertility* **73:** 559–566.

O'Neil C (1985b) Examination of the cause of early pregnancy associated thrombocytopenia in mice. *Journal of Reproduction and Fertility* **73:** 567–577.

O'Neil C (1985c) Partial characterization of the embryo-derived in mice. *Journal of Reproduction and Fertility* **75:** 375–380.

O'Neil C, Gidley-Baird AA, Pike IL et al (1985) Maternal blood platelet physiology and luteal phase endocrinology as a means of monitoring pre- and post-implantation embryo viability following in vitro fertilization. *Journal of In-Vitro-Fertilization and Embryo Transfer* **2:** 87–93.

O'Neil C, Ryan JP, Collier M et al (1989) Supplementation of in-vitro fertilisation culture medium with platelet-activating factor. *Lancet* **ii:** 769–772.

Orlicky DJ, Silio M, Williams C, Gorden J & Gerschenson LE (1986) Regulation of inositol phosphate levels by prostaglandins in cultured endometrial cells. *Journal of Cellular Physiology* **128:** 105–112.

Pai JK, Siegel MI, Egan RW & Billah MM (1988) Phospholipase D catalyzes phospholipid metabolism in chemotactic peptide-stimulated HL-60 granulocytes. *Journal of Biological Chemistry* **263:** 12472–12477.

Pakrasi PL, Cheng HC & Dey SK (1983) Prostaglandins in the uterus: modulation by steroid hormones. *Prostaglandins* **26:** 991–1009.

Phillips CA & Poyser NL (1981) Studies on the involvement of prostaglandins in implantation in the rat. *Journal of Reproduction and Fertility* **62:** 73–81.

Psychoyos A & Martel D (1985) Embryo-endometrial interaction at implantation. In Edwards RC, Purdy JM & Steptoe PC (eds) *Implantation of the Human Embryo*, pp 197–219. London: Academic Press.

Randall RW, Bonser RW, Thompson NT, Garland LG (1990) A novel and sensitive assay for phospholipase D in intact cells. *FEBS Letters* **264:** 87–90.

Rees MCP, Parry DM, Anderson ABM & Turnbull AC (1982) Immunohistochemical localisation of cyclooxygenase in the human uterus. *Prostaglandins* **23:** 207–214.

Rhee SG, Suh PG, Ryu SH & Lee SY (1989) Studies of inositol phospholipid-specific phospholipase C. *Science* **244:** 546–550.

Roberts TK, Adamson LM, Smart YC, Stanger JD & Murdoch RN (1987) An evaluation of peripheral blood platelet enumeration as a monitor of fertilization and early pregnancy. *Fertility and Sterility* **47:** 848–854.

Ross CA, Meldolesi J, Milner TA et al (1989) Inositol 1,4,5-trisphosphate receptor localized to endoplasmic reticulum in cerebellar Purkinje neurons. *Nature* **339:** 468–470.

Ryan JP, O'Neil C & Wales RG (1990a) Oxidative metabolism of energy substrates by preimplantation mouse embryos in the presence of platelet-activating factor. *Journal of Reproduction and Fertility* **89:** 301–307.

Ryan JP, Spinks NR, O'Neil C & Wales RG (1990b) Implantation potential and fetal viability of mouse embryos cultured in media supplemented with platelet-activating factor. *Journal of Reproduction and Fertility* **89:** 309–315.

Saito M, Bourque E & Kanfer JN (1975) Phosphatidohydrolase and base-exchange activity of commercial phospholipase D. *Archive of Biochemistry and Biophysics* **164:** 420–428.

Saksena SK, Lau IF & Chang MC (1976) Relationship between oestrogen, prostaglandin $F_{2\alpha}$ and histamine in delayed implantation in the mouse. *Acta Endocrinologica* **42:** 225–232.

Samuelsson B, Goldyne M, Granstrom E et al (1978) Prostaglandins and thromboxanes. *Annual Review of Biochemistry* **47:** 997–1029.

Schrey MP, Cornford PA, Read AM & Steer PJ (1988) A role for phosphoinositide hydrolysis in human uterine smooth muscle during parturition. *American Journal of Obstetrics and Gynecology* **159:** 964–970.

Seilhamer JJ, Pruzanski W, Vadas P et al (1989a) Cloning and recombinant expression of phospholipase A_2 present in rheumatoid arthritic synovial fluid. *Journal of Biological Chemistry* **264:** 5335–5338.

Seilhamer JJ, Randall TL, Johnson LK et al (1989b) Novel gene exon homologous to pancreatic phospholipase A_2: sequence and chromosomal mapping of both human genes. *Journal of Cellular Biochemistry* **39:** 327–337.

Shukla SD (1985) Platelet-activating factor stimulated formation of inositol trisphosphate in platelets and its regulation by various agents including Ca^{2+}, indomethacin, CV3988 and forskolin. *Archive of Biochemistry and Biophysics* **240:** 674–681.

Singh EJ, Baccarini IM & Zuspan FP (1975) Levels of prostaglandins $F_{2\alpha}$ and E_2 in human endometrium during the menstrual cycle. *American Journal of Obstetrics and Gynecology* **121**: 1003–1006.

Slivka SR, Meier KE & Insel PA (1988) α_1-adrenergic receptors promote phosphatidylcholine hydrolysis in MDCK-D1 cells. *Journal of Biological Chemistry* **263**: 12242–12246.

Smith SK & Kelly RW (1988) Effect of platelet-activating factor on the release of $PGF_{2\alpha}$ and PGE_2 by separated cells of human endometrium. *Journal of Reproduction and Fertility* **82**: 271–276.

Snyder F (1990) Platelet-activating factor and related acetylated lipids as potent biologically active cellular mediators. *American Journal of Physiology* **259**: C697–C708.

Streb H, Bayerdorffer E, Hasse W, Irvine RF & Schulz I (1984) Effect of inositol-1,4,5-trisphosphate on isolated subcellular fractions of rat pancreas. *Journal of Membrane Biology* **81**: 241–253.

Tawfik OW & Dey SK (1988) Further evidence for role of leukotrienes as mediators of decidualization in the rat. *Prostaglandins* **35**: 379–402.

Thompson NT, Bonser RW & Garland LG (1991) Receptor-coupled phospholipase D and its inhibition. *Trends in Pharmacological Science* **12**: 404–408.

Tsai MH, Yu CL & Stacey DW (1990) A cytoplasmic protein inhibits the GTPase activity of H-Ras in a phospholipid-dependent manner. *Science* **250**: 982–985.

Ukena D, Dent G, Birke FW et al (1988) Radioligand binding of antagonists of platelet-activating factor to intact human platelets. *FEBS Letters* **228**: 285–289.

Varol FG, Hadjiconstantinou M, Travers JB & Neff NH (1989) Platelet-activating factor stimulates phosphoinositol hydrolysis in the rat myometrium. *European Journal of Pharmacology* **159**: 97–98.

Whittle BJR, Oren-Wolman N & Guth PH (1985) Gastric vasoconstrictor action of leukotriene C_4, $PGF_{2\alpha}$ and thromboxane mimetic U-46619 on rat submucosal microcirculation in vivo. *American Journal of Physiology* **248**: G580–G586.

4

Biochemistry of myometrial contractility

C. H. EGARTER
P. HUSSLEIN

The human uterus is almost inactive during early and mid-pregnancy. As pregnancy advances, the uterus becomes increasingly active and, at or near term, labour starts. Despite much research effort, the factors regulating uterine contractility during pregnancy as well as the precise order of events leading to the initiation of parturition in the human female are only partly known. During pregnancy, the myometrium relaxes to accommodate the developing infant and products of conception and, with the onset of labour, it provides the rhythmic tonic contractions which lead to the expulsion of the uterine contents. The cervical tissue, however, is hard and firmly holds the uterine contents during the first part of pregnancy. At about the 34th week of pregnancy a biochemical process of cervical maturation commences, finally leading to the fully dilatated cervix at delivery (Huszar, 1984; Huszar and Naftolin, 1984). An important point in the understanding of uterine function was the recognition that the myometrium and the cervix are functionally interrelated and act in close co-operation during pregnancy and labour.

PHYSIOLOGICAL REGULATION OF UTERINE CONTRACTILITY

Unlike skeletal muscle, the myometrial smooth muscle cells are not a homogenous tissue, but are embedded in extracellular material composed mainly of collagen fibres, which facilitates the transmission of contractile forces generated by individual muscle cells. The muscle cells communicate with one another through connections called gap junctions. These junctions are believed to synchronize myometrial function by conduction of electro-physiological stimuli during labour. In both human and animal myometria it has been shown that in the final weeks of pregnancy, when irregular contractions increase and cervical maturation occurs, the myometrial gap junctions increase in number until the commencement of labour (Garfield et al, 1982). The formation of myometrial gap junctions has been studied in in vitro organ cultures, and regulatory roles for oestrogen, progesterone and prostaglandins have been established (Garfield, 1984). Furthermore, a relationship between electrical activity, the conductivity properties of the myometrium and the density of gap junctions has been shown (Verhoeff et al, 1984). This indicates that the various related components of myometrial cellular regulation, including the formation of gap junctions, enhance electrical activity and the response to oestrogen, oxytocin and prosta-glandins are simultaneous events which collectively contribute to the increased myometrial activity of labour.

The subcellular structure of smooth muscle is also different from striated skeletal muscle. In the longitudinal axis of the latter contractile unit, the so-called sarcomere, repeating patterns of dense and light bands between the so-called Z lines, represents the filaments of myosin and actin, respectively. Each thick myosin filament is surrounded by thin actin filaments (Figure 1a). The sliding motion of these filaments against each other is the basis of contraction and force generation process (Huxley, 1971a). The organization of smooth muscle cells is different in that the thick myosin and thin actin filaments occur in long, random bundles throughout the smooth muscle cells and the continuity of these filaments is not interrupted by Z lines. Analogous in function to the Z lines of striated muscle (Small, 1977) are intermediate filaments, which form a network that links protein structures known as dense bodies. The intermediate filaments and dense bodies do not play an active part in the contractile process, but they are associated with the cell membrane and are generally distributed throughout the cytoplasm in groups to form a network with attachment sites located over the entire cell. They link the individual fibrils, composed of actin and myosin, into integrated mechanical units (Figure 1b). Whereas in skeletal muscle the direction of contraction is always aligned with the axis of muscle fibres, smooth muscle can exert pulling

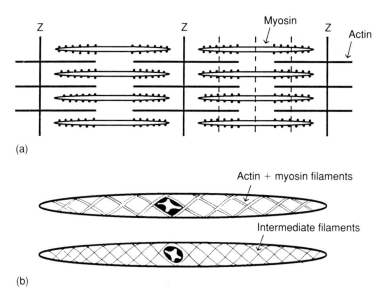

(a)

(b)

Figure 1. (a) Schematic diagram of striated muscle. Overlapping actin and myosin filaments. (b) Schematic diagram of smooth muscle. Bundles of actin and myosin filaments connecting opposing sides on the cell surface. Intermediate filaments form a network between the actin–myosin filament groups. Modified from Stephans (1977), with permission.

forces in any direction due to its organization. This enables the uterus to generate forces in any axis necessary and to assume virtually any shape to accommodate fetuses of various sizes during labour (Huszar and Roberts, 1982). It is well established in both smooth and skeletal muscle that contraction is based on a sliding of actin and myosin filaments without any internal change in the length of either filament (Huxley, 1971b; Bagby, 1983). The sliding action is caused by the cyclic formation of cross-bridges when myosin heads interact with actin monomers, conformational changes in the myosin heads which effectively move the myosin filament along the actin filament, and detachment of the myosin heads from the actin filaments at the end of each cycle.

MYOSIN AND ACTIN

A principal component of muscle contraction is the myosin molecule. It is both an enzyme that hydrolyses ATP during contraction and relaxation as well as a structural protein which is organized in thick filaments to optimize the actin–myosin interaction and conduct the forces of contraction. In smooth muscles, the myosin molecule is composed of two heavy chains of about 200 kDa and two pairs of light chains of 15 and 20 kDa. The head of the myosin molecule carries three important sites (Figure 2): (1) the actin-combining site, where myosin and actin interact; (2) the ATPase site, where

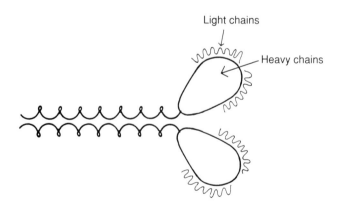

Figure 2. Schematic structure of myosin filaments.

ATP is hydrolysed; and (3) the 20 kDa light chains, which provide an element of contractile regulation through reversible phosphorylation. The other major muscle protein is actin, a globular protein of 45 kDa. The actin monomers polymerize into long, thin filaments. When the actin and myosin filaments slide past one another during uterine contractions the myosin heads and actin molecules form cross-bridges that generate the contractile force of labour.

The actin–myosin interaction in smooth muscle is regulated through enzymatic phosphorylation or dephosphorylation of the 20 kDa myosin light chain (Adelstein and Eisenberg, 1980). The actin–myosin interaction can take place only if myosin light chains have been phosphorylated, and this can be measured in vitro as the level of actomyosin ATPase, as this enzyme activity can be shown to be about three- or four-fold higher when the myosin light chains are completely phosphorylated (Figure 3) (Huszar and Bailey, 1979; Janis et al, 1981).

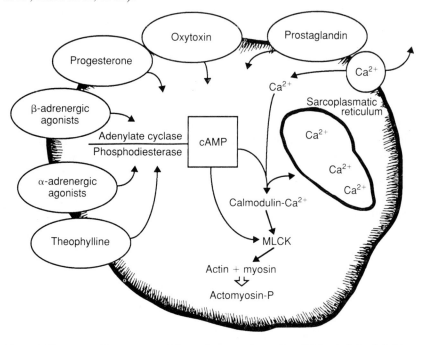

Figure 3. The contractile apparatus of the uterine smooth muscle cell. Myosin light chain kinase (MLCK) is regulated through the calcium and cyclic AMP (cAMP) pathways. Calcium and cAMP levels in the cell are modulated by various drugs and hormones. Modified from Huszar (1984), with permission.

Myosin light chain phosphorylation depends on the activity of a special enzyme, myosin light chain kinase (MLCK). This enzyme can be regarded as the key regulator of contractility in smooth muscles. Relaxation of smooth muscles occurs when another enzyme, myosin light chain phosphatase, removes the phosphate group from the myosin light chains (Pato and Adelstein, 1980). Thus, the contractile state of smooth muscle is defined by the relative activities of MLCK and myosin light chain phosphatase.

CALCIUM

Calcium of smooth muscles, such as myometrium, originates in the intra-cellular as well as in the extracellular areas. The sarcoplasmic reticulum represents the major intracellular store for calcium (Somlyo et al, 1985). Smooth muscles contain a well-developed sarcoplasmic reticulum and this releases enough calcium to fulfil the contractile needs of these cells. The membranes of the sarcoplasmic reticulum contain an intracellular ATP-dependent calcium transport pump which is an important regulator of cytoplasmic calcium levels and thus the contractile state of the muscle. Inositol 1,4,5-triphosphate has been shown to be involved in this release of calcium from the sarcoplasmic reticulum into the cytosol (Michell, 1975). The products of phosphatidylinositol by phospholipase C have recently been recognized as second messengers which act as intracellular molecules that transmit the extracellular signals to bring about the desired physiological response. Studies with smooth muscle tissues suggest an important role for inositol 1,4,5-triphosphate in opening a calcium channel of the sarcoplasmic reticulum which is either a receptor for inositol 1,4,5-triphosphate itself or may be coupled to this receptor.

But calcium may also enter the cytoplasm from extracellular sources by appropriate stimulation. Two main routes exist for calcium entry: the voltage-operated calcium channels and the receptor-operated calcium channels (Hurwitz, 1986). Eicosanoids facilitate the entry of calcium into the cell, perhaps through specific calcium channels or by activation of the receptor-operated channels. Calcium channelling is based on a complex of membrane-bound glycoproteins with an aqueous pore at the centre. Calcium channels are thought to exist in different states: the open or activated state and the closed or deactivated state. When the membrane is depolarized to an appropriate level, voltage-operated calcium channels convert to the activated state, thus allowing a substantial calcium influx to the cell. Receptor-operated calcium channels are opened in response to activating ligands such as hormones or neurotransmitters, which bind to specific receptors associated with the channel. Voltage-operated calcium channels have been divided into long, transient and neuronal types according to their conductance properties. The long and transient types are important in smooth muscle activation. Furthermore, the long-type calcium channels are blocked by a variety of so-called calcium channel blockers or activated by structural analogues (Janis and Triggle, 1986; Triggle and Janis, 1987).

In the resting cell, the cytoplasmic free calcium level is about 130 nM. Physiological stimuli, such as membrane depolarization or contractile agents like acetylcholine or noradrenaline, may cause a transient increase in the cellular free calcium to about 500–700 nM, which is detected by the 'calcium sensor protein' calmodulin. Calmodulin can bind calcium with high affinity (Potter et al, 1983). Calcium binding induces a dramatic change in calmodulin conformation which exposes a hydrophobic domain of interaction with target enzymes such as MLCK (Stull et al, 1986). The phosphorylated myosin interacts with actin and causes a higher level of contractility in the myometrium. Further experiments on the regulation of smooth muscle cells were based on pharmacological agents, including phenothiazines which bind to calmodulin in a calcium-dependent manner and inhibit its interaction with MLCK. In an animal model these compounds inhibited both phosphorylation of the myosin light chain and actin-activated Mg^{2+} ATPase of myosin (Hidika et al, 1980). The calmodulin antagonists also inhibited tension development or induced relaxation of smooth muscle fibres. These studies strongly support the idea that myosin phosphorylation and dephosphorylation are key events in the 'on–off' switch in actin activation of the myosin Mg^{2+} ATPase and smooth muscle contractility.

MYOSIN LIGHT CHAIN KINASE

The key enzyme MLCK has so far been shown to be affected by three different cellular regulatory systems. Intracellular free calcium in a concentration of about 10^{-6}–10^{-7} M is necessary for MLCK activity. Furthermore, MLCK is active only when calmodulin, the calcium-dependent regulatory protein, is associated with the enzyme (Yagi et al, 1978). Finally, cyclic AMP (cAMP) has at least two important actions towards decreasing myometrial contractility. cAMP stimulates the calcium pump of the sarcoplasmic reticulum, and this leads to a lower level of cytoplasmic free calcium. On the other hand, cAMP may cause phosphorylation of MLCK itself by a cAMP-dependent protein kinase (Adelstein et al, 1978). This phosphorylation inhibits enzymatic activity by reducing the affinity of the MLCK for the calmodulin–calcium complex.

The connection between oestrogen and progesterone and between enzymes of cAMP synthesis and cAMP degradation was also investigated. In addition to the well-known adenylate cyclase stimulation by β-adrenergic agonists, α-adrenergic influence caused a decrease in cellular cAMP levels, most likely due to activation of phosphodiesterase (Berg et al, 1986). This may explain why the concentration of α-adrenergic receptors and myometrial contractility increase after oestrogen treatment in rabbits. However, when progesterone was administered to oestrogen-treated rabbits there was an inhibition of the contractile activity mediated by a β-adrenergic response (Roberts et al, 1986). This mechanism does not appear to be the dominant regulator, because there was no decline in the myometrial β-adrenergic binding or β-adrenergic receptor concentrations during term and preterm labour (Dattel et al, 1986). Experiments directed to the contractile and electrical properties of myometrial strips of parturient rats demonstrated that the characteristic changes in electrical and contractile activity during pregnancy and labour are related to the endocrine events that cause calcium modulation of the action potential (Bengtsson et al, 1984).

OXYTOCIN

Oxytocin is known to be a potent uterotonic hormone that is secreted from the posterior pituitary gland. Although increased concentrations of oxytocin before and during labour could not clearly be demonstrated (Dawood et al, 1978; Mitchell et al, 1980), the potential importance of oxytocin as a trigger for parturition is obvious (Alexandrova and Soloff, 1980). The effect of oxytocin is mediated by myometrial oxytocin receptors, which are modulated by various factors. After the administration of oestrogens, for instance, an increase occurs in the number of uterine receptors sensitive to oxytocin and also α-adrenergic agonists (Roberts et al, 1977; Nissenson et al, 1978). This increase can be prevented by the concurrent administration of progesterone. The phenomenon further illustrates the importance of the oestrogen–progesterone ratio in the sensitivity of the uterus to uterotonic agents. In binding to the receptor, oxytocin has been shown to inhibit the Ca^{2+} ATPase of the myometrial cell membrane which pumps calcium from the inside to the extracellular milieu and promotes the influx of calcium both from the sarcoplasmic reticulum and from the extracellular area (Kao, 1977). Whether this mechanism is predominant in maintaining the intracellular calcium milieu is not yet clear. However, as discussed earlier the increase in the cytoplasmic concentration of calcium activates the contractile process. Furthermore, oxytocin may have another central regulatory function. At term, decidua parietalis shows a high concentration of oxytocin receptors (Fuchs et al, 1984). Theoretically, the binding of oxytocin to its receptor in the decidua may be a stimulus for prostaglandin synthesis since prostaglandins are found in high concentration in uterine decidual tissues obtained from women in labour (Karim, 1972). So oxytocin may act via prostaglandins as a trigger of uterine contractility.

In another interesting hypothesis, the gap junctions represent oxytocin receptors. Indeed, oxytocin receptors appear at the same time as gap junctions. If oxytocin is bound to gap junction proteins in the cell membrane this could lead via structural changes to an increase in permeability of the gap junctions (Husslein, 1984; Verhoeff and Garfield, 1986).

PROGESTERONE

The effects of progesterone on the myometrium are characterized by a relative quiescence and uncoupling of the excitation–contraction process. Progesterone action may be due to a combination of reduced activities of cell membrane function and reduced cell-to-cell communication. This diminishes permeability for calcium, sodium and potassium, as well as modulating the intracellular calcium binding that makes less calcium available for the calmodulin–MLCK system. Progesterone may also influence the phospholipids of the myometrial cells attenuating phosphatidylinositol and prostaglandin biosynthesis (Garfield, 1984) (Figure 4). Also, progesterone action is clearly related to the postreceptor events. For instance, in the rabbit myometrium, progesterone increased the cellular response to β-adrenergic receptor stimulation, and the rate of cAMP synthesis was much higher under the influence of progesterone compared with that of oestrogen (Riemer et al, 1986). Indirect clinical evidence also indicates that regulation of uterine contractility is mediated by steroid compounds. Oestrogens stimulate or increase sensibility of α-adrenergic receptors, leading to an increased production of prostaglandin $F_{2\alpha}$ ($PGF_{2\alpha}$), whereas progesterone stimulates

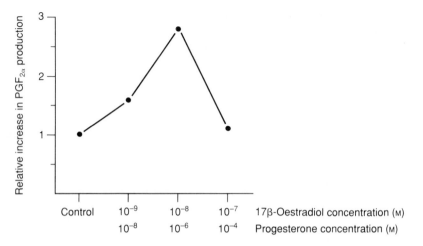

Figure 4. Dose-dependent influence of 17β-oestradiol/progesterone on relative $PGF_{2\alpha}$ concentrations in human monolayer cultures of proliferative endometrium (picograms of $PGF_{2\alpha}$ per millilitre of medium per 24 hours per 50 000 cells). Modified from Zahradnik (1988), with permission.

β-adrenergic receptors, leading to the preponderance of prostacyclin synthase and, via cAMP, to the relaxation of smooth muscle cells (Omini et al, 1978) (Figure 5).

That the local influence of progesterone is of importance for the regulation of myometrial contractility has recently gained further support. Treatment with mifepristone, a steroid acting as an antiprogesterone at the receptor level, results in increased uterine activity as well as an increased sensitivity to prostaglandins (Swahn and Bygdeman, 1988). However, it is unclear whether withdrawal of progesterone will also result in increased endogenous prostaglandin production. A dose-dependent stimulation of $PGF_{2\alpha}$ and PGE_2 synthesis with mifepristone on human endometrial and decidual tissue cultures has been demonstrated (Smith and Kelly, 1987).

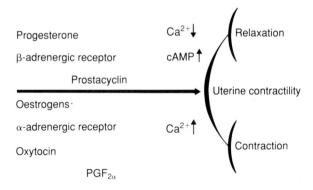

Figure 5. Schematic diagram of steroid–catecholamine–prostaglandin interaction on the human uterus.

However, since treatment during early pregnancy resulted in a high frequency of incomplete abortions and an increased risk of vaginal bleeding, prostaglandin production may not be stimulated in vivo or the release is impaired and delayed (Bygdeman and Van Look, 1989). Furthermore, when mifepristone was administered to non-human primates in late pregnancy, labour was induced in some but not all animals and the increase in prostaglandin concentration in amniotic fluid was delayed in comparison with spontaneous delivery (Haluska et al, 1987). These data indicate that withdrawal of progesterone influence, at least when caused by progesterone receptor blockage, was not sufficient to induce the orderly sequence of changes in prostaglandin production necessary for the development of co-ordinated and totally effective myometrium contractility.

PROSTAGLANDINS AND THEIR ROLE IN SPONTANEOUS OR INDUCED ABORTION AND LABOUR

It is generally accepted that prostaglandins play an important role in the physiology of reproduction and gestation. The regulation of uterine contractility during pregnancy by these components of the eicosanoid system is recognized increasingly (Mitchell, 1987). Prostaglandins and the related acidic lipids all arise from the principal precursor, arachidonic acid, via three different pathways catalysed by the enzymes of cyclooxygenase, leading to prostaglandins, prostacyclin and thromboxane, and lipoxygenase, leading to leukotrienes (Figure 6). The exact regulation of prostaglandin metabolism in

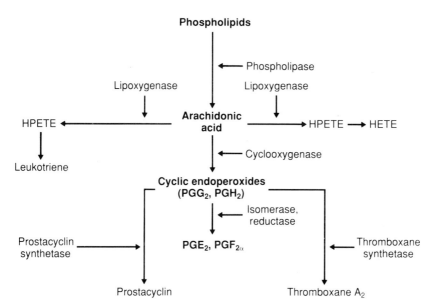

Figure 6. Prostaglandin pathways. HPETE, hydroperoxyeicosatetraenoic acid; HETE, hydroxyeicosatetraenoic acid.

the uterus as well as in the cervix, however, is not yet known definitely. There may also be several protein and protein factors which are implicated in the modulation of the various pathways (Wilson et al, 1985). Human amnion and chorion produce mostly PGE_2, while the decidua produces PGE_2 and $PGF_{2\alpha}$. The amnion, which has no blood supply, receives arachidonic acid from the fetus via amniotic fluid, whereas the chorion, which also lacks blood supply, receives arachidonic acid from the decidua.

PGE_2 and $PGF_{2\alpha}$ are thought to be important factors in the initiation of human parturition for the following reasons:

1. exogenous administration of prostaglandins is able to induce uterine activity at all stages of gestation;
2. production of prostaglandins by intrauterine tissues increases during pregnancy;
3. the concentration of prostaglandins in amniotic fluid and maternal blood increases, as does the concentration in the urine.

It is presently thought likely that the last step in the complicated series of interconnected events resulting in regular uterine contractions is increased prostaglandin production. Major events seem to occur in the following order: degeneration of the decidua, release of lysosomal enzymes and synthesis of prostaglandins, followed by cervical ripening, uterine contractions and expulsion of the uterine contents. This association can also be extended to chorioamnionitis-related preterm labour, which stimulates prostaglandin biosynthesis (Romero et al, 1986). What initiates the increased release of prostaglandins is also still unclear. It has been suggested that an increased synthesis of PGE_2 is the key event in the onset of regular contractions and that the increase in prostaglandin synthesis results from the fetus (Strickland et al, 1983). The fetal factor may be synthesized in the fetal kidney and reach amniotic fluid by way of fetal urine. This fetal signal may act to cause an increase in the rate of release of arachidonic acid from glycerophospholipids or else to cause an increase in the activity of prostaglandin synthetase in amnion, or both (Casey and MacDonald, 1986).

Prostaglandins also cause increased myometrial contractility in vitro, and it appears that there is even a regional sensitivity of the uterus in response to various prostaglandins which may be mediated by additional factors like α- and β-adrenergic innervation (Figure 5). As could be shown, for example (Bryman et al, 1986), PGE_2 as well as $PGF_{2\alpha}$ causes relaxation rather than contraction of cervical smooth muscle cells.

In contrast to other hormones, prostaglandins are synthesized at the site of action by the amnion, decidua and myometrium of parturient women (Giannopoulis et al, 1985). PGE_2 and $PGF_{2\alpha}$ are known to stimulate myometrial contractility, most likely by acting as calcium ionophores, and they increase intracellular calcium. At the present time this can be best explained as due to modulation to calcium fluxes (Ohnishi and Devlin, 1979), but the exact action is still under investigation. The relationship between calcium and prostaglandins is rather complex because prostaglandins apparently increase the calcium permeability of the cell membrane and intracellular free calcium. However, for the synthesis of prostaglandins, calcium is necessary. In fact, in cell cultures calcium channel blockers decreased prostaglandin synthesis whereas calcium ionophores increased prostaglandin production (Olson et al, 1983).

Furthermore, the action of prostaglandins appears to be mediated by specific receptors located on the plasma membranes of target cells. Although very little is known about such receptors it seems that neither their density nor affinity changes during parturition (Okazaki et al, 1981). The increased contractile activity during labour is directly related to the rise of PGE_2 and $PGF_{2\alpha}$ and to the production of other eicosanoids by the feto-placental unit (Huszar and Naftolin, 1984). The relationship between the major pathways of eicosanoid synthesis is dynamic, and the occurrence of various prostaglandins, thromboxanes and leukotrienes may change according to the phases of the reproduction cycle (Moonen et al, 1986). It has been shown that in certain conditions the pathway in a specific organ may also be manipulated (McGiff, 1979). Local concentrations of enzymes may determine whether thromboxane, a potent platelet-aggregating and smooth-muscle-contracting agent, or prostacyclin, which inhibits platelet aggregation and smooth muscle contraction, may arise from the common precursor.

These observations, together with the finding of a striking increase of arachidonic acid concentration in amniotic fluid during labour, are suggestive of a unique role for the fetal membranes in the initiation of regular uterine contractions. Presently the precise nature of this role must remain speculative. However, the role of fetal membranes in the initiation process that ends in parturition or abortion may be formulated as follows. First, a relatively large amount of arachidonic acid is released from glycerophospholipid stores in the amnion, a small portion of which serves as the precursor of PGE_2 in the fetal membranes; another portion may serve as the precursor of PGE_2 and $PGF_{2\alpha}$ in the decidua. Secondly, PGE_2 produced in the amnion may facilitate the release of arachidonic acid in either the chorion laeve or the uterine decidua and thereby facilitate the production of PGE_2 in the chorion and PGE_2 and $PGF_{2\alpha}$ in the decidua. It has already been shown that in other tissues PGE_2 acts to facilitate the release of arachidonic acid, for example in the adrenal cortex. The earlier increase in the level of PGE_2 over that of $PGF_{2\alpha}$ in amniotic fluid before labour commences and the earlier increase of PGE_2 metabolites over those of $PGF_{2\alpha}$ in maternal blood during labour are consistent with this postulate. The administration of vaginal suppositories containing PGE_2 to women in the second trimester of pregnancy may facilitate the production of $PGF_{2\alpha}$. It could be demonstrated that $PGF_{2\alpha}$ metabolites in plasma increased strikingly after such treatment (Figure 7). Thus, it can be seen that any stimulus which would facilitate PGE_2 synthesis in the fetal membranes, e.g. hypoxia, infection, exposure to oxytocin, hypertonic solutions, prostaglandins or arachidonic acid, or as yet unidentified stimuli, could serve to initiate the series of steps which result in the formation of $PGF_{2\alpha}$ in the decidua and/or in the myometrium.

The major role of prostaglandins in labour of spontaneous onset as well as in several forms of induced labour seems to be the three-fold action of these compounds: the influence on cervical softening; the induction of gap

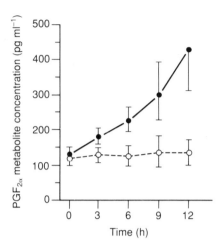

Figure 7. Plasma concentration of $PGF_{2\alpha}$ metabolites after PGE_2 vaginal suppository. ●——●, PGE_2 vaginally; ○---○, control. Modified from Husslein (1984).

junctions; and the direct stimulation of myometrial contractions. Moreover, prostaglandins produced in the placenta play a major role in the mechanism of placental separation and expulsion.

Due to the unique action of prostaglandins the development of pharmacologically produced prostaglandins offers the hope of an effective alternative to surgical abortion as well as labour induction. The naturally occurring PGE_2 and $PGF_{2\alpha}$ are potent stimulants of myometrial contractility in vivo at any stage of pregnancy, depending only on the dose applied. The basic response of the early and mid-pregnant uterus to intravenous injection of the primary prostaglandins is characterized by a rapid elevation of uterine tonus that declines gradually towards the resting level. Continuous intravenous administration maintains uterine activity, with a gradual development of labour-like contractions (Wiqvist et al, 1971). However, primary prostaglandins are very rapidly metabolized and the half-life of these compounds in the circulation is less than a minute. But a more prolonged duration of action can be obtained if these compounds are administered either extra- or intra-amniotically.

The rapid metabolism of natural prostaglandins was also the reason why a number of analogues have been developed which are not substrates for the initial step of the enzymatic degradation by 15-dehydrogenase. Some of these, such as 16,16-dimethyl-*trans*-Δ^2-PGE_1 methyl ester (gemeprost; May & Baker, Dagenham, UK), 16-phenoxy-17,18,19,20-tetranor-PGE_2 (sulprostone; Schering, Berlin, FRG) and 15(S)-15-methyl-$PGF_{2\alpha}$ (minprostin; Upjohn, Kalamazoo, USA) are presently in routine clinical use in several countries. Generally, these derivatives are more potent than the corresponding parent compound and their action is prolonged or more specific on uterine rather than on other smooth muscle tissue. In conclusion, PGE_2 and $PGF_{2\alpha}$, as well as the different analogues, all have a direct stimulatory effect on myometrial smooth muscle cells, lead to specific changes in the cervical tissue (see Chapter 5), and may also act partially through a stimulation of the endogenous production of various local prostaglandins.

REFERENCES

Adelstein RS & Eisenberg E (1980) Regulation and kinetics of the actin–myosin–ATP interaction. *Annual Review of Biochemistry* **49:** 921.

Adelstein RS, Conti MA, Hathaway DR & Klee CB (1978) Phosphorylation of smooth muscle myosin light chain kinase by the catalytic subunit of adenosine 3'5'-monophosphate-dependent protein kinase. *Journal of Biological Chemistry* **253:** 8347.

Alexandrova M & Soloff MS (1980) Oxytocin receptors and parturition. I. Control of oxytocin receptor concentration in the rat myometrium at term. *Endocrinology* **106:** 730.

Bagby RM (1983) Organisation of contractile/cytoskeletal elements. In Stephens NL (ed.) *Biochemistry of Smooth Muscle*, p 1. Boca Raton: CRC Press.

Bengtsson B, Chow EM & Marshall JM (1984) Calcium dependency of pregnant rat myometrium: comparison of circular and longitudinal muscle. *Biology of Reproduction* **30:** 869.

Berg G, Andersson RGG & Ryden G (1986) β-Adrenergic receptors in human myometrium during pregnancy. *American Journal of Obstetrics and Gynecology* **154:** 601.

Bryman I, Norström A & Lindblom B (1986) Influence of prostaglandins and adrenoceptor agonists on contractile activity in the human cervix at term. *Obstetrics and Gynecology* **67:** 574.

Bygdeman M & Van Look PFA (1989) The use of prostaglandins and antiprogestins for pregnancy termination. *International Journal of Gynaecology and Obstetrics* **29:** 5.

Casey ML & MacDonald PC (1986) Initiation of labor in women. In Huszar G (ed.) *The Physiology and Biochemistry of the Uterus in Pregnancy and Labor*. Boca Raton: CRC Press.

Dattel BJ, Lam F & Roberts JM (1986) Failure to demonstrate decreased β-adrenergic receptor concentration or decreased agonist efficacy in term or preterm human parturition. *American Journal of Obstetrics and Gynecology* **154:** 450.

Dawood MY, Raghavan KS, Pociask C & Fuchs F (1978) Oxytocin in human pregnancy and parturition. *Obstetrics and Gynecology* **51:** 138.

Fuchs AR, Fuchs F, Husslein P, Fernström M & Soloff S (1984) Oxytocin receptors in pregnant human uterus and the regulation of oxytocin action during pregnancy and parturition. *American Journal of Obstetrics and Gynecology* **150:** 734.

Garfield RE (1984) Myometrial ultrastructure and uterine contractility. In Bottari S, Thomas JP, Vokaer A & Vokaer R (eds) *Uterine Contractility*, p 81. New York: Masson.

Garfield RE, Puri CP & Csapo AI (1982) Endocrine, structural, and functional changes in the uterus during premature labor. *American Journal of Obstetrics and Gynecology* **142:** 21.

Giannopoulis G, Jackson K, Kredentser J & Tulchinsky D (1985) Prostaglandin E_2 and $F_{2\alpha}$ receptors in human myometrium during the menstrual cycle and in pregnancy and labor. *American Journal of Obstetrics and Gynecology* **153:** 904.

Haluska GJ, Stanczyk FZ, Cook MJ & Novy MJ (1987) Temporal changes in uterine activity and prostaglandin response to RU-486 in rhesus macaques in late gestation. *American Journal of Obstetrics and Gynecology* **157:** 1487.

Hidika H, Yamaki T, Naka M, Tanaka T, Hayashi H & Kobayashi R (1980) Calcium-regulated modulator protein interacting agents inhibit smooth muscle calcium-stimulated protein kinase and ATPase. *Molecular Pharmacology* **17:** 66.

Hurwitz L (1986) Pharmacology of calcium channels and smooth muscle. *Annual Review of Pharmacology and Toxicology* **26:** 225.

Husslein P (1984) Die Bedeutung von Oxytocin und Prostaglandinen für den Geburtsmechanismus beim Menschen. *Wiener Klinische Wochenschrift* **96(supplement 155):** 10–13.

Huszar G (1984) Physiology of myometrial contractility and of cervical dilatation. In Fuchs F & Stubblefield P (eds) *Preterm Birth: Causes, Prevention, Management*, p 21. MacMillan.

Huszar G & Bailey P (1979) Relationship between actin–myosin interactions and myosin light chain phosphorylation in human placental smooth muscle. *American Journal of Obstetrics and Gynecology* **135**: 718.

Huszar G & Naftolin F (1984) The myometrium and uterine cervix in normal and preterm labor. *New England Journal of Medicine* **311**: 571.

Huszar G & Roberts JR (1982) Biochemistry and pharmacology of the myometrium and labor: Regulation at the cellular and molecular levels. *American Journal of Obstetrics and Gynecology* **142**: 225.

Huxley HE (1971a) The Croonian Lecture 1970. The structural basis of muscular contraction. *Proceedings of the Royal Society of London, Series B* **178**: 131.

Huxley HE (1971b) The structural basis of muscular contraction. *Proceedings of the Royal Society of London, Series B* **178**: 131.

Janis R & Triggle DJ (1986) Effects of calcium channel antagonists on the myometrium. In Huszar G (ed.) *The Physiology and Biochemistry of the Uterus*, p 201. Boca Raton: CRC Press.

Janis RA, Barany K, Barany M & Sarmiento JG (1981) Association between myosin light chain phosphorylation and contraction of rat uterine smooth muscle. *Molecular Physiology* **1**: 3.

Kao CY (1977) Electrophysiological properties of the uterine smooth muscle. In Wynn RM (ed.) *Biology of the Uterus*, pp 423–496. New York: Plenum Press.

Karim SMM (1972) Prostaglandins and human reproduction. *The Prostaglandins*, pp 71–164. New York: Wiley Interscience.

McGiff JC (1979) New development in prostaglandin and thromboxane research. *Federal Proceedings* **38**: 64.

Michell RH (1975) Inositol phospholipids and cell surface receptor function. *Biochimica et Biophysica Acta* **415**: 81.

Mitchell MD (1987) Regulation of eicosanoid biosynthesis during pregnancy and parturition. In Hillier K (ed.) *Eicosanoids and Reproduction*. Lancaster: MTP Press.

Mitchell MD, Mountford LA, Natale R & Robinson JS (1980) Concentrations of oxytocin in the plasma and amniotic fluid of rhesus monkeys during the latter half of pregnancy. *Journal of Endocrinology* **84**: 473.

Moonen P, Klok G & Keirse MJ (1986) Distribution of prostaglandin endoperoxide synthase and prostacyclin synthase in the late pregnant uterus. *Journal of Obstetrics and Gynecology* **93**: 255.

Nissenson R, Flouret G & Hechter O (1978) Opposing effects of estradiol and progesterone on oxytocin receptors in rabbit uterus. *Proceedings of the National Academy of Sciences of the USA* **75**: 2044.

Ohnishi ST & Devlin TM (1979) Calcium ionophore activity of a prostaglandin B1 derivative. *Biochemical and Biophysical Research Communications* **89**: 240.

Okazaki T, Casey ML, Okita JR, MacDonald PC & Johnston JM (1981) Initiation of human parturition. XII. Biosynthesis and metabolism of prostaglandins in human fetal membranes and uterine decidua. *American Journal of Obstetrics and Gynecology* **139**: 373.

Olson DM, Opavsky MA & Challis JRG (1983) Prostaglandin synthesis by human amnion is dependent upon extracellular calcium. *Canadian Journal of Physiology and Pharmacology* **6**: 1089.

Omini C, Pasargiklian R, Folco GC, Fano M & Berti F (1978) Pharmacological activity of PGI2 and its metabolite 6-oxo-PGF$_{1\alpha}$ on human uterus and fallopian tubes. *Prostaglandins* **15**: 1045.

Pato MD & Adelstein RS (1980) Dephosphorylation of the 20,000-dalton light chain of myosin by two different phosphatases from smooth muscle. *Journal of Biological Chemistry* **225**: 6535.

Potter JD, Strag-Brown P, Walker PL & Iida S (1983) Ca^{2+} binding to calmodulin. *Methods in Enzymology* **102**: 135.

Riemer RK, Jacobs MM, Wu YY & Roberts JM (1986) Progesterone-induced rabbit myometrial β-adrenergic response is accompanied by increased concentration and expression of stimulatory adenylate cyclase coupling protein (Gs). *Program of the 33rd Annual Meeting of the Society for Gynecologic Investigation* Toronto, Canada, p 171 (abstract 274P).

Roberts JM, Insel PA, Goldfein RD & Goldfein A (1977) Alpha-adrenoreceptors but not beta-adrenoreceptors increase in rabbit uterus with estrogen. *Nature* 270: 624.

Roberts JM, Insel PA & Goldfein A (1986) Regulation of myometrial adrenoceptors and adrenergic response by sex steroids. *Molecular Pharmacology* 20: 52.

Romero R, Emamian M, Quintero R, Wan M, Hobbins JC & Mitchell M (1986) Amniotic fluid prostaglandin levels and intra-amniotic infections. *Lancet* i: 1380.

Small JV (1977) The contractile apparatus of the smooth muscle cell: structure and composition. In Stephans NL (ed.) *The Biochemistry of Smooth Muscle*, p 379. Baltimore: University Park Press.

Smith SK & Kelly RW (1987) The effect of antiprogestins RU-486 and ZK 98,734 on the synthesis and metabolism of $PGF_{2\alpha}$ and E_2 in separated cells from early human decidua. *Journal of Clinical Endocrinology and Metabolism* 65: 527.

Somlyo AV, Bond M, Somlyo AP & Scarpa A (1985) Inositol triphosphate induced calcium release and contraction in vascular smooth muscle. *Proceedings of the National Academy of Sciences of the USA* 82: 5231.

Stephans NL (1977) *The Biochemistry of Smooth Muscle*. Baltimore: University Park Press.

Strickland DM, Saeed SA, Casey ML & Mitchell MD (1983) Stimulation of prostaglandin synthesis by urine of the human fetus may serve as a trigger of parturition. *Science* 220: 521.

Stull JT, Nunnally MH & Michnoff CH (1986) *The Enzymes*, vol. XVII, p 113. New York: Academic Press.

Swahn ML & Bygdeman M (1988) The effect of the antiprogestin RU-486 on uterine contractility and sensitivity to prostaglandin and oxytocin. *British Journal of Obstetrics and Gynecology* 95: 126.

Triggle DJ & Janis RA (1987) Calcium channel ligands. *Annual Review of Pharmacology and Toxicology* 27: 347.

Verhoeff A, Garfield RE, Ramondt J, van Kooten C & Wallenburg HC (1984) *Electrical and Mechanical Uterine Activity in Relation to Gap Junction Area in Estrogen-Treated Ovariectomised Sheep*, p 179a. Washington, DC: Society for Gynecologic Investigation.

Verhoeff A & Garfield RE (1986) Ultrastructure of the myometrium and the role of gap junctions in myometrial function. In Huszar G (ed.) *The Physiology and Biochemistry of the Uterus in Pregnancy and Labor*. Boca Raton: CRC Press.

Wilson T, Liggins GC, Aimer GP & Skinner SJM (1985) Partial purification and characterisation of two compounds from amniotic fluid which inhibit phospholipase activity in human endometrial cells. *Biochemical and Biophysical Research Communications* 131: 22.

Wiqvist N, Bygdeman M & Toppozada M (1971) Induction of abortion by the intravenous administration of $PGF_{2\alpha}$. *Acta Obstetrica et Gynecologica Scandinavica* 50: 381.

Yagi K, Yazawa M, Katiuchi S, Woshima M & Uenishi K (1978) Identification of an activator protein for myosin light chain kinase as the Ca^{2+} dependent modulator protein. *Journal of Biological Chemistry* 253: 1338.

Zahradnik HP (1988) In Haller U, Kubli F & Husslein P (eds) *Prostaglandine in Geburtshilfe und Gynäkologie*. Berlin: Springer-Verlag.

5

Prostaglandins and the cervix

A. A. CALDER
I. A. GREER

INTRODUCTION

The cervix divides the upper genital tract from the lower. The principal biological activities of the upper genital tract are ovulation, ovum transport, menstruation, pregnancy and parturition, while the lower genital tract is more concerned with sexual function, reception of semen, and the outward passage of menses, fetuses and their secundines. The cervix has a vital role in regulating and controlling many of these functions and is perhaps best regarded as the frontier post between those two parts of the genital tract. Thus, it can be seen to have an important role in remaining closed to prevent either the access of pathogenic organisms and other harmful influences to the upper genital tract or the untimely expulsion of pregnancy. Equally, however, it must facilitate the reception and transport of spermatozoa and the outward passage of menstrual fluid and the mature fetus. The last mentioned of these processes represents the most dramatic performance in the life of the cervix. It is required relatively infrequently and never occurs if the woman remains childless.

In addition to participating in these basic reproductive functions of menstruation, conception, pregnancy maintenance and parturition, the cervix is a prime target for techniques aimed at prevention of conception in order to control fertility and for therapeutic processes which aim to interrupt the pregnancy at any stage along its course. In addition, the clinician may often require to effect dilatation of the non-pregnant cervix in order to allow diagnostic or therapeutic manipulations to take place in the upper genital tract. These include such procedures as endometrial biopsy, diagnostic curettage, hysteroscopy and endometrial resection.

The changing patterns of reproductive behaviour which have accompanied the advance of civilization have led to marked changes in the frequency with which the cervix participates in its different biological activities. Thus, women who lived before the era of effective contraception had more pregnancies than their contemporary equivalents. Nevertheless, a shorter reproductive lifespan and the influence of lactational amenorrhoea on birth spacing meant that she might have had on average six or seven pregnancies. The woman of the industrialized West abandoned lactation in

Baillière's Clinical Obstetrics and Gynaecology—
Vol. 6, No. 4, December 1992
ISBN 0–7020–1694–2

the last century and in consequence had more menstrual cycles and more pregnancies. It was not uncommon for a Victorian woman to have 15 or 16 live births; in addition, she probably had a number of spontaneous abortions and might also have experienced criminal abortion. Today's woman benefits from advances in contraceptive technology and the availability of safe therapeutic abortion and rarely has more than three or four term pregnancies. The cost of this, however, is a multiplicity of menstrual cycles. We might therefore estimate that the primitive cervix witnessed an average of six or seven episodes of parturition at term, perhaps one or two spontaneous miscarriages and 30 or 40 episodes of menstruation. The Victorian cervix saw eight or 12 term births, several abortions—either spontaneous or criminal—and perhaps a 100 menstrual cycles. In marked contrast, today's cervix usually participates in fewer than four term births, but may be required to dilatate for a small number of miscarriages and therapeutic abortions while playing a role in as many as 300 or 400 menstrual cycles. In consequence, today's woman requires her cervix to act efficiently in ensuring the success of her small number of planned pregnancies while from time to time it will require to be dilatated for purposes of therapeutic abortion or for the investigation and diagnosis of the increasing array of menstrual disturbances which have accompanied these changing reproductive patterns.

Prostaglandins are believed to play a critical biological role in the control of cervical function. An enhanced knowledge of this role allows greater scope for the clinician to influence most, if not all, of the above processes for the benefit of the individual woman. In this chapter consideration will first be given to the current state of knowledge of the role of prostaglandins in the normal function of the female genital tract before attention is turned to the clinical and therapeutic applications of the prostaglandins and their inhibitors.

BIOLOGICAL CONTROL OF CERVICAL FUNCTION

The functions of the cervix may be simply summarized as opening or remaining closed depending on the needs of the moment. The principal role of prostaglandins appears to be to provoke cervical softening and dilatation (Amy et al, 1985). Before considering how these mechanisms operate, it is however necessary to address the physical composition of the cervix.

It is of paramount importance to recognize at the outset the fundamental structural difference between the uterine corpus and the uterine cervix. Although these are both components of the same organ, namely the uterus, they could hardly be more different in their composition. Whereas the corpus is almost entirely composed of smooth muscle fibres (the myometrium), the cervix contains little muscle and is predominantly composed of connective tissue in which collagen is the most abundant element (Danforth, 1947). There is a small amount of elastic tissue and some smooth muscle but the latter is sparse and tends to be limited to the periphery of the cervical stroma. In the non-pregnant state the collagen fibres are organized into dense bundles with a relatively small amount of ground substance which effectively acts as the cement which binds the individual collagen fibrils. This ground substance is mainly made up of large proteoglycan complexes which incorporate a variety of glycosaminoglycans (GAGs). These include such substances as keratan sulphate, heparan sulphate and hyaluronic acid, but the principal cervical GAGs are condroitin sulphate and its epimer, dermatan sulphate (von Maillot et al, 1979; Uldbjerg et al, 1983). The structural arrangement of the proteoglycan complex shows a hyaluronic acid chain linked to core proteins which incorporate glycosaminoglycans as side chains. The protein cores and their associated GAGs lie in intimate contact with the collagen fibres within the cervix. This arrangement is thought to be vital for the appropriate alignment of the collagen fibrils within the tissue which is necessary to confer on the cervix its mechanical rigidity (Lindahl and Hook, 1978; Golichowski, 1980; Scott and Orford, 1981). The longer the chain length of the GAGs and the greater their charged density, the more avidly they bind to collagen. The different GAGs vary markedly in this regard so that those which contain iduronic acid, such as dermatan sulphate, bind very strongly and bring stability to the tissue, in contrast to those which contain glucuronic acid and which have the opposite effect of destabilizing the tissue and increasing its compliance (Obrink, 1973).

The profound change known as cervical ripening which must take place in late pregnancy to facilitate rapid effacement and dilatation during labour is believed to result, at least in part, from a qualitative change in the GAGs of the cervical ground substance. In addition, the water content of the cervix increases as pregnancy advances and this may result from an increased cervical content of those GAGs which are generally more hydrophilic (Junqueira et al, 1980). A greater degree of hydration of the tissue during cervical ripening may contribute to a change in the biophysical quality of the collagen. The absolute concentration of collagen within the tissue seems to be reduced during ripening and this may represent either active removal of collagen from the tissue or, alternatively, an increase in the relative amount of ground substance (GAGs and water).

Control of cervical ripening

As we have seen there are two possible mechanisms by which the physical properties of cervical tissue may be altered and indeed it seems probable that these two mechanisms operate in concert. The cervical tissue may be softened as a result of changes within the binding 'cement' of the cervix, namely the ground substance, which allow a loosening of the bonds between individual collagen fibres. This may be considered to resemble the reduction in the strength of a metal hawser when its component wires lose their tightly woven structure. The second possibility might then be seen to resemble the rusting or removal of the wires from the hawser, i.e. the degradation and absolute loss of collagen from the tissue under the influence of lytic enzymes.

The main lytic enzymes within the cervix are collagenase, which may come from the cervical fibroblasts, and also elastase, which may be produced by infiltrating white cells such as neutrophils (Uldbjerg et al, 1983). This concept is in line with the proposal by Liggins (1981) that cervical ripening is akin to an inflammatory process. Indeed, in several experimental circumstances cervical ripening has been observed to be associated with an inflammatory infiltrate.

The fundamental changes in cervical tissue which are required for cervical softening and dilatation may thus be seen to be under the control of cellular elements which are either intrinsic to the cervical tissue (fibroblasts) or which infiltrate and modify the tissue as required. The fibroblasts are thought to be important for the manufacture and secretion into the tissue not only of collagen but also of the proteoglycan complexes and they, together with infiltrating white cells, are probably the main source of those lytic enzymes which modify both cervical collagen and ground substance (Calder and Greer, 1991).

In general the rigidity of connective tissue is determined by the age of the collagen and the degree to which individual collagen fibrils are cross-linked. Older collagen with many cross-links tends to be tougher than younger collagen. There may also be qualitative changes in the type of collagen expressed within cervical tissue, although this remains to be examined in detail. Danforth et al (1974) showed that there were clear differences between the tightly bound collagen of the non-pregnant and early pregnant cervix in which the ground substance is sparse and the widely scattered and dissociated collagen fibrils and abundant ground substance which characterize the cervix at term. An overall loss of collagen from the cervix has been demonstrated biochemically (Danforth et al, 1974; Uldbjerg et al, 1981; Granstrom et al, 1989) and also histologically (Junqueira et al, 1980). The latter investigators employed picrosirius red, a stain specific for polymerized collagen, and their findings suggest an even greater reduction in collagen in the ripe term cervix than biochemical investigations would seem to suggest. One possible explanation for this may be that collagen remains in the cervix in a non-polymerized state rather than as the intact fibres, which take up the specific stain. The absolute concentration of collagen within the tissue does seem to be related to the degree of cervical ripeness assessed clinically at term (Ekman et al, 1986) and this finding corresponds with the observations of Uldbjerg et al (1983), who showed a clear relationship between increasing activities of leukocyte elastase and collagenase and the falling concentration of collagen in the cervix as pregnancy progresses towards term. Thus, as pregnancy progresses and moves towards parturition a dynamic remodelling of the collagen may take place such that mature collagen is replaced by younger collagen with fewer cross-links so that it may be more readily broken down during parturition. These processes are well developed before the onset of labour during that phase of pregnancy which occupies its last 4 or 5 weeks and which is best described as 'pre-labour' and a further and very dramatic increase in collagenase activity is seen once labour becomes properly established (Rajabi et al, 1988).

Endocrine control

In its non-pregnant condition, the cervix is known to display a varying degree of compliance at different phases of the menstrual cycle (Anthony et al, 1982). It is also known to be more rigid before the menarche and after the menopause. Such observations point clearly to an influence on the cervical tissue of those endocrine changes which characterize the ovarian cycle. The markedly more dramatic cervical changes associated with pregnancy and parturition are also thought to be largely under endocrine control and the same hormones probably represent the most important players. These endocrine changes of pregnancy have been extensively reviewed by Turnbull (1989), Calder and Greer (1991) and Challis et al (1991).

Progesterone appears to exert an inhibitory role on cervical ripening. This may be partly attributable to its potent anti-inflammatory properties (Sitteri et al, 1977), which may prevent the influx and activation of neutrophils, or it may alternatively or additionally exert this influence by inhibiting collagenase activity within uterine tissues (Jeffrey et al, 1971; Jeffrey and Koob, 1980). This concept of progesterone exerting an important role in the inhibition of cervical ripening is further supported by the observation that antiprogestins promote cervical softening in early pregnancy (Gupta and Johnston, 1990; Radestad et al, 1990). In animal studies (Chwalisz, 1988) this effect was seen to be accompanied by an influx of neutrophils into the cervical tissue, lending further support to the mechanisms postulated above.

Oestrogens, especially oestradiol, are thought to have an effect more or less opposite to that of progesterone. They have been shown to provoke cervical ripening in clinical studies (Gordon and Calder, 1977; Allan et al, 1989) and this may reflect a biological role for these hormones. The sheep, which is often taken as a model for human pregnancy, demonstrates rapid and dramatic cervical softening immediately prior to parturition and this is associated with very acute changes in these placental hormones in the form of a rapid rise in oestradiol secretion and a sharp decline in progesterone. No such dramatic changes have been convincingly demonstrated in human pregnancy in association with parturition but there may be more subtle and gradual alterations, if not in the circulating levels of these hormones, then at least in their tissue activities during the phase of prelabour cervical ripening.

Another candidate as an endocrine influence on cervical ripening is relaxin. Both experimental (von Maillot et al, 1977) and clinical (MacLennan, 1981) studies appear to support the view that relaxin favours cervical ripening.

Whatever the precise roles of such endocrine changes in late pregnancy are, and precisely how they operate, it seems very likely that their influence is mediated by the local activity of prostaglandins within the cervical tissues.

Role of prostaglandins

The prostaglandins probably represent the final link which translates endocrine messages which have their origin in the ovary in the non-pregnant condition and predominantly in the fetus during pregnancy into the funda-mental changes at tissue level. At least three prostaglandins may participate in these processes, namely prostaglandin E_2 (PGE_2), prostaglandin $F_{2\alpha}$ ($PGF_{2\alpha}$) and prostacyclin (PGI_2). All these prostanoids are produced within the uterine tissues and appear to be activated in association with cervical ripening (Ellwood et al, 1980). The role of prostacyclin is rather uncertain in this regard, and since it has not as yet attained any clinical importance in the management of cervical function it will not be further discussed here. Of the other two prostaglandins, PGE_2 is probably much more important than $PGF_{2\alpha}$. The latter, which is principally produced in the decidua, is probably more important in the control of myometrial contractility than of cervical ripening (Greer et al, 1990).

Prostaglandins clearly play a role in the control of cervical ripening. Clinical and experimental studies have shown that prostaglandins (especially PGE_2) produce dramatic cervical softening, effacement and dilatation (Calder, 1980) and it now seems certain that this represents a biological phenomenon. Inhibition of prostaglandin synthesis with drugs such as aspirin (Lewis and Schulman, 1973) is known not only to delay parturition but also to inhibit cervical ripening. The precise mechanism whereby prostaglandins influence the cervical tissue is not yet clear although it seems likely that this is mediated by the activity of the fibroblasts and infiltrating white cells within cervical tissue.

The mechanisms whereby circulating hormones influence prostaglandin activities are not fully elucidated although progesterone probably inhibits prostaglandin synthesis and enhances its catabolism in the light of the observation that the antiprogestins exert exactly opposite effects (Kelly et al, 1986; Kelly and Buckman, 1990). Oestradiol on the other hand has been shown to be capable of stimulating prostaglandin production within uterine tissues (Liggins et al, 1977) while Fitzpatrick and Dobson (1981) have demonstrated that the cervical softening which can be induced in the sheep cervix by the infusion of oestradiol is associated with an increased pro-duction of prostaglandins from the cervix.

The changes which take place in the activity of these steroid hormones during the course of the menstrual cycle and also during pregnancy and parturition may therefore modify the activity of prostaglandins within the stroma of the cervix in order to influence its biophysical properties. Pregnancy, however, represents a more complex set of circumstances, not only in relation to these steroid hormones and relaxin, but also in the potential sources of the prostaglandins. While production within the cervix itself is probably very important, it should also be recognized that the most potent sources of these prostaglandins in pregnancy are the decidua ($PGF_{2\alpha}$) and the amniotic membrane (PGE_2). The PGE_2 which derives from the fetal membranes may be as important as the endogenous PGE_2 which is released within the cervix. This would imply a migration of such PGE_2 across the chorion to provoke softening at the internal cervical os and while this has not yet been shown to take place in vivo there are theoretical grounds for believing that it might do so (Calder and Elder, 1992).

CLINICAL SITUATIONS

The clinical circumstances in which prostaglandins may be employed to produce cervical softening and dilatation are as follows:

1. To facilitate induction of labour at term.
2. To increase the ease and safety of therapeutic abortion.
3. To facilitate access to the non-pregnant uterus for diagnostic or therapeutic purposes.

In contrast, there may be an increasing benefit from understanding and manipulating prostaglandin activity during the course of pregnancy in order to prevent preterm delivery. One important aspect of this is the clinical phenomenon of cervical incompetence.

Cervical ripening to facilitate labour induction at term

Human labour often seems to those most closely concerned to be a very sudden event. Thus, the parents, perhaps sitting quietly at home anticipating the birth of their baby, may suddenly find themselves collecting together the necessary items and hurriedly arranging transport to hospital because they have recognized that the great event has begun. Equally, midwives and obstetricians are accustomed to the sound of ambulance sirens and to the sight of mothers in labour being rapidly transported on trolleys to the labour ward. In the light of such common experience it might be expected that artificial induction of the birth process might be quickly and efficiently accomplished in every case. That it is not owes as much to the fact that the transition from pregnancy to parturition is in physiological terms not nearly as rapid as it might appear, as it does to our imperfect understanding of the biological processes concerned.

The earlier part of this chapter described the processes which bring about that transition from pregnancy to parturition and it will be readily appreciated that these processes occupy a protracted period covering several weeks of what is appropriately described as 'prelabour'. Thus, clinical procedures aimed at advancing the timing of spontaneous delivery must reproduce not only the events of parturition proper but also those of prelabour.

The clinical procedures which have been employed by obstetricians in order to induce labour are many and varied and are by no means universally successful. Some of these have employed the rational use of naturally occurring substances which are known to participate in the control of normal parturition, while others represent a myriad of bizarre assaults on the mother, both pharmacological and mechanical. The longest established of these is surgical amniotomy. This was introduced in the mid-18th century by Thomas Denman of the Middlesex Hospital with the object of avoiding problems of cephalopelvic disproportion by the induction of the premature delivery of a smaller baby. Although fraught with a variety of complications it was almost invariably eventually successful and it became known as the 'English method'. The most troublesome of the complications, however, was intrauterine sepsis, the risk of which increased the longer the delay between amniotomy and delivery, and this complication was not uncommonly fatal for mother or baby or both. Because of this the clinicians of yesteryear searched for methods whereby amniotomy might be avoided or at least deferred until a stage when it might be more reliably and safely performed. These other methods included the introduction into the lower genital tract and cervix of such devices as balloons, such as those favoured by Tarnier in Paris in 1862 (Speert, 1958). This was a soft rubber bag the size of a hen's egg which was inserted through the cervix on the end of a male catheter. This was later superseded by the better known bag which is associated with the name of Tarnier's pupil, Champetier de Ribes. It consisted of a conical-shaped silk balloon which was covered in rubber and was introduced beyond the cervix with forceps prior to its distension with fluid. Such devices, which came to be known as metreurynters (from the Greek, literally meaning 'to dilate the womb'), enjoyed considerable vogue and were further modified by such as James Voorhees in the USA at the turn of the century (Speert, 1958). It is interesting to reflect that the success, such as it was, of such devices was probably largely attributable to the endogenous prostaglandins which are released following such manipulations (Mitchell et al, 1977), as a result either of the direct physical effect they exert or of a degree of low-grade infection which they provoke.

A variant on the use of inflatable balloons was the use of bougies made usually of gum elastic. These were also introduced through the cervix and probably acted in a similar fashion. This allowed the option of beginning with a single bougie and increasing the number introduced as the degree of dilatation increased. Most of these physical techniques fell out of favour in the early years of this century although more recently, perhaps as a result of the improvement in the quality of manufacture of catheters and particularly such types as the Foley catheter which incorporate a rubber balloon, they have returned into favour (Embrey and Mollison, 1968).

An equally bizarre approach to labour induction was the fondly remembered 'OBE' which was still in vogue as late as 1970 (Donald, 1966). This consisted of an oral dose of castor oil followed by a hot bath and a soap and water enema. This combination was undoubtedly an extremely efficient method of stimulating the contractility of the smooth muscle within the gastrointestinal tract but had a less reliable influence on the genital tract! It did, however, succeed in a minority of cases and had the attraction for the clinicians of those days that it incurred no significant dangers, albeit it did nothing for the dignity of the recipient mothers.

Hormonal methods

The hormone which has been most widely employed for labour induction is oxytocin. In the first half of this century its use was fraught with problems of impurity and varying potency of the crude preparations which were available; however, since 1955 (Boissonas et al, 1955) a reliable synthetic preparation has been available. It was not until 1968, however, that the optimal method of exploiting oxytocin for this purpose was described. Prior to that time many clinicians favoured the use of buccal administration, which, while being an effective route of absorption, was less satisfactory in terms of fine control than was the intravenous route. This became firmly established as the route of choice following the work of Turnbull and Anderson (1968). They pointed to the need to perform amniotomy as a prelude to the administration of oxytocin, the dose of which needs to be titrated against the uterine response. Thus, the past 25 years have seen the availability of a method of labour induction which is generally efficient and reliable and the principle of amniotomy and intravenous oxytocin infusion has been applied almost universally in maternity hospitals. The same quarter century has, however, also witnessed the introduction of prostaglandins in clinical practice and they have also been found to offer important clinical options for labour induction (Karim et al, 1969, 1970).

The history of induction of labour has shown very clearly that we cannot always anticipate the results of clinical intervention. Undoubtedly, the passing years have seen steady improvements in the efficiency, reliability and acceptability of the methods available but even with the best techniques the response is not always satisfactory. The reasons for this are worthy of careful consideration.

The establishment of human labour might be considered to resemble the means by which an aircraft becomes airborne. The point at which it leaves the runway is the culmination of a process which involved careful preparation, starting and warming up the engines and the generation of forward momentum from a standing start to a point where the velocity is sufficient for take-off. In contrast, however, to the roar of the engines and the obvious speed of an aircraft, human labour reaches the point of take-off in the quietest and most surreptitious fashion and the equivalent of its journey along the runway occupies several days during prelabour. The objective observer has almost nothing on which to base an assessment of when a particular pregnancy might reach the point of take-off.

The majority of labour inductions are carried out at term (i.e. beyond 37 completed weeks of pregnancy) and because prelabour occupies several weeks it is inevitable that very few labour inductions are attempted from what might be considered 'a standing start'. It has become abundantly clear, however, that the success of labour induction will depend above all else on the point the individual pregnancy has reached within prelabour or in other words, using the aircraft analogy, it will depend on the amount of runway velocity already generated. Thus, most labours at the time induction is attempted are already very close to the point of take-off and require comparatively little additional persuasion to become established. A minority, however, are required to be accomplished from 'a standing start' and this is by no means only determined by the gestational age of the pregnancy.

A number of clinical measures will reflect the condition of the individual pregnancy. For instance, the sensitivity of the uterus to oxytocin is known to increase steadily as we travel through prelabour from pregnancy to parturition. A second and more easily made observation is the condition of the uterine cervix. The degree of cervical ripeness may be assessed using a scoring system such as that described by Bishop (1964), who showed that a very ripe cervix presaged the onset of spontaneous labour within a few days whereas a very unripe cervix heralded a delay of several weeks before labour. This was independent of gestational age.

The clinical importance of these concepts is reinforced by the observation that while amniotomy followed by the intravenous titration of oxytocin is a highly efficient means of labour induction, its success declines in parallel to the degree of cervical ripeness (Calder, 1977). This is particularly true of primigravid subjects, in whom amniotomy and intravenous oxytocin titration when the cervix is unripe is a recipe for a most unsatisfactory outcome. Although titration of oxytocin will produce powerful uterine contractility in such circumstances the resultant labour is almost invariably protracted with unsatisfactory cervical effacement and dilatation and an unacceptable incidence of complications such as fetal hypoxia, maternal pyrexia and the need to resort to delivery by caesarean section. It is in such cases that the need for cervical ripening prior to induction of labour is paramount and to date the agents most capable of accomplishing this are the prostaglandins, especially PGE_2.

The use of prostaglandins to ripen the cervix at term

Several years of painstaking research have clarified the optimal way in which prostaglandins may be used to ripen the term cervix. This subject has recently been reviewed by Calder and Elder (1992). The current situation may be summarized as follows:

1. The prostaglandin of choice is PGE_2 ($PGF_{2\alpha}$ may be usefully employed if PGE_2 is not available but the latter is greatly superior on grounds of efficacy and safety).
2. Local routes of administration within the genital tract offer important advantages over systemic therapy (oral or intravenous).
3. The preferred vehicle for administration of PGE_2 within the genital tract is a gel formulation which allows rapid and reliable absorption of the small doses which are necessary.
4. There is a choice of three different routes for local administration. The extra-amniotic route (Calder et al, 1977) which is most effectively employed by means of a small balloon Foley catheter is probably the most effective, although less agreeable to the mothers concerned. A dose of as little as 300–500 μg of PGE_2 in gel is generally sufficient. Most mothers find vaginal administration more acceptable, and this route using a five-fold larger dose (approximately 2 mg of PGE_2) is effective for cervical ripening in the majority of cases (McKenzie and Embrey, 1977) although it is perhaps less successful in the most unripe cases. A third option is presented by the intracervical administration advocated by Ulmsten and colleagues (1979), and although this is favoured in many countries in continental Europe it has not yet found wide favour in the UK. The evidence suggests that it is more complicated to administer than vaginal therapy and may be no more effective (Keirse et al, 1987).

The approach to be recommended, therefore, is that as a first attempt at cervical ripening a dose of 2 mg of PGE_2 gel should be instilled into the posterior vaginal fornix. A time interval should then be allowed for this to take effect and labour induction should only be embarked upon when the Bishop score has improved to 5 or 6. Indeed, our own policy is to repeat prostaglandin therapy at intervals of no less than 6 hours until the cervix has attained complete effacement and a dilatation of at least 3 cm. Amniotomy carried out at that stage will generally be followed by a satisfactory and successful labour.

In the most resistant of cases an alternative to repeated vaginal PGE_2 administration lies in resort to extra-amniotic therapy and we favour this approach. In the future, however, it is likely that more sophisticated delivery systems may be developed which will allow intracervical therapy to be employed with greater reliability.

Regardless of which of these routes is employed, however, it is apparent that the clinical benefits in the form of shorter and more successful labours with less stress to the fetus can be anticipated.

All have been shown to reduce the duration of induced labours, the need for caesarean delivery and the incidence of maternal, fetal and neonatal complications. It is now widely accepted that amniotomy and oxytocin therapy before the cervix has ripened (either spontaneously or in response to prostaglandins) is against the best interests of both mother and offspring.

The use of prostaglandins to modify the cervix in association with therapeutic abortion

The stage of gestation at which therapeutic abortion is performed varies between the earliest weeks of pregnancy and the latter part of the second trimester. Prostaglandin therapy is effective throughout this period and is commonly applied either as the primary method of abortion or as an adjunct to other methods, especially surgical techniques.

The techniques which are applied for therapeutic abortion can be neatly divided into four categories as follows:

1. Less than 8 weeks' gestation.
2. Eight to 12 weeks' gestation.
3. Twelve to 16 weeks' gestation.
4. Beyond 16 weeks' gestation.

Within each of these groups there are options of medical or surgical techniques.

Less than 8 weeks' gestation

At this stage, the choice lies between surgical termination by uterine curettage or medical termination, which is often termed 'menstrual induction'. If the choice is medical termination, the primary prostaglandins (PGF_2 and $PGE_{2\alpha}$) may be effective but less so than analogues such as 16-phenoxy-tetranor-PGE_2-methylsulphonamide (sulprostone, Schering AG) or 16,16-dimethyl-*trans*-Δ^2-PGE_1 methyl ester (gemeprost, Rhone-Poulenc). The latter has the advantage of being effective by vaginal administration and a dose of 1 mg in the form of a pessary repeated at three-hourly intervals will yield complete abortion in greater than 90% of cases. However, side effects including severe uterine pain, nausea and vomiting may limit the attractiveness of this technique (Bygdeman et al, 1983).

8 to 12 weeks' gestation

At this stage most, if not all, abortions are best performed by suction curettage or a similar surgical approach. It is generally considered, however, that preoperative therapy to soften and dilatate the cervix is advantageous and again the synthetic analogues sulprostone and gemeprost are the agents of choice. These are generally more effective than the alternative use of laminaria (Christensen et al, 1983) but gastrointestinal side effects and pain are not infrequently troublesome. They do, however, produce cervical dilatation adequate to allow the surgical procedure to be completed. This has been demonstrated by placebo-controlled studies using techniques to measure the force necessary for dilatation (Fisher et al, 1981; Chen and Elder, 1983).

Such therapy does not only reduce the forces required for cervical dilatation but also results in a reduction in the blood loss associated with pregnancy termination. The overall reduction in such complications has led to a recommendation by the Medical Advisory Committee of the International Planned Parenthood Federation in 1984 that such therapy should be a routine preliminary to vacuum aspiration.

12 to 16 weeks' gestation

Termination at this stage of gestation may be accomplished either by surgical dilatation and evacuation ('D & E') or by prostaglandin therapy alone. With either option, the advantages of prostaglandin therapy in increasing cervical compliance will increase the facility and safety of the procedure. Vaginal therapy with gemeprost pessaries may be employed as a single dose before cervical dilatation or alternatively on a repeated basis of 3-hourly dosing with the effect of causing abortion to take place within an interval of 12–18 hours. This approach has been widely adopted as an alternative to the previously favoured technique of extra-amniotic PGE_2 infusion (Cameron and Baird, 1984).

Beyond 16 weeks' gestation

Most of the considerations referred to in the foregoing sections continue to apply beyond 16 weeks. Although therapeutic abortion is rarely required at these gestations, the use of either extra-amniotic PGE_2 infusion or vaginal gemeprest pessaries will facilitate cervical maturation and uterine contractility to ensure that the duration of the procedure and consequently the woman's ordeal is kept to a minimum.

THE NON-PREGNANT CERVIX

Hitherto there has been no substantial attempt to explore the potential value of prostaglandins or other agents in modifying the non-pregnant cervix. One study showed no significant difference in cervical dilatation between placebo and Cervagem (gemeprost) pessaries. It is of interest to note that the placebo caused some cervical dilatation (Elder and Lewis, 1991). Such an approach may in the future be found to be of value in order to facilitate diagnostic or therapeutic procedures by increasing the gynaecologist's access to the uterine cavity in the conscious patient.

SUMMARY

The dramatic capabilities of prostaglandins to modify the condition of the uterine cervix have been exploited to the considerable benefit of patients who require therapeutic interventions for labour induction and termination of pregnancy. This will continue to be an important facet of clinical obstetric and gynaecologic practice, although further refinements and improvements in techniques seem certain to continue.

REFERENCES

Allen J, Uldbjerg N, Petersen LK et al (1989) Intracervical 17-β-oestradiol before induction of second trimester abortion with a prostaglandin E_1 analogue. *European Journal of Obstetrics, Gynecology and Reproductive Biology* **32:** 123–127.

Amy JJ, Calder AA & Kelly RW (1985) Prostaglandins and human reproduction. In Macdonald RR (ed.) *Scientific Basis of Obstetrics and Gynaecology*, 3rd edn, pp 255–303. Edinburgh: Churchill Livingstone.

Anthony GS, Fisher J, Coutts JRF et al (1982) Forces required to surgical dilatation of the pregnant and nonpregnant human cervix. *British Journal of Obstetrics and Gynaecology* **89:** 913–916.

Bishop EH (1964) Pelvic scoring for elective induction. *Obstetrics and Gynecology* **24:** 266–268.

Boissonas RA, Guttmanns & Jaquenand PA (1955) A new synthesis of oxytocin. *Helvetica Chima Acta* **38:** 1491–1495.

Bygdeman M, Christensen MJ, Green K et al (1983) Termination of early pregnancy—future developments. *Acta Obstetrica et Gynaecologica Scandinavica* **113(supplement):** 125–129.

Calder AA (1977) The unripe cervix. *57th William Blair Bell Memorial Lecture, June 1977*. London: Royal College of Obstetricians and Gynaecologists.

Calder AA (1980) Pharmacological management of the unripe cervix in the human. In Naftolin F & Stubblefield PG (eds) *Dilatation of the Uterine Cervix*, pp 317–333. New York: Raven Press.

Calder AA & Elder MG (1992) Prostaglandins for cervical ripening and labour induction. In Vane JR & Grady J (eds) *Clinical Application of Prostaglandins*, in press. Sevenoaks: Arnold.

Calder AA & Greer IA (1991) Pharmacological modulation of cervical compliance. *Seminars in Perinatology* **15:** 162–172.

Calder AA & Greer IA (1992) Cervical physiology and induction of labour. In Bonnar J (ed.) *Recent Advances in Obstetrics and Gynaecology*, pp 33–56. Edinburgh: Churchill Livingstone.

Calder AA, Embrey MP & Tait T (1977) Ripening of the cervix with extraamniotic prostaglandin E_2 in viscous gel before induction of labour. *British Journal of Obstetrics and Gynaecology* **84:** 264–268.

Cameron IT & Baird DT (1984) The use of 16,16-dimethyl-*trans*-Δ^2-prostaglandin E_1 methyl ester (gemeprost) vaginal pessaries for termination of pregnancy in the early second trimester. *British Journal of Obstetrics and Gynaecology* **191:** 1136–1140.

Challis JRG, Riley SC & Yang K (1991) Endocrinology of labour. *Fetal Medicine Review* **3:** 47–66.

Chen JK & Elder MG (1983) Preoperative cervical dilatation by vaginal pessaries containing a prostaglandin E_1 analogue (gemeprost). *Obstetrics and Gynecology* **62:** 399–404.

Christensen NJ, Bygdeman M & Green K (1983) Comparison of different prostaglandin analogues and laminaria for pre-operative dilatation of the cervix in late first trimester abortion. *Contraception* **27:** 51–61.

Chwalisz R (1988) Cervical ripening and induction of labour with progesterone antagonists. *XI European Congress of Perinatal Medicine—Rome*, p 60. Rome: CIC Edizioni Internaziolini.

Danforth DN (1947) The fibrous nature of the human cervix and its relation to the isthmic segment in gravid and nongravid uteri. *American Journal of Obstetrics and Gynaecology* **53:** 541–560.

Danforth DN, Veis A, Breen M et al (1974) The effect of pregnancy and labor on the human cervix: changes in collagen, glycoproteins and glycosaminoglycans. *American Journal of Obstetrics and Gynecology* **120:** 641–649.

Donald I (1966) *Practical Obstetric Problems*, p 356. London: Lloyd-Luke.

Ekman G, Malmstrom A & Uldbjerg N (1986) Cervical collagen: an important regulator of cervical function in term labour. *Obstetrics and Gynecology* **67:** 633–636.

Elder MG & Lewis G (1991) Randomised double blind placebo controlled trial of gemeprost pessaries for cervical dilatation in non-pregnant women. *Acta Obstetrica et Gynecologica Scandinavica* **70:** 149–152.

Ellwood DA, Mitchell MD & Anderson ABM (1980) The in vitro production of prostanoids by the human cervix during pregnancy: preliminary observations. *British Journal of Obstetrics and Gynaecology* **87:** 210–214.

Embrey MP & Mollison BG (1967) The unfavourable cervix and induction of labour using a cervical balloon. *Journal of Obstetrics and Gynaecology of the British Commonwealth* **74:** 44–48.

Fisher J, Anthony GS, McManus TJ et al (1981) Use of a force measuring instrument during cervical dilatation. *Journal of Medical Engineering Technology* **5:** 194–195.

Fitzpatrick RJ & Dobson H (1981) Softening of the ovine cervix at parturition. In Ellwood DA & Anderson ABM (eds) *The Cervix in Pregnancy and Labour: Clinical and Biochemical Investigations*, pp 40–56. Edinburgh: Churchill Livingstone.

Golichowski A (1980) Cervical stroma interstitial polysaccharide metabolism in pregnancy. In Naftolin F & Stubblefield PG (eds) *Dilatation of the Uterine Cervix: Connective Tissue Biology and Clinical Management*, pp 99–112. New York: Raven Press.

Gordon AJ & Calder AA (1977) Oestradiol applied locally to ripen the unfavourable cervix. *Lancet* **ii:** 1319–1321.

Granstrom L, Ekman G, Ulmsten U et al (1989) Changes in the connective tissue of corpus and cerix uteri during ripening and labour in term pregnancy. *British Journal of Obstetrics and Gynaecology* **96:** 1198–1202.

Greer IA, McLaren M & Calder AA (1990) Plasma prostaglandin E_2 and prostaglandin $F_{2\alpha}$ metabolite levels following vaginal administration of prostaglandin E_2 for induction of labor. *Acta Obstetrica et Gynecologica Scandinavica* **69:** 621–625.

Gupta JK & Johnson N (1990) Effect of mifepristone on dilatation of the pregnant and non-pregnant cervix. *Lancet* **i:** 1238–1240.

Jeffrey JJ & Koob TJ (1980) Endocrine control of collagen degradation in the uterus. In Naftolin F & Stubblefield PG (eds) *Dilatation of the Uterine Cervix*, pp 135–145. New York: Raven Press.

Jeffrey JJ, Coffey RJ & Eizen AZ (1971) Studies of uterine collagenase in tissue culture II: effect of steroid hormones on enzyme production. *Biochimica et Biophysica Acta* **252:** 143.

Junqueira LCU, Zugaib M & Montes GS et al (1980) Morphologic and histochemical evidence for the occurrence of collagenolysis and for the role of neutrophilic polymorphonuclear leukocytes during cervical dilatation. *American Journal of Obstetrics and Gynecology* **138:** 273–281.

Karim SMM, Trussell RR, Hillier K et al (1969) Induction of labour with prostaglandin $F_{2\alpha}$. *Journal of Obstetrics and Gynaecology of the British Commonwealth* **76:** 769–782.

Karim SMM, Hillier K, Trussell RR et al (1970) Induction of labour with prostaglandin E_2. *Journal of Obstetrics and Gynaecology of the British Commonwealth* **77:** 200–210.

Keirse MJNC, Schulpen MAGT, Borbeij RSACM et al (1987) The Dutch experience in cervical ripening with prostaglandin gel. In Keirse MJNC & de Koning Gans HJ (eds) *Priming and Induction of Labour by Prostaglandins. 'A State of the Art'*, pp 53–71. Leiden: Boerhaave Cursus.

Kelly RW & Bukman A (1990) Antiprogestagenic inhibition of uterine prostaglandin inactivation: a permissive mechanism for uterine stimulation. *Journal of Steroid Biochemistry and Molecular Biology* **37:** 97–101.

Kelly RW, Healy DL, Cameron IT et al (1986) The stimulation of prostaglandin production by two antiprogesterone steroids in human endometrial cells. *Journal of Clinical Endocrinology and Metabolism* **62:** 1116–1123.

Lewis RB & Schulman JD (1973) Influence of acetylsalicylic acid, an inhibitor of prostaglandin synthesis, on duration of human gestation and labour. *Lancet* **ii:** 1159.

Liggins GC (1981) Cervical ripening as an inflammatory reaction. In Liggins DA & Anderson ABM (eds) *The Cervix in Pregnancy and Labour: Clinical and Biochemical Investigations*, pp 1–9. Edinburgh: Churchill Livingstone.

Liggins GC, Forster CS, Grieves SA, Forster CS & Knox BS (1977) Parturition in the sheep. In Knight J & O'Connor M (eds) *The Fetus and Birth*, pp 5–25. Amsterdam: Elsevier/Excerpta Medica/North Holland.

Lindahl U & Hook M (1978) Glycosaminoglycans and their binding to biological macromolecules. *Annual Review of Biochemistry* **47:** 385.

MacKenzie IZ & Embrey MP (1977) Cervical ripening with intravaginal PGE_2 gel. *British Medical Journal* **ii:** 1981.

MacLennan AH (1981) Cervical ripening and the induction of labour by vaginal prostaglandin $F_{2\alpha}$ and relaxin. In Ellwood DA & Anderson ABM (eds) *The Cervix in Pregnancy and Labour: Clinical and Biochemical Investigations*, pp 187–196. Edinburgh: Churchill Livingstone.

Mitchell MD, Flint APF, Bibby J et al (1977) Rapid increases in plasma prostaglandin concentrations after vaginal examination and amniotomy. *British Medical Journal* **2:** 1183–1185.

Obrink B (1973) A study of the interactions between monomeric tropocollagen and glycosaminoglycans. *European Journal of Biochemistry* **33:** 387–400.

Radestad A, Bygdeman M & Green K (1990) Induced cervical ripening with mifepristone (RU486) and bioconversion of arachidonic acid in human pregnant uterine cervix in the first trimester. *Contraception* **41:** 283–292.

Rajabi MR, Dean DD, Beydoon SN et al (1988) Elevated tissue levels of collagenase during dilatation of uterine cervix in human parturition. *American Journal of Obstetrics and Gynecology* **41:** 283–292.

Scott JE & Orford CR (1981) Dermatan sulphate rich proteoglycan associates with rat tail tendon collagen at the d band in the gap region. *Biochemical Journal* **197:** 213.

Sitteri PK, Febres F, Clemens LE et al (1977) Progesterone and maintenance of pregnancy: is progesterone nature's immunosuppressant? *Annals of the New York Academy of Sciences* **286:** 384–397.

Speert H (1958) *Obstetric and Gynecologic Milestones*, pp 518–524. New York: Macmillan.

Turnbull AC & Anderson ABM (1968) Induction of labour; results with amniotomy and oxytocin titration. *Journal of Obstetrics and Gynaecology of the British Commonwealth* **75:** 32–41.

Turnbull AC (1989) The endocrine control of labour. In Turnbull A & Chamberlain G (eds) *Obstetrics*, pp 189–204. Edinburgh: Churchill Livingstone.

Uldbjerg N, Ekman G & Malmstrom A (1981) Biochemical and morphological changes of human cervix after local application of prostaglandin E_2 in pregnancy. *Lancet* **i:** 267–268.

Uldbjerg N, Ekman G & Malmstrom A (1983) Ripening of the human uterine cervix related to changes in collagen, glycosaminoglycans and collagenolytic activity. *American Journal of Obstetrics and Gynecology* **147:** 662–666.

Ulmsten U (1979) A new gel for intracervical application of PGE_2. *Lancet* **i:** 377.

von Maillot K, Stuhlsatz HW, Mohanaradhkrishan V et al (1979) Changes in the glycos-aminoglycan distribution pattern in the human uterine cervix during pregnancy and labour. *American Journal of Obstetrics and Gynecology* **135:** 503–506.
von Maillot K, Weiss M, Nagelschmidt M et al (1977) Relaxin and cervical dilatation during parturition. *Archiv für Gynakologie* **223:** 323–331.

6

Therapeutic uses of prostaglandins

M. J. N. C. KEIRSE

Therapeutic uses of prostaglandins in obstetrics are derived from two associated, but distinctly different, properties of prostaglandins: the stimulation of uterine smooth muscle and the remodelling of connective tissue. These two properties are often differentiated as myometrial and cervical effects of prostaglandins, because smooth muscle is predominantly present in the myometrium and connective tissue predominantly in the cervix. While this differentiation corresponds reasonably well with clinical observation, it is not entirely correct. Indeed, prostaglandin induced connective tissue changes, although clinically most obvious in the cervix, occur throughout the uterus. Similarly, the effects on smooth muscle, which are most obvious in the myometrium, probably occur also in the small proportion of smooth muscle within the cervix. It is worth being aware of this when contemplating whether prostaglandins are required for their cervical effects or for their myometrial effects. Myometrial and cervical effects cannot be separated entirely either pharmacologically or clinically. Nevertheless, a diligent choice of routes, vehicles and doses of administration may go a long way in helping to accentuate any one of these clinical aims of prostaglandin administration.

In practice, the therapeutic use of prostaglandins is further determined by whether these cervical and myometrial effects should result in the birth of a healthy baby or in the evacuation of a pregnant uterus. This, along with the difference in gestational age associated with the difference in cervical rigidity and myometrial sensitivity to prostaglandins, determines to a large extent what compounds and methods of administration are appropriate for which indication. Thus, where excellent prostaglandin analogues are available, natural prostaglandins will have a minimal role to play in second trimester abortions or in terminating pregnancies because of fetal death or gross fetal anomaly. Unfortunately, clinicians wishing to use prostaglandins are still hampered by large differences in the availability of prostaglandin preparations from one country to another. This problem is even greater for prostaglandin analogues. Limitations in the availability of such compounds may thus dictate the use of a natural prostaglandin, when a suitable analogue would be a more appropriate option.

Baillière's Clinical Obstetrics and Gynaecology—
Vol. 6, No. 4, December 1992
ISBN 0–7020–1694–2

INDUCTION OF LABOUR IN VIABLE PREGNANCIES

In order to be successful, induction of labour must fulfil three aims. First, it should result in what is defined as 'labour', namely adequate uterine contractions and progressive dilatation of the cervix. Second, this labour must result in vaginal delivery, as there is little purpose in bringing about labour as a mere preparation for caesarean section. Third, in viable pregnancies, these aims must be achieved with a minimum of discomfort and risk to both the mother and the baby.

It has been known for at least 30 years that the achievement of these goals is largely dependent on the condition of the cervix. A firm and rigid cervix requires a total quantity of uterine work that may be three to four times greater than what is needed when the cervix is softer and more yielding (Burnhill et al, 1962; Arulkumaran et al, 1985). Realization of the import-ance of the cervix has resulted in the development of various scores to assess cervical 'ripeness' and to predict the likely outcome of induction of labour by conventional means (reviewed by Keirse and van Oppen, 1989a). It has also resulted in a search for methods that decrease cervical resistance in preparation for formal attempts to induce labour by stimulation of uterine contractility. They are commonly referred to as methods for 'pre-induction', 'cervical ripening' or 'cervical softening' (Table 1).

Table 1. Summary of methods for cervical ripening of which con-trolled evaluations have been reported in the literature since 1950.

Type of intervention	Route of administration
Prostaglandins (PGE$_2$, PGE$_1$ and PGF$_{2\alpha}$)	Oral Vaginal Endocervical Extra-amniotic Intracervical
Oestradiol	Intramuscular Vaginal Endocervical Extra-amniotic
Oestriol	Extra-amniotic
Dehydroepiandrosterone sulphate	Intravenous
Oxytocin	Buccal Intravenous
Relaxin	Vaginal Endocervical
Non-medicated gels	Extra-amniotic
Foley catheter	Extra-amniotic
Bougie	Endocervical
Laminaria	Endocervical
Lamicel, Dilapan	Endocervical
Nipple stimulation	Breasts

Pre-induction or cervical ripening

An 'unripe', firm and rigid cervix fails to dilate as well as a ripe cervix in response to myometrial contractility. This results not only in a greater quantity of uterine work during induction, but also in high rates of failed induction. Failed induction is characterized by protracted and exhausting labour, unusually large analgesic requirements, high incidence of instrumental delivery and caesarean section, and a variety of other complications (Calder, 1979). Foremost among these are intrauterine infection, when amniotomy is part of the induction procedure, and uterine hyperstimulation or hypertonus with concomitant effects on fetal oxygenation.

A few years after the introduction of prostaglandins for inducing labour in the late 1960s, it was found that doses of prostaglandins, which by themselves were insufficient to induce labour successfully, had a marked effect on softening the cervix (Calder and Embrey, 1973). From then onwards, a large number of investigations have been conducted on the effects of prostaglandins for ripening the cervix prior to induction of labour. In 1989, Keirse and van Oppen reviewed all the evidence from clinical studies on cervical ripening, which had used a randomized or quasi-randomized design, and the review has been updated (Keirse, 1990).

Overall effects of prostaglandins

Regularly updated systematic analyses of controlled evaluations of methods used to enhance cervical compliance (Table 1) are now available in the Oxford Database of Perinatal Trials (Chalmers, 1992). The most recent analyses indicate that the pharmacological use of prostaglandins is currently the most effective means to enhance cervical ripening. It is also the only approach to cervical ripening that is reasonably supported by evidence from controlled evaluations. For instance, controlled evaluations of oxytocin have clearly established that this agent is of no value for enhancing cervical ripening, even when administered for many hours (Keirse and van Oppen, 1989a). Similarly, the most recent data on oestrogen administration, an approach that appeared promising in the past (Keirse and van Oppen, 1989a), now indicate that this has little to offer in clinical practice (Keirse, 1992). A variety of devices, such as laminaria, Foley catheters and balloons, have been applied to the problem of the unripe cervix. Their effects are likely to be—at least partially—prostaglandin mediated, since the insertion of these devices is known to stimulate endogenous prostaglandin synthesis in the uterus (Manabe et al, 1982; Keirse et al, 1983). There is no adequate evidence today, however, that the effects of these devices are large enough to confer real benefit. This may be due to the limited amount of prostaglandins released in comparison to that used pharmacologically, to the limited number of women included in controlled trials of these methods, or to both.

Controlled evaluations comparing prostaglandins with either placebo formulations or no prostaglandin treatment have clearly demonstrated that prostaglandins are effective agents to ripen the cervix. This is true to the extent that further placebo or no treatment controlled comparisons are superfluous for establishing the effects of prostaglandins on cervical ripening, although such studies are still being reported (Rayburn et al, 1992; Troostwijk et al, 1992). Most of the individual trials show clear effects of prostaglandins in terms of enhanced cervical ripeness and shorter induction to delivery intervals during subsequent induction of labour. Individually, however, most of them fail to demonstrate statistically significant differences in more substantive outcome measures. This has led some to conclude that prostaglandin-induced cervical ripening has little effect on labour induction and no effect on the incidence of caesarean section (Owen et al, 1991), but these conclusions are not supported by the results of systematic overviews of all placebo and no treatment-controlled evaluations of prostaglandin treatment for cervical ripening (Keirse and van Oppen, 1989a). Since such overviews were reported there have been several further controlled comparisons with placebo or no active treatment (Curet and Gauger, 1989; Prasad et al, 1989; Buttino and Garite, 1990; Chatterjee et al, 1990; Bernstein, 1991; Owen et al, 1991; Rayburn et al, 1992; Troostwijk et al, 1992). Although they merely confirm the conclusions from earlier analyses (Keirse and van Oppen, 1989a), new data published before 1991 as well as the data of Bernstein (1991), which were previously available, have been amalgamated with those of previous trials (reviewed by Keirse and van Oppen, 1989a) in a formal and systematic meta-analysis.

Cumulative effects derived from almost 50 reports dealing with controlled evaluations of prostaglandins against placebo or no prostaglandin treatment are summarized visually in Figures 1–3. When interpreting these figures, it should be realized that the studies incorporated in this analysis have used different prostaglandins in a wide range of doses, vehicles and routes of administration. In some studies, the prostaglandin preparation was administered only once. In others, administration was repeated either once or several times. The studies also vary widely in terms of entry criteria: some involved only nulliparous women, others both nulliparous and parous women. Several cervical scoring systems were applied to define the need for cervical ripening, and within these scoring systems different cut-off points were used to select candidates for participation in the studies. The time interval allowed for ripening the cervix also differed between studies. Furthermore, there are differences in the manner of implementing induction of labour after cervical ripening and in the criteria used to decide whether and when ripening should be followed by formal induction. In some of the trials induction of labour was conducted routinely after ripening irrespective of its effect; in others induction was implemented only if an adequate degree of cervical ripening had been achieved. However, trials were incorporated in the overview summarized in Figures 1–3 only if the policy for subsequent induction was the same for prostaglandin treated women as for those receiving no prostaglandin treatment.

The heterogeneity of these studies is, therefore, nearly as large as the heterogeneity that exists among individual women for whom induction of labour is contemplated in the presence of an unripe cervix. Obviously, this heterogeneity may limit the scientific merit of the meta-analysis on which

OUTCOMES

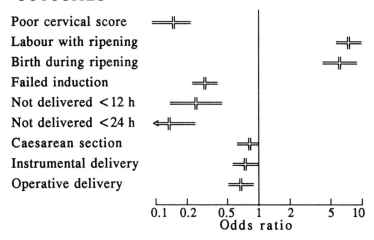

Figure 1. Effects of prostaglandins versus the effects of no treatment or placebo treatment for cervical ripening on labour and delivery outcomes as evident from controlled evaluations of any prostaglandin administered by any route for ripening the cervix before formal induction of labour. The data are shown as typical odds ratios with their 95% confidence intervals and are based on all controlled evaluations reported from 1975 up to 1990. Not all outcomes, however, were available for each trial. Odds ratios below 1 indicate that the outcome was less frequent in prostaglandin-treated women than in women receiving placebo or no treatment and odds ratios above 1 indicate the reverse. Confidence intervals that do not cross the line drawn at unity indicate that the difference is statistically significant at least at the 5% level.

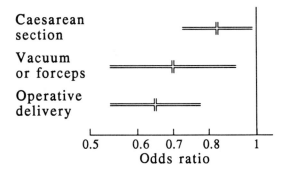

Figure 2. Effects of prostaglandins versus the effects of no treatment or placebo treatment for cervical ripening before the induction of labour on the rates of caesarean section, instrumental vaginal delivery, and operative delivery. Data relate to all controlled evaluations of any prostaglandin administered by any route for ripening the cervix that were reported between 1975 and 1990. All odds ratios and all confidence intervals are below 1 indicating that all of these outcomes were less frequent with prostaglandin treatment than in the control groups.

OUTCOMES

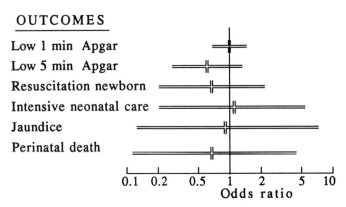

Figure 3. Effects of prostaglandins versus the effects of no treatment or placebo treatment for cervical ripening on infant outcomes as evident from controlled evaluations. The data are shown as typical odds ratios with their 95% confidence intervals and are based on all controlled evaluations of any prostaglandin administered by any route for ripening the cervix reported from 1975 up to 1990. Several outcomes, however, were available for only few trials as indicated by the large confidence intervals. None of these and other infant outcomes studied showed differential effects (good or bad) between the prostaglandin treatment and no treatment or placebo treatment. For further interpretation of the figure see Figure 1.

these figures are based. On the other hand, it may increase the clinical relevance of this approach in two respects. First, in clinical practice, women requiring induction in the presence of an unripe cervix present with a wide variety of indications and individual differences. All of these need to be taken into account when deciding on appropriate treatment. Yet the literature rarely provides reliable data that will suit the particular requirements of an individual woman or an individual clinician. Heterogeneous data and broad generalizations, provided these are comprehensive, accurate, and quality controlled, provide an overall estimate within which clinical decisions can be made. Secondly, the availability of prostaglandin preparations regrettably differs among countries and institutions. While expected to make appropriate choices among preparations, clinicians rarely have adequate control over what is available. Detailed information on a wide range of preparations, doses and administration techniques is therefore only worth considering if there are general merits in the use of prostaglandins. Moreover, as the various trials clearly indicate, conclusions related to a particular form of administration are notoriously prone to α and β error. This is because there is no evidence of a clear and consistent research strategy among these trials; there are too many variations among trials and virtually always too few patients in each trial.

In terms of labour and delivery outcomes there is no doubt that prostaglandin-induced cervical ripening confers considerable benefits (see Figure 1). These benefits include a marked and statistically significant reduction in the rate of failed induction, a greater likelihood of being delivered within a reasonable time interval once induction is started, and an increased likelihood of having a spontaneous vaginal delivery. The latter is the result of a reduction in the rates of both caesarean section and instrumental vaginal delivery (Figure 2).

These effects are observed with both prostaglandin E_2 (PGE_2) and $PGF_{2\alpha}$. Although there is less information on $PGF_{2\alpha}$ than there is on PGE_2, both the indirect (from placebo or no treatment controlled evaluations of $PGF_{2\alpha}$) and direct (from controlled comparisons of PGE_2 and $PGF_{2\alpha}$) evidence available suggests that PGE_2 and $PGF_{2\alpha}$ are equally effective, provided that they are given in approximately equipotent doses. Equipotency in vivo cannot be determined exactly from the data that are available, but doses of $PGF_{2\alpha}$ need to be roughly ten times higher than those of PGE_2 in order to obtain similar effects (Keirse and van Oppen, 1989a). This ratio between $PGF_{2\alpha}$ and PGE_2 is similar or perhaps slightly higher than that observed for the myometrial effects of these two prostaglandins (Keirse and Chalmers, 1989). Since the same potency ratio does not apply to other organ systems, it follows that equipotent doses in terms of uterine and cervical effects expose other organ systems to a five- to ten-fold higher dose when $PGF_{2\alpha}$ is used instead of PGE_2. This explains the greater likelihood of side-effects with $PGF_{2\alpha}$ than with PGE_2. Therefore, after the instability of PGE_2 preparations was resolved, PGE_2 quickly superseded $PGF_{2\alpha}$ and is now virtually the only natural prostaglandin used both for cervical ripening and for induction of labour. Yet recent publications indicate that $PGF_{2\alpha}$ is still being used in some countries, especially for midtrimester abortions or for ending pregnancy after fetal death (Papaeorgiou et al, 1991; Peat, 1991; Jaschevatzky et al, 1992). If other prostaglandins are available this would seem to be inappropriate in the light of current evidence.

When all trials are combined there is a tendency, though not statistically significant, for fetal heart rate abnormalities to occur more frequently with than without prostaglandin treatment. Apparently this does not result in a greater likelihood of operative delivery, which shows an overall decrease with prostaglandin treatment, or of poor Apgar scores at birth (see Figure 3). Almström and colleagues (1991) recently reported on the endocervical administration of PGE_2 for cervical ripening and labour induction in 80 women with ultrasonically diagnosed intrauterine growth retardation (defined as less than 2 SD below the mean) and an unripe cervix. Although 33% of these women also had other complications, 64% of the infants with growth retardation confirmed at birth were born spontaneously. Operative delivery, by caesarean section or vacuum extraction, for fetal distress occurred in 28% (95% confidence interval: 16–40%) of the cases with a birthweight less than 2 SD below the mean and in only 10% (95% confidence interval: 2–26%) of those with higher birthweight. Along with the data from controlled evaluations, these data would suggest that cervical ripening is a reasonable option when there is a risk of fetal distress provided that adequate surveillance of fetal and maternal condition is instituted.

There is only limited information about uterine hyperstimulation or uterine hypertonus in the many controlled trials as this outcome is reported in less than a third of the controlled trials. There are no internationally agreed definitions of either hypertonus or hyperstimulation and these outcomes are, therefore, often vaguely and variably defined. In addition, it is not always clear whether such occurrences had any consequences in terms of either potential fetal compromise or use of additional interventions. Nevertheless, it would appear that there is an increased risk of hyper-stimulation and/or hypertonus, although this is not statistically significant. Overall, during ripening and subsequent induction this occurred in 5.3% (95% confidence interval: 3.8 to 6.8%) of prostaglandin-treated women as compared with 3.3% (95% confidence interval: 2.0–4.5%) in controls. It should be noted that these conditions, which are to some extent subjective and prone to observer bias, are reported more frequently from institutions without prior experience of prostaglandins than from those accustomed to their use. For example, Noah and his colleagues (1987) reported an incidence of 7.7% among 416 women treated with endocervical PGE_2 (0.5 mg in triacetin gel) when this treatment was introduced in various European centres, while Egarter and his colleagues (1990) recorded an incidence of only 0.5% among 394 women treated at the Vienna University hospital, where prostaglandins had been used for some time. There are indications that some preparations are more prone to cause hyperstimu-lation than others. Particularly worrying in this respect has been a controlled release polymer pessary containing as much as 10 mg of PGE_2 for which, contrary to expectation (Taylor et al, 1990a, 1991), incidences of uterine hyperstimulation and fetal heart rate abnormalities have been reported that are roughly two to three times higher than with other prostaglandin preparations (Khouzam and Ledward, 1990; Miller et al, 1991; Rayburn et al, 1992; Witter et al, 1992). From several studies it would appear that the risk of myometrial hyperstimulation for similar efficacy is lowest with the use of endocervical PGE_2 (Egarter et al, 1990; Granström et al, 1990; Zanini et al, 1990; Keirse et al, 1991; Lopes et al, 1991), but this only applies if insertion beyond the internal os and into the extra-amniotic space is avoided (Keirse et al, 1985). It may be noted that uterine hypertonus or hyper-stimulation whether during ripening or during labour is readily controlled by administration of a β-mimetic agent (Egarter et al, 1990). This treatment is equally effective whether the excessive contractility is due to prostaglandin or to oxytocin administration, but it should rarely be needed during cervical ripening.

There is a difference of opinion as to whether cervical ripening may lead to increased uterine contractility or not. On the one hand, cervical ripening is undertaken because the cervix is considered to be insufficiently compliant to respond adequately to uterine contractions. It thus seems logical to avoid such contractions until greater cervical compliance has been achieved, especially if the contractions are uncomfortable or painful for the mother. Considered from this point of view, the onset of labour during cervical ripening and especially before sufficient cervical change has occurred can be seen as an undesirable side-effect. On the other hand, cervical ripening aims to promote successful labour and delivery and there is no point in applying this procedure if there is no need to bring the pregnancy to an end. Judged from this point of view, an increase in uterine contractility to the extent that labour and delivery occur without the need for further intervention may be desirable. This would apply especially if the procedure is safe for mother and baby, and if maternal discomfort is less than it would be when a further induction procedure is needed. Whichever point of view one favours, it is an established fact that enhancing cervical compliance with prostaglandins without increasing myometrial contractility is currently impossible. This is clearly demonstrated by the increased frequency of the onset of labour and even delivery during the time allocated for cervical ripening, which is a consistent feature in virtually all trials reported thus far. This is illustrated by the results of all placebo- and no treatment-controlled trials reported in the first 12 years that such trials were conducted (Figure 4). Attempts to achieve uterine quiescence during ripening by the combined use of β mimetics and prostaglandins have proved to be rather futile, in that any possible gain from the addition of a β mimetic agent was offset by reduced cervical ripening (Insull et al, 1989; Taylor et al, 1990b).

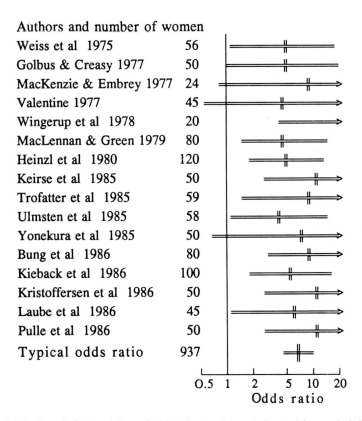

Figure 4. Likelihood of being delivered within the time interval allocated for cervical ripening with prostaglandins compared with placebo treatment or no treatment. Results are shown for all controlled evaluations of prostaglandins for cervical ripening reported between 1975 and 1986. All trials show that women receiving prostaglandin pretreatment were more likely to be delivered during the ripening period than controls. In most of the trials that effect was statistically significant. For further interpretation of the figure see Figure 1.

Regrettably, it is unclear to what extent, if any, the baby shares in the improvements in labour and delivery outcomes. Obstetricians who conducted or reported the studies reviewed have apparently been too preoccupied with appropriate management of labour and delivery and, albeit to a lesser extent, with recording data on labour and delivery outcomes. There is clear evidence that there has been inadequate attention to infant outcomes in most of the controlled clinical research on cervical ripening. For example, more than half of the trial reports fail to mention specifically whether there were any perinatal deaths or not. Substantive data on infant outcomes, such as resuscitation of the newborn, defined morbidity, and admission to special care nurseries, are notoriously lacking in the large majority of the reports. Considering the traditional obstetric preoccupation with perinatal mortality and morbidity, this may be interpreted as a strong belief in the perinatal safety of prostaglandin administration for cervical ripening. Nevertheless, such belief is no adequate substitute for evidence. All that can be said on the basis of the limited evidence available is that the use of prostaglandins for cervical ripening is unlikely to have marked effects, good or bad, on the fetus or infant (see Figure 3). There is currently no evidence that the use of prostaglandins for cervical ripening improves perinatal outcome nor is there any evidence that it will jeopardize perinatal health. Due to the excessive underreporting of infant outcome, the precision of the estimates of 'no difference' in neonatal outcome measures is very poor (see Figure 3).

Effects of different routes of administration

Extra-amniotic administration was the first route of PGE_2 administration to be explored for cervical ripening (Calder and Embrey, 1973), but few controlled evaluations of this approach have been reported and they were based on exceedingly small numbers of women. Overall there are too few data from well-controlled research for an adequate judgement of the merits and hazards of this approach. The latter include its invasiveness, the fact that many women find insertion of the extra-amniotic catheter unpleasant, the small risk of infection and of excessive uterine stimulation due to an occasional rapid uptake of the prostaglandin from the choriodecidual space. Trials which compared extra-amniotic with vaginal or with endocervical administration showed that the extra-amniotic route was more likely to result in the onset of labour than either of the other two routes of administration (Wilson, 1978; Toplis and Sims, 1979; Stewart et al, 1983; Greer and Calder, 1989). The extra-amniotic route has now been replaced almost entirely by vaginal and endocervical administration. If there is still a place for it, it must be small and should be reserved for women with a very unripe cervix in whom immediate induction of labour is warranted. In such circumstances it may still be better to introduce a commercially available 0.5 mg PGE_2 gel at the level of the internal os, to find its way in the extra-amniotic space around the cervix, rather than to rely on variable extemporaneous preparations administered higher into the extra-amniotic space.

With the availability of oral PGE_2 for induction of labour in the late 1970s, five trials, each involving between 30 and 60 women, compared this approach with either placebo or no treatment for cervical ripening (Friedman and Sachtleben, 1975; Weiss et al, 1975; Golbus and Creasy, 1977; Pearce, 1977; Valentine, 1977). It was soon established that oral PGE_2 needed to be administered repeatedly over a period of several hours in order to have any effect at all. This approach is now abandoned as not suitable for cervical ripening, although it is still being used for inducing labour in women with a favourable cervix or with prelabour rupture of the membranes (Davies et al, 1991).

The two main approaches currently in use involve the vaginal and the endocervical routes of administration. The earliest controlled evaluation of vaginal PGE_2 for cervical ripening used a dose of 2 mg in a self-prepared gel (MacKenzie and Embrey, 1977). Doses were later increased to as much as 5 mg in homemade gels (MacKenzie and Embrey, 1979; Prins et al, 1983) or to 3 mg PGE_2 pessaries. Since the advent of commercially available PGE_2 gel preparations for vaginal use, it is now generally accepted that a dose of 2 mg is adequate (Keirse and Elder, 1991). This may well be because the gel preparations provide more rapid and more reliable release of PGE_2 than the tablets, resulting in greater bioavailability and efficacy (Mahmood, 1989; Greer et al, 1990; Greer, 1992). It is also possible that the biological strength of homemade preparations was considerably less than its alleged prostaglandin content, due to instability, hydrolysis of PGE_2 to PGA_2 (which occurs readily in acid aqueous media, especially at relatively high temperatures) or characteristics of absorption. Such events would be the logical explanation for the findings in American studies that slices of 20 mg PGE_2 wax pessaries, named 'chips', are more active than homemade preparations of gels medicated by the melting down of the same PGE_2 pessaries (Smith et al, 1990).

For endocervical administration, the commonly used and best evaluated form consists of 0.5 mg of PGE_2 in a viscous gel. Two such gels are commercially available in Europe. One of these, based on 2.5 ml triacetin gel, is marketed as Prepidil (Upjohn); the other is starch based by a combination of dextran and polydextrin particles and is marketed as Cerviprost (Organon). There has been much argument on optimal gel formulations in the belief that the degree of viscosity of the gel is the main factor that determines endocervical as opposed to extra-amniotic or vaginal administration. The main determinant, however, is not gel viscosity, but the volume of space in the endocervical canal. When the cervix is very unripe, this volume is very small and part of the medicated gel, which is usually 2–3 ml, is bound to disappear beyond the internal os or to flow back into the vagina. Suggested differential effects of various gel formulations (Skajaa et al, 1991) probably depend more on how much of the PGE_2 is deposited beyond the internal os than on gel properties, as has been observed with different injection techniques using the same gel (Keirse et al, 1985, 1987). This may also be the reason that comparative studies between endocervical and vaginal administration have thus far failed to indicate a clear superiority of either one of these methods. On balance the endocervical approach may offer a slight advantage. Especially if enough of the gel can be introduced in the cervical canal without spilling over in the extra-amniotic space, there is likely to be a greater ripening effect with less concomitant uterine contractility (Ekman et al, 1983; Thiery et al, 1984; Ulmsten et al, 1985; Egarter et al, 1990; Granström et al, 1990; Zanini et al, 1990; Lopes et al, 1991; M. J. N. C. Keirse et al, unpublished findings). However, with extremely unfavourable cervical scores (Bishop scores 0–2) little of the gel is likely to remain within the cervical canal. In such circumstances, one may deliberately opt for administering some of the gel beyond the internal os, or for vaginal administration of the larger 2 mg dose, if repeated applications are to be kept to a minimum. It should be realized, though, that the total dose of PGE_2 necessary to prime the cervix for induction may vary between individuals, even if they appear to have comparable cervical scores.

There is reasonable consensus that an inadequate response of the cervix to a first dose of PGE_2 is best dealt with by repeating the PGE_2 administration. There is less consensus on the most appropriate approach if a second attempt does not meet with success. On the one hand, there are some who will continue repeat administrations against all odds. Milliez and his colleagues (1991), for example, reported repeat endocervical instillations of 0.25 mg PGE_2 every 48 hours up to nine times. For women requiring more than one instillation (half of their patients) they reported delays between the first procedure and delivery ranging from 2.4 to 16 days with an average of 9 days. On the other hand, there are those who feel that women who require early delivery and fail to respond to two sequential PGE_2 doses may benefit more from immediate caesarean section than from the prospects of a prolonged induction (Karaiskakis et al, 1991). As is often the case, the most reasonable approach would appear to be somewhere in between. First, delays of 48 hours between successive instillations are unnecessarily long compared with more appropriate intervals of about 6 hours. Second, among women who fail to respond adequately to two doses, a significant proportion will still achieve an increase in cervical compliance after a third dose provided that an appropriate preparation is used in an adequate dose. The latter may not necessarily be the case with the use of extemporaneous preparations. If three doses fail to have any effect, it becomes very unlikely that further treatment will drastically alter cervical resistance and the choices for ending the pregnancy then become either to abandon the wish to end the pregnancy, proceed to formal induction of labour or proceed to caesarean section. The most fundamental concept behind this, however, should be that cervical ripening is not a trivial intervention and requires a clear indication in order to be justified.

Formal induction of labour

From 1971 onwards, 3 years after the introduction of prostaglandins for induction of labour (Karim et al, 1968), a large number of controlled evaluations of the use of prostaglandins for inducing labour have been reported. At first, these involved controlled comparisons between intravenous prostaglandins and intravenous oxytocin. Later, with the advent of other routes of prostaglandin administration, the controlled comparisons have been with placebo treatments, with intravenous and buccal oxytocin, between PGE_2 and $PGF_{2\alpha}$, and between different routes, formulations and doses of prostaglandins (Table 2). In some of the comparisons amniotomy was part of the procedure; in others it was not; in still others amniotomy was applied in one group but not in the other. This has resulted in a large amount of literature. Comprehensive reviews of that literature up to 1989 are available elsewhere (Keirse and Chalmers, 1989; Keirse and van Oppen, 1989b) and only the salient points need to be considered here.

Table 2. Forms of prostaglandin administration for induction of labour which have been used in controlled trials with random or quasi-random allocation of women to different treatments.

Type of drug	Form of administration
PGE_2	Intravenous (infusion)
	Oral (tablets, solutions)
	Buccal (tablets)
	Rectal (tablets)
	Vaginal (tablets, pessaries, gels)
	Endocervical (various gels)
	Extra-amniotic (solutions, gels)
$PGF_{2\alpha}$	Intravenous (infusion)
	Oral (tablets)
	Vaginal (gels)
	Endocervical (gels)
	Extra-amniotic (solutions, gels)

Although differential effects of PGE_2 and $PGF_{2\alpha}$ are confounded by changes in the routes of administration that have occurred during the history of their use, by differences in their oxytocic potencies, and by limited data on direct controlled comparisons between them, it is fair to conclude that $PGF_{2\alpha}$, which was the first compound to be introduced, should no longer be used for induction of labour. Also, the earliest route of administration, intravenous infusion, has fallen into disrepute. Eight controlled comparisons with intravenous oxytocin, reported between 1971 and 1973, provided no evidence in support of intravenous prostaglandin administration (for a review see Keirse and van Oppen, 1989b). It was only through the introduction of oral administration in 1971 (Karim and Sharma, 1971) that prostaglandins became a feasible option and a real alternative to the more conventional methods of labour induction. The later exploration of extra-amniotic and, especially, vaginal routes of administration followed by greater attention to women's comfort during labour finally established PGE_2 as having the potential to be more than a mere alternative to the traditional oxytocin infusion.

Comparison with oxytocin

Results are available from several systematic meta-analyses of controlled comparisons between various prostaglandin and various oxytocin regimens for inducing labour (Keirse and van Oppen, 1989b). Although a few other such trials have been reported since (e.g. MacLennan et al, 1989; Rayburn et al, 1989; Lyndrup et al, 1990), the wide body of evidence available from controlled studies conducted between 1971 and 1988 has hardly changed.

When the membranes in oxytocin-induced and prostaglandin-induced women are treated in the same fashion, either by rupture or by leaving them intact, fewer women remain undelivered 24 and 48 hours after prostaglandin induction than after oxytocin induction (Figure 5). These differences, which are based on large numbers of women participating in a variety of such trials, are even more marked when the likelihood of not being delivered vaginally is examined. These data, shown in Figure 5, indicate that there is little difference in the likelihood of being delivered either vaginally or by any route within 12 hours between prostaglandin and oxytocin inductions. However, women who are undelivered after 12 hours are more likely to remain undelivered after 24 hours and after 48 hours if they were induced with oxytocin than if they were induced with prostaglandins. They also have a considerably greater chance of not being delivered vaginally within 24 or 48 hours if they were induced with oxytocin than if they were induced with prostaglandins.

Nevertheless, these data, based on some 29 controlled trials, do not show a difference in the rates of caesarean section between prostaglandin and oxytocin inductions (Figure 6). The rate of instrumental vaginal delivery, on

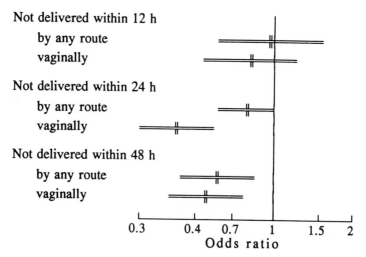

Figure 5. Likelihood of not being delivered within specified time intervals after starting induction of labour with either prostaglandins or oxytocin. Odds ratios and 95% confidence intervals are based on data from the controlled comparisons between (any) prostaglandin(s) and (any) oxytocin that were published between 1971 and 1990 and for which the appropriate outcome measure was available either in the published report or in the additional information requested from the authors. Data on vaginal deliveries within 12, 24 and 48 hours, respectively, relate to more than 700, 1100 and 1500 women participating in controlled trials of prostaglandins versus oxytocin. Data on delivery by any route in the same time intervals relate to some 500, 2000 and 2100 women, respectively. (See Figure 1 for interpretation of the figure.)

the other hand, is markedly lower after prostaglandin than after oxytocin induction. This effect is based on fewer trials because several authors of the earlier studies did not consider instrumental delivery to be sufficiently interesting in order to report its frequency. Nevertheless, the difference is statistically significant (odds ratio 0.77, 95% confidence interval 0.60–0.99, see Figure 6). As a consequence, there is also a statistically significant reduction in the odds of operative delivery with some 25% (odds ratio 0.74, 95% confidence interval 0.59–0.92, see Figure 6). The reduction in the odds of operative delivery is roughly similar to that seen in controlled evaluations of prostaglandins used for cervical ripening. This may well be an indication that this effect is not due to selective reporting of prostaglandin-favourable outcomes in the trial reports that provide information on both caesarean section and instrumental vaginal delivery. Another indication that this is likely to be a true effect, and not due to publication bias, is that only one of the individual trials (Ulstein et al, 1979) failed to show a statistically significant difference in this outcome.

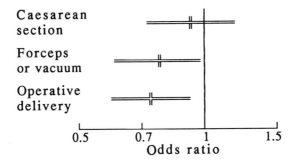

Figure 6. Odds ratio and 95% confidence intervals for the rates of caesarean section, instrumental vaginal delivery, and operative delivery derived from the controlled comparisons of prostaglandins with oxytocin for formal induction of labour published between 1971 and 1990. An odds ratio less than 1 indicates a lower rate of this type of delivery with prostaglandins than with oxytocin while a confidence interval that does not cross the line drawn at unity indicates that the difference is statistically significant.

A recent randomized study, conducted by Lamont and his colleagues (1991), provides important clues to the mechanisms that may explain these findings. They showed that women with a Bishop score of 4 or more required less uterine effort to achieve the same degree of cervical dilatation if labour was induced with vaginal PGE_2 gel than if labour was induced by amniotomy and oxytocin. This would indicate that, even with a relatively favourable cervix, gain in cervical compliance during labour may still be an important factor in determining the success of induction. Not surprisingly, the striking differences between PGE_2 and oxytocin were found predominantly in nulliparous women (Lamont et al, 1991). Indeed, more than 30 years ago Turnbull (1957) had suggested that parous women have a reduced cervical resistance, which he attributed to their previous labours and deliveries. It has also been demonstrated, both in spontaneous and in induced labours, that parous women require less uterine effort to achieve delivery than nulliparous women (Arulkumaran et al, 1984, 1985; Steer et al, 1985).

There is now clear evidence that oxytocin has little, if any, effect on cervical compliance. Such evidence, suggested as early as 1973 (Calder and Embrey, 1973) now comes from placebo- and no treatment-controlled trials of oxytocin for cervical ripening and from controlled comparisons between oxytocin and prostaglandins for cervical ripening (Keirse and van Oppen, 1989a). It is also supported by evidence from studies conducted by Arulkumaran and his colleagues (1985), which indicate that the amount of uterine contractility and the amount of oxytocin required to achieve delivery is directly proportional to the degree of cervical and pelvic tissue resistance. The effects of PGE_2 on connective tissue resistance, have been well established from the many cervical ripening studies conducted both in and outside pregnancy.

The differential effects of PGE_2 and oxytocin on connective tissue resistance are likely to be the explanation for the lower total uterine effort required during PGE_2 as opposed to oxytocin inductions. This along with an increased freedom of movement, which has its own beneficial effects (Roberts, 1989), may explain women's preference for PGE_2 induction rather than for the traditional amniotomy plus oxytocin induction (Kennedy et al, 1982; Lamont, 1990). It would also result in a lower need for and use of analgesia, a finding that is consistent with the data of the few controlled trials between prostaglandin and oxytocin for which use of analgesia has been reported (Keirse and van Oppen, 1989b). The effects on connective tissue resistance, greater freedom of movement and lower use of analgesia may all be mechanisms, which contribute to the lower incidence of instrumental vaginal delivery achieved with prostaglandins as compared with oxytocin (see Figure 6).

These same findings would support the view that the use of PGE_2 is a more appropriate method than oxytocin for inducing labour in women previously delivered by caesarean section (MacKenzie, 1991). Such women are likely to have a less favourable cervix than other parous women, especially if they had elective caesarean sections as their only previous deliveries. Even if they have a ripe cervix, they are also likely to benefit from the lower total uterine activity needed to achieve cervical dilatation. In the largest series reported to date (MacKenzie, 1991) the use of PGE_2 carried a risk of scar rupture equal to that observed during spontaneous labour (0.2%, 95% confidence interval <0.01–1.2%). The overall incidence of scar damage (dehiscence and rupture) was 1% (95% confidence interval 0.35–2.4%) with all cases of such damage occurring among women who had received oxytocin augmentation after PGE_2 administration. There is clearly an increased risk of scar damage when more than one oxytocic agent is required or used and other series (e.g. Gordon, 1988) testify to that.

Similarly, current evidence, although far from conclusive and under intensive investigation to date, may suggest that PGE_2 would be a more logical choice than oxytocin if induction of labour is deemed to be appropriate in women with prelabour rupture of the membranes. On the whole, however, such women are more likely to benefit from an initially expectant rather than an interventionist approach (M. J. N. C. Keirse et al, unpublished data).

Choice of prostaglandin preparation

There are obviously major differences between different PGE_2 preparations. Thus, the combined evidence from controlled comparisons involving the use of oral PGE_2 indicates that gastrointestinal side-effects may occur in about 10% of women in whom labour is induced in this manner (Keirse and van Oppen, 1989b). The combined evidence from controlled and observational studies clearly suggests that vaginal PGE_2 administration is the most logical approach and the method that is most acceptable for the mother (Keirse and Chalmers, 1989; Lamont, 1990). Among the preparations currently available in Europe, PGE_2 in triacetin gel (available in doses of 1 and 2 mg of PGE_2) would appear to be the best option. These gel preparations appear to provide more rapid and more reliable release of PGE_2 than tablets or pessaries, resulting in greater bioavailability and efficacy (Mahmood, 1989; Greer et al, 1990; Greer, 1992). Consequently and contrary to views expressed a few years ago (Keirse and Chalmers, 1989; Keirse and van Oppen, 1989b), the balance between oral and vaginal administration of PGE_2 has now clearly shifted in favour of the latter.

INDUCTION OF LABOUR IN PREGNANCIES WITH A DEAD OR NON-VIABLE FETUS

Induction of labour when the fetus is considered to be non-viable either because it is dead, suffers from major structural or chromosomal anomalies, or is subjected to second trimester abortion, differs from other inductions in two respects. First, these indications present themselves within a much wider range of gestational age than is applicable for other indications for induction. The earlier the gestational age, the higher the cervical resistance and the lower the myometrial sensitivity to prostaglandins is likely to be. Both of these effects tend to result in higher prostaglandin requirements at earlier gestational ages. Second, there is no need to take fetal well-being into account. Among other effects, this implies not only that prostaglandin analogues can be used as an alternative to natural prostaglandins, but also that worries about side-effects, such as hypertonus, need only be considered in terms of their maternal effects.

Consequently, in several institutions, the use of natural prostaglandins for non-viable pregnancies has been almost entirely replaced by the use of prostaglandin analogues. These include intravenous infusion of sulprostone (a synthetic PGE_2 analogue) at a rate of $1 \, \mu g \, min^{-1}$ (Kanhai and Keirse, 1989, 1992) and gemeprost (a PGE_1 analogue) administered by vaginal pessary for late abortions. Moreover, with the availability of the anti-progestin mifepristone, this whole area of indications ranging from second trimester terminations to the management of fetal abnormality and fetal death is likely to introduce drastic changes in current prostaglandin protocols (Chapter 10).

In the UK, the extra-amniotic approach with a single injection of 1.5–2.5 mg of PGE_2 in a gel, routinely followed by oxytocin augmentation after 6 hours, has been a main method for terminating pregnancies in the second trimester, although it is associated with high rates of side-effects, including vomiting in 45% and diarrhoea in 17% of women (Hill et al, 1989). In recent years, this approach as well as the intra-amniotic approach reserved for the later gestations and involving the use of a single intra-amniotic injection of 5–10 mg of PGE_2 followed by oxytocin augmentation is losing its popularity in favour of the use of prostaglandin analogues, which on the whole provide much safer treatment options (Hill et al, 1991; MacKenzie, 1992). In any case, it is to be anticipated that natural prostaglandins will become of decreasing interest for the termination of non-viable pregnancies as and when the better prostaglandin analogues become more widely available.

REFERENCES

Almström H, Ekman G & Granström L (1991) Preinductive cervical ripening with PGE_2 gel in term pregnant women with ultrasonically diagnosed intra-uterine growth-retarded fetuses. *Acta Obstetrica et Gynecologica Scandinavica* **70:** 555–559.

Arulkumaran S, Gibb DMF, Lun KC, Heng SH & Ratnam SS (1984) The effect of parity on uterine activity in labour. *British Journal of Obstetrics and Gynaecology* **91:** 843–848.

Arulkumaran S, Gibb DMF, Ratnam SS, Lun KC & Heng SH (1985) Total uterine activity in induced labour—an index of cervical and pelvic resistance. *British Journal of Obstetrics and Gynaecology* **92:** 693–697.

Bernstein P (1991) Prostaglandin E_2 gel for cervical ripening and labour induction: a multi-centre placebo-controlled trial. *Canadian Medical Association Journal* **145:** 1249–1254.

Bung P, Baer S, Djahanschahi D, Huch R, Huch A, Huber JF, Extermann P, Beguin F, Delaloye JF, Germond M, Bossart H, De Grandi P, Pfister A, Ehrsam A & Haller U (1986) Multizentrische Erfahrungen bei intrazervikaler Applikation eines neuen PGE_2-Gels bei Geburtseinleitung. *Geburtshilfe und Frauenheilkunde* **46:** 93–97.

Burnhill MS, Danezis J & Cohen J (1962) Uterine contractility during labor studied by intra-amniotic fluid pressure recordings. *American Journal of Obstetrics and Gynecology* **83:** 561–571.

Buttino LJ & Garite TJ (1990) Intracervical prostaglandin in postdate pregnancy. A randomized trial. *Journal of Reproductive Medicine* **35:** 155–158.

Calder AA (1979) The management of the unripe cervix. In Keirse MJNC, Anderson ABM & Bennebroek Gravenhorst J (eds) *Human Parturition. New Concepts and Developments*, pp 201–217. The Hague: Leiden University Press.

Calder AA & Embrey MP (1973) Prostaglandins and the unfavourable cervix. *Lancet* **ii:** 1322–1323.

Chalmers I (ed.) (1992) *Oxford Database of Perinatal Trials*, Version 1.3, Disk Issue 7, Spring 1992. Oxford: Oxford University Press.

Chatterjee MS, Ramchandran K, Ferlita J & Mitrik ML (1991) Prostaglandin E_2 (PGE_2) vaginal gel for cervical ripening. *European Journal of Obstetrics, Gynecology and Reproductive Biology* **38:** 197–202.

Curet LB & Gauger LJ (1989) Cervical ripening with intravaginal prostaglandin E_2 gel. *International Journal of Gynaecology and Obstetrics* **28:** 221–228.

Davies NJ, Martindale E & Haddad NG (1991) Cervical ripening with oral prostaglandin E_2 tablets and the effect of the latent period in patients with premature rupture of the membranes at term. *Journal of Obstetrics and Gynaecology* **11:** 405–408.

Egarter CH, Husslein PW & Rayburn WF (1990) Uterine hyperstimulation after low-dose prostaglandin E_2 therapy: tocolytic treatment in 181 cases. *American Journal of Obstetrics and Gynecology* **163:** 794–796.

Ekman G, Forman A, Marsal K & Ulmsten U (1988) Intravaginal versus intracervical application of prostaglandin E_2 in viscous gel for cervical priming and induction of labor at term in patients with an unfavorable cervical state. *American Journal of Obstetrics and Gynecology* **147:** 657–661.

Friedman EA & Sachtleben MR (1975) Preinduction priming with oral prostaglandin E_2. *American Journal of Obstetrics and Gynecology* **121:** 521–523.

Golbus MS & Creasy RK (1977) Uterine priming with oral prostaglandin E_2 prior to elective induction with oxytocin. *Prostaglandins* **14:** 577–581.

Gordon H (1988) Uterine rupture and its association with oxytocic drugs: the Northwick Park Hospital experience. *Journal of Obstetrics and Gynaecology* **8** (supplement 1): 16–17.

Granström L, Ekman G & Ulmsten U (1990) Myometrial activity after local application of prostaglandin E_2 for cervical ripening and term labor induction. *American Journal of Obstetrics and Gynecology* **162:** 691–694.

Greer IA (1992) Cervical ripening. In Drife JO & Calder AA (eds) *Prostaglandins and the Uterus*, pp 191–205. London: Springer-Verlag.

Greer IA & Calder AA (1989) Pre-induction cervical ripening with extra-amniotic and vaginal prostaglandin E_2. *Journal of Obstetrics and Gynaecology* **10:** 18–22.

Greer IA, McLaren M & Calder AA (1990) Vaginal administration of PGE_2 for induction of labor stimulates endogenous $PGF_{2\alpha}$ production. *Acta Obstetrica et Gynecologica Scandinavica* **69:** 621–625.

Hill NCW & MacKenzie IZ (1989) 2308 second trimester terminations using extraamniotic or intraamniotic prostaglandin E_2: an analysis of efficacy and complications. *British Journal of Obstetrics and Gynaecology* **96:** 1424–1431.

Hill NCW, Selinger M, Ferguson J & MacKenzie IZ (1991) Management of intra-uterine fetal death with vaginal administration of gemeprost or prostaglandin E_2: a random allocation controlled trial. *Journal of Obstetrics and Gynaecology* **11:** 422–426.

Insull GM, Cooke I & MacKenzie IZ (1989) Tocolysis during cervical ripening with vaginal PGE_2. *British Journal of Obstetrics and Gynaecology* **96:** 179–182.

Jaschevatzky OE, Dascalu S, Noy Y, Rosenberg RP, Anderman S & Ballas S (1992) Intrauterine $PGF_{2\alpha}$ infusion for termination of pregnancies with second-trimester rupture of membranes. *Obstetrics and Gynecology* **79:** 32–34.

Kanhai HHH & Keirse MJNC (1989) Induction of labour after fetal death: a randomized controlled trial of two prostaglandin regimens. *British Journal of Obstetrics and Gynaecology* **96:** 1400–1404.

Kanhai HHH & Keirse MJNC (1992) Low dose sulprostone for pregnancy termination in case of fetal abnormality. *Prenatal Diagnosis*. In press.

Karaiskakis PT, Rayburn WF, Smith CV & Woods RE (1991) Failed induction of labor despite sequential prostaglandin E-2 therapy. *American Journal of Perinatology* **8:** 128–130.

Karim SMM & Sharma SD (1971) Oral administration of prostaglandins for the induction of labour. *British Medical Journal* **i:** 260–262.

Karim SMM, Trussell RR, Patel RC & Hillier K (1968) Response of pregnant human uterus to $PGF_{2\alpha}$—induction of labour. *British Medical Journal* **iv:** 621–623.

Keirse MJNC (1990) Clinical use of eicosanoids for cervical ripening before induction of labour. In Mitchell MD (ed.) *Eicosanoids in Reproduction*, pp 223–247. Boca Raton: CRC Press.

Keirse MJNC (1992) Oestrogens for cervical ripening. In Chalmers I (ed.) *Oxford Database of Perinatal Trials*, Version 1.3, Disk Issue 7, Spring 1992, Record 3869. Oxford: Oxford University Press.

Keirse MJNC & Chalmers I (1989) Methods for inducing labour. In Chalmers I, Enkin M & Keirse MJNC (eds) *Effective Care in Pregnancy and Childbirth*, pp 1057–1079. Oxford: Oxford University Press.

Keirse MJNC & Elder MG (1991) *Induction of Labour: Special Issues*, pp 49–52. Amsterdam: Excerpta Medica.

Keirse MJNC & van Oppen ACC (1989a) Preparing the cervix for induction of labour. In Chalmers I, Enkin M & Keirse MJNC (eds) *Effective Care in Pregnancy and Childbirth*, pp 988–1056. Oxford: Oxford University Press.

Keirse MJNC & van Oppen ACC (1989b) Comparison of prostaglandins and oxytocin for inducing labour. In Chalmers I, Enkin M & Keirse MJNC (eds) *Effective Care in Pregnancy and Childbirth*, pp 1080–1111. Oxford: Oxford University Press.

Keirse MJNC, Thiery M, Parewijck W et al (1983) Chronic stimulation of uterine prostaglandin synthesis during cervical ripening before the onset of labor. *Prostaglandins* 25: 671–682.

Keirse MJNC, Kanhai HHH, Verwey RA & Bennebroek Gravenhorst J (1985) European multi-centre trial of intra-cervical PGE_2 in triacetin gel. Report on the Leiden data. In Wood C (ed.) *The Role of Prostaglandins in Labour*, pp 93–100. London: Royal Society of Medicine.

Keirse MJNC, Schulpen MAGT, Corbeij RSACM & Oosterbaan HP (1987) The Dutch experience in cervical ripening with prostaglandin gel. In Keirse MJNC & de Koning Gans HJ (eds) *Priming and Induction of Labour by Prostaglandins 'A State of the Art'*, pp 53–77. Leiden: Boerhaave Committee for Postacademic Medical Education.

Kennedy JH, Stewart P, Barlow DH & Calder AA (1982) Induction of labour: a comparison of a single prostaglandin E_2 vaginal tablet with amniotomy and intravenous oxytocin. *British Journal of Obstetrics and Gynaecology* 89: 704–707.

Khouzam MN & Ledard RS (1990) Difficulties with controlled-release prostaglandin E_2 pessaries. *Lancet* ii: 119.

Kieback DG, Zahradnik HP, Quaas L, Kroner-Fehmel EE & Lippert TH (1986) Clinical evaluation of endocervical prostaglandin PGE_2-triacetin-gel for preinduction cervical softening in pregnant women at term. *Prostaglandins* 32: 81–85.

Kristoffersen M, Sande HA & Sande OS (1986) Ripening of the cervix with prostaglandin E_2-gel. A randomized study with a new ready-to-use compound of triacetin-prostaglandin-E_2-gel. *International Journal of Gynaecology and Obstetrics* 24: 297–300.

Lamont RF (1990) Induction of labour: oxytocin compared with prostaglandins. *Contemporary Reviews in Obstetrics and Gynaecology* 2: 16–20.

Lamont RF, Neave S, Baker AC & Steer PJ (1991) Intrauterine pressures in labours induced by amniotomy and oxytocin or vaginal prostaglandin gel compared with spontaneous labour. *British Journal of Obstetrics and Gynaecology* 98: 441–447.

Laube DW, Zlatnik FJ & Pitkin RM (1986) Preinduction cervical ripening with prostaglandin E_2 intracervical gel. *Obstetrics and Gynecology* 68: 54–57.

Lopes P, Besse O, Sagot P, Dantal F, De Morel P, Panel N & Lerat MF (1991) Effectiveness of prostaglandin E_2 administered on a biodegradable support for cervical ripening and induction of labour. *Journal of Gynecology, Obstetrics and Biology of Reproduction* 20: 827–832.

Lyndrup J, Legarth J, Dàhl C, Philipsen T, Sindberg Eriksen P & Weber T (1990) Induction of labour: The effect of vaginal prostaglandin or i.v. oxytocin—a matter of time only? *European Journal of Obstetrics, Gynecology and Reproductive Biology* 37: 111–119.

MacKenzie I (1991) Prostaglandin induction and the scarred uterus. Data. In Keirse MJNC & Elder MG (eds) *Induction of Labour: Special Issues*, pp 29–39. Amsterdam: Excerpta Medica.

MacKenzie I (1992) Prostaglandins and midtrimester abortion. In Drife JO & Calder AA (eds) *Prostaglandins and the Uterus*, pp 119–133. London: Springer-Verlag.

MacKenzie I & Embrey MP (1977) Cervical ripening with intravaginal prostaglandin PGE_2 gel. *British Medical Journal* ii: 1381–1384.

MacKenzie I & Embrey MP (1979) A comparison of PGE_2 and $PGF_{2\alpha}$ vaginal gel for ripening the cervix before induction of labour. *British Journal of Obstetrics and Gynaecology* 86: 167–170.

MacLennan AH & Green RC (1979) Cervical ripening and induction of labour with intra-vaginal prostaglandin $F_{2\alpha}$. *Lancet* i: 117–119.

MacLennan A, Fraser I, Jakubowicz D, Murray Arthur F, Quinn M & Trudinger B (1989) Labour induction with low dose PGE_2 vaginal gel: result of an Australian multicentre randomized trial. *Australian and New Zealand Journal of Obstetrics and Gynaecology* 29: 124–128.

Mahmood TA (1989) A prospective comparative study on the use of prostaglandin E_2 gel (2 mg) and prostaglandin E_2 tablet (3 mg) for the induction of labour in primigravid women with unfavourable cervices. *European Journal of Obstetrics, Gynecology and Reproductive Biology* 33: 169–175.

Manabe Y, Manabe A & Sagawa N (1982) Stretch-induced cervical softening and initiation of labor at term. A possible correlation with prostaglandins. *Acta Obstetrica et Gynecologica Scandinavica* **61:** 279–280.

Miller AM, Rayburn WF & Smith CV (1991) Patterns of uterine activity after intravaginal prostaglandin E_2 during preindication cervical ripening. *American Journal of Obstetrics and Gynecology* **165:** 1006–1009.

Milliez JM, Jannet D, Touboul C, El Medjadji M & Paniel BJ (1991) Maturation of the uterine cervix by repeated intracervical instillation of prostaglandin E_2. *American Journal of Obstetrics and Gynecology* **165:** 523–528.

Noah ML, De Coster JM, Fraser TJ & Orr JD (1987) Preinduction cervical softening with endocervical PGE_2 gel. *Acta Obstetrica et Gynecologica Scandinavica* **66:** 3–7.

Owen J, Winkler CL, Harris BAJ, Hauth JC & Smith MC (1991) A randomized, double-blind trial of prostaglandin E_2 gel for cervical ripening and meta-analysis. *American Journal of Obstetrics and Gynecology* **165:** 991–996.

Papageorgiou I, Minaretzis D, Tsionou CH & Michalas S (1991) Late midtrimester medical pregnancy terminations: three different procedures with prostaglandin $F_{2\alpha}$ and laminaria tents. *Prostaglandins* **41:** 487–493.

Pearce DJ (1977) Pre-induction priming of the uterine cervix with oral prostaglandin PGE_2 and a placebo. *Prostaglandins* **14:** 571–576.

Peat B (1991) Second trimester abortion by extra-amniotic $PGF_{2\alpha}$ infusion: experience of 178 cases. *Australian and New Zealand Journal of Obstetrics and Gynaecology* **31:** 47–51.

Prasad RNV, Adaikan PG, Arulkumaran S & Ratnam SS (1989) Preinduction cervical priming with PGE_2 vaginal film in primigravidae—a randomised, double blind, placebo controlled study. *Prostaglandins, Leukotrienes and Essential Fatty Acids* **36:** 185–188.

Prins RP, Bolton RN, Mark C, Neilson DR & Watson P (1983) Cervical ripening with intravaginal prostaglandin E_2 gel. *Obstetrics and Gynecology* **61:** 459–462.

Pulle C, Granese D, Panama S & Celona A (1986) Cervical ripening and induction of labour by single intracervical PGE_2 gel application. *Acta Therapeutica* **12:** 5–12.

Rayburn W, Woods R, Eggert J & Ramadei C (1989) Initiation of labor with a moderately favorable cervix: A comparison between prostaglandin E_2 gel and oxytocin. *International Journal of Gynaecology and Obstetrics* **30:** 225–229.

Rayburn WF, Wapner RJ, Barss VA, Spitzberg E, Molina RD, Mandsager N & Yonekura ML (1992) An intravaginal controlled-release prostaglandin E_2 pessary for cervical ripening and initiation of labor at term. *Obstetrics and Gynecology* **79:** 374–379.

Roberts J (1989) Maternal position during the first stage of labour. In Chalmers I, Enkin M & Keirse MJNC (eds) *Effective Care in Pregnancy and Childbirth*, pp 883–892. Oxford: Oxford University Press.

Skajaa K, Mamsen A & Secher NJ (1991) Influence of vehicle form on efficiency of prostaglandin E_2 gel for cervical ripening. *European Journal of Obstetrics, Gynecology and Reproductive Biology* **42:** 177–180.

Smith CV, Rayburn WF, Connor RE, Fredstrom GR & Phillips CB (1990) Double-blind comparison of intravaginal prostaglandin E_2 gel and 'chip' for preinduction cervical ripening. *American Journal of Obstetrics and Gynecology* **163:** 845–847.

Steer PJ, Carter MC, Choong K, Hanson M, Gordon AJ & Pradhan P (1985) A multicentre prospective randomized controlled trial of induction of labour with an automatic closed-loop feedback controlled oxytocin infusion system. *British Journal of Obstetrics and Gynaecology* **92:** 1127–1133.

Stewart P, Kennedy JH, Hillan E & Calder AA (1983) The unripe cervix: management with vaginal or extra-amniotic prostaglandin E_2. *Journal of Obstetrics and Gynaecology* **4:** 90–93.

Taylor AVG, Boland J & MacKenzie IZ (1990a) The concurrent in vitro and in vivo release of PGE_2 from a controlled-release hydrogel polymer pessary for cervical ripening. *Prostaglandins* **40:** 89–98.

Taylor AVG, Boland JC & MacKenzie IZ (1990b) Prostaglandin induced cervical ripening under tocolytic cover in primiparae: results of a double blind placebo controlled trial. *British Journal of Obstetrics and Gynaecology* **97:** 827–831.

Taylor AVG, Boland J, Bernal AL & MacKenzie IZ (1991) Prostaglandin metabolite levels during cervical ripening with a controlled-release hydrogel polymer prostaglandin E_2 pessary. *Prostaglandins* **41:** 585–594.

Thiery M, Decoster JM, Parewijck W, Noah ML, Derom R, Van Kets H, Defoort P, Aertsens

W, Debruyne G, De Geest K & Vandekerckhove F (1984) Endocervical prostaglandin E_2 gel for preinduction cervical softening. *Prostaglandins* **27**: 429–439.

Toplis PJ & Sims CD (1979) Prospective study of different methods and routes of administration of prostaglandin E_2 to improve the unripe cervix. *Prostaglandins* **18**: 127–136.

Trofatter K, Bowers D, Gall SA & Killam AP (1985) Preinduction cervical ripening with prostaglandin E_2 (prepidil) gel. *American Journal of Obstetrics and Gynecology* **153**: 268–271.

Troostwijk AL, Van Veen JBC & Doesburg WH (1992) Pre-induction intracervical application of a highly viscous prostaglandin E_2 gel in pregnant women with an unripe uterine cervix: a double-blind placebo-controlled trial. *European Journal of Obstetrics, Gynecology and Reproductive Biology* **43**: 105–111.

Turnbull AC (1957) Uterine contractions in normal and abnormal labour. *Journal of Obstetrics and Gynaecology of the British Empire* **64**: 321–332.

Ulmsten U, Ekman G, Belfrage P, Bygdeman M & Nyberg C (1985) Intracervical versus intravaginal PGE_2 for induction of labor at term in patients with an unfavorable cervix. *Archives of Gynecology* **236**: 243–248.

Ulstein M, Sagen N & Eikhom SN (1979) A comparative study of labor induced by prostaglandin E_2 and buccal tablets of demoxytocin. *International Journal of Gynaecology and Obstetrics* **17**: 243–245.

Valentine BH (1977) Intravenous oxytocin and oral prostaglandin E_2 for ripening of the unfavourable cervix. *British Journal of Obstetrics and Gynaecology* **84**: 846–854.

Weiss RR, Tejani N, Israeli I, Evans MI, Bhakthavathsalan A & Mann LI (1975) Priming of the uterine cervix with oral prostaglandin E_2 in the term multigravida. *Obstetrics and Gynecology* **46**: 181–184.

Wilson PD (1978) A comparison of four methods of ripening the unfavourable cervix. *British Journal of Obstetrics and Gynaecology* **85**: 941–944.

Wingerup L, Andersson KE & Ulmsten U (1978) Ripening of the uterine cervix and induction of labour at term with prostaglandin E_2 in viscous gel. *Acta Obstetrica et Gynecologica Scandinavica* **57**: 403–406.

Witter FR, Rocco LE & Johnson RB (1992) A randomized trial of prostaglandin E_2 in a controlled-release vaginal pessary for cervical ripening at term. *American Journal of Obstetrics and Gynecology* **166**: 830–834.

Yonekura ML, Songster G & Smith-Wallace T (1985) Preinduction cervical priming with PGE_2 intracervical gel. *American Journal of Perinatology* **2**: 305–310.

Zanini A, Ghidini A, Norchi S, Beretta E, Cortinovis I & Bottino S (1990) Pre-induction cervical ripening with prostaglandin E_2 gel: intracervical versus intravaginal route. *Obstetrics and Gynecology* **76**: 681–683.

7

The role of prostaglandins in obstetrical disorders

OLAVI YLIKORKALA
LASSE VIINIKKA

INTRODUCTION

Pregnancy and parturition are characterized by extensive changes in maternal physiology including, for example, cardiovascular adaptation to the appearance of a new circulatory organ, the placenta, which receives one-fifth of the maternal minute volume during the last weeks of gestation, and to the huge growth of the uterus to permit the development and growth of the placenta and fetus. During pregnancy, the smooth muscle cells, whether in blood vessels or in the uterus, are relaxed, whereas during parturition the cells in the myometrium exhibit rhythmic contractions. If maternal adaptation fails or remains deficient, various complications of pregnancy may ensue. How is this regulated? Maternal adaptation to pregnancy requires several endocrine and humoral factors, among which the rapidly released and promptly acting prostaglandins are an important group.

NORMAL PREGNANCY

Of the large prostaglandin family, compounds of the D, E or F series, or the vasodilator, platelet antiaggregatory compound prostacyclin (prostaglandin I_2, PGI_2) and its endogenous antagonist, the vasoconstrictor, platelet pro-aggregatory compound thromboxane A_2 (TXA_2) have been most often studied in relation to pregnancy. These are all produced through the metabolism of arachidonic acid via the cyclooxygenase pathway, whereas leukotrienes, which are produced via the lipoxygenase pathway, have been studied less in pregnancy.

Intrauterine tissues, especially the placenta, produce huge amounts of classic prostaglandins of the D, E and F series. Despite this fact, concentrations of prostaglandins in maternal plasma increase only moderately, if at all, with advancing gestational age (e.g. see Friedman, 1988; Noort, 1989; Erwich, 1991). This may either mean that prostaglandins are not released from fetoplacental tissues to the maternal compartment, or, more likely, that rises in circulating prostaglandin levels cannot be detected due to methodological problems involved with the measurement of prostaglandins in plasma. Prostaglandin metabolites are assayable in urine, and increase during pregnancy, possibly reflecting renal prostaglandin production.

Because changes in vascular or platelet behaviour are associated with many pregnancy disorders the role of the most vasoactive and platelet-active compounds, PGI_2 and TXA_2, in regard to the initiation of complications of pregnancy, may be more important than that of other prostaglandins. These prostanoids, or their balance, is probably of greatest significance in the regulation of blood circulation and coagulation.

All intrauterine pregnancy-associated tissues produce PGI_2 and TXA_2 in vitro (see Ylikorkala and Mäkilä, 1985), although placental capacity to produce PGI_2 seems to be a controversial issue (see Erwich, 1991). The exact source of fetoplacental PGI_2/TXA_2 is not known but, since PGI_2 is the main product of endothelial cells, we may assume that PGI_2 originates mainly from the blood vessels of pregnancy tissues. Platelets are the main source of TXA_2 in vivo, and contaminating platelets may have been one source of TXA_2 in in vitro experiments involving various fetoplacental tissues. However, since non-vascular amnion also produces both these compounds (see Ylikorkala and Mäkilä, 1985), it is evident that in the tissues of pregnancy, some extravascular and extraplatelet apparatus for the synthesis of PGI_2 and TXA_2 exists.

Contradictory data exist as to the concentrations of the metabolites of PGI_2 and TXA_2 in maternal plasma (see Ylikorkala and Mäkilä, 1985; Friedman, 1988; Fitzgerald and FitzGerald, 1990; Erwich, 1991), a problem which, at least partly, is due to analytical difficulties. The increased concentration of TXB_2 (a metabolite of TXA_2) in serum (Ylikorkala and Viinikka, 1980) suggests that during pregnancy the capacity of platelets to produce TXA_2 increases. This may also explain the findings that urinary excretion of TXA_2 metabolites increases two- to five-fold during pregnancy, most of this rise coming from platelets (Ylikorkala et al, 1986a; Fitzgerald et al, 1987a,b, 1990). Urinary excretion of PGI_2 metabolites increases even more (five- to eight-fold) than does TXA_2 (Ylikorkala et al, 1986a; Fitzgerald et al, 1987a). Thus, during normal pregnancy there is a predominance of vasodilatory PGI_2 which contributes to low vascular resistance and to a fall in blood pressure. This may also diminish the vascular response to angiotensin II and perhaps also to other vasoconstrictors (Everett et al, 1978; Mastrogiannis et al, 1991).

Since an adequate blood flow is essential for normal fetal development, much attention has been focused on the role of PGI_2 and TXA_2 in flow regulation. As regards PGI_2 in the regulation of blood flow in pregnancy, no correlation was found between the concentrations of the metabolites of PGI_2 in the maternal circulation and the blood flow in the placenta or umbilical vessels (Ylikorkala et al, 1983, 1984). The opposite was also found: the production of PGI_2 by the umbilical artery ex vivo correlated with umbilical flow, as assessed by Doppler measurement before labour (Mäkilä et al, 1983). Moreover, high placental flow was associated with high PGI_2 and low TXA_2 production ex vivo by placental pieces (Mäkilä et al, 1986). These data strongly suggest that placental PGI_2 and TXA_2 production serves as an important regulator of the fetal blood supply.

PRE-ECLAMPSIA

Pre-eclampsia, which has been known for more than 4000 years (Griffith, 1893), is still one of the major pregnancy complications; it occurs in 7% of primigravidae, and recurs in 25% of affected cases (see Rubin and Horn, 1988; Lindheimer and Katz, 1989). Pre-eclampsia is characterized by one or more changes such as maternal vasoconstriction, elevated blood pressure, microthrombosis, oedema and proteinuria. In light of this it is understandable that the blood flow in the fetoplacental unit tends to decrease and, as a result, intrauterine fetal growth retardation (IUGR) is common in babies born to pre-eclamptic women.

These pre-eclamptic signs and symptoms are precisely those which could be expected if the balance between PGI_2 and TXA_2 was shifted towards the dominance of the latter. Much attention has therefore been focused on possible changes in their production in pre-eclampsia.

At the beginning of the 1980s, data accumulated rapidly on decreased in vitro PGI_2 production by intrauterine tissues of pre-eclamptic patients (Bussolino et al, 1980; Downing et al, 1980; Remuzzi et al, 1980). The first in vivo results demonstrated in amniotic fluid the reduction of PGI_2-like biological activity and decreased concentration of 6-keto-$PGF_{1\alpha}$, the non-enzymatic metabolite of PGI_2 (Bodzenta et al, 1980; Ylikorkala et al, 1981a). At the moment there is a consensus of opinion that fetoplacental PGI_2 production is lower in pre-eclampsia.

The data on maternal PGI_2 production were for a long time less conclusive—partly due to the uncertainties of the measurement of PGI_2 production in vivo. With the advent of reliable measurement of maternal systemic production of PGI_2, i.e. the measurement of urinary 2,3-dinor-6-keto-$PGF_{1\alpha}$, it has become evident that PGI_2 deficiency also occurs in pre-eclamptic mothers (Ylikorkala et al, 1986b; Fitzgerald et al, 1987a). This decreased excretion of PGI_2 metabolites may even precede the appearance of the clinical signs of pre-eclampsia (Fitzgerald et al, 1987a). We must, however, remember that, even if the excretion of PGI_2 metabolites by the pre-eclamptic mother is lower, we do not know whether this reflects decreased PGI_2 production in maternal or in fetoplacental tissues. The early finding that dermal PGI_2 production also decreases in pre-eclamptic mothers (Bussolino et al, 1980) suggests, however, that maternal PGI_2 production may be diminished. There is also a theory that in pre-eclamptic pregnancies leukotrienes possibly in excess in pregnancy-associated tissues could inhibit PGI_2 synthesis (Turk et al, 1980; Saeed and Mitchell, 1983).

Among other theories, increased lipid peroxidation (see Broughton-Pipkin, 1990; Wisdom et al, 1991), or even increased progesterone production in pre-eclampsia (Walsh and Coulter, 1989), have been suggested as the reason for decreased PGI_2 production. In addition, precursor fatty acids may have a role in the regulation of PGI_2 production. Eicosapentaenoic acid (EPA) may replace arachidonic acid in the prostanoid synthesis cascade (see Chapter 1). This leads to the formation of biologically active PGI_3 but inactive TXA_3, i.e. to the dominance of vasodilation and platelet anti-aggregatory activity, which should restrict the development of pre-eclampsia.

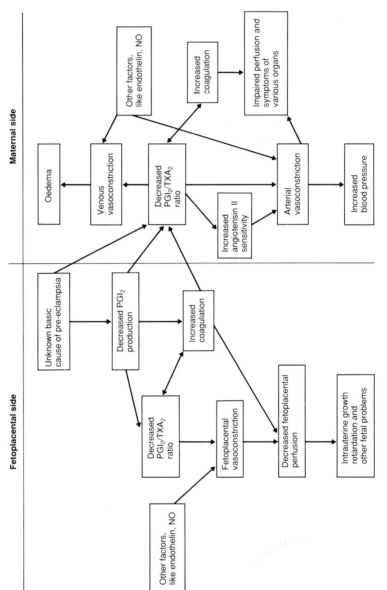

Figure 1. The role of PGI_2 and TXA_2 as well as of related factors in the aetiology of pre-eclampsia. NO, nitric oxide.

The diet of Eskimos is rich in EPA, and among them pre-eclampsia is a very rare disease (Dyerberg and Bang, 1985). Experimental data show that dietary supplementation with EPA and docosahexaenoic acid lowers blood pressure in patients with essential hypertension (Bønaa et al, 1990), which would also support this view. At present, the realistic conclusion is, however, that we do not know whether PGI_2 deficiency is a primary change or is secondary to faulty development of spiral arteries or to endothelial cell injury (Musci et al, 1988; Roberts et al, 1989). It may further be possible that not only PGI_2 but also other vasoactive agents, such as vasoconstrictory endothelin, contribute to the development of vascular changes characteristic of pre-eclampsia, perhaps in concert with prostaglandin changes (Mitchell et al, 1990; Mastrogiannis et al, 1991; Myatt et al, 1991).

Increase in TXA_2 production would also favour coagulation and vaso-constriction, i.e. the typical symptoms of pre-eclampsia. The data on TXA_2 production in pre-eclampsia are more scanty, but there are findings suggesting increased production of TXA_2 in pre-eclamptic women. The authors showed that placentae of pre-eclamptic or hypertensive women produce increased amounts of TXB_2 in vitro (Mäkilä et al, 1984a), but that the mean urinary excretion of TXB_2 is normal (Ylikorkala et al, 1986b). In another study, the excretion of the other two TXA_2 metabolites, 2,3-dinor-TXB_2 and 11-dehydro-TXB_2, shows very large variations, but both are clearly higher in pre-eclamptic patients (Fitzgerald et al, 1990). It is obvious that an increase in TXA_2 production is largely dependent on the degree of platelet activation. Moreover, the platelet-inhibitory activity in serum is reduced in pre-eclampsia (Benedetto et al, 1989).

The biochemical chain leading to pre-eclampsia is summarized in Figure 1. For some unknown reason, fetoplacental PGI_2 production is deficient. This results in a low PGI_2/TXA_2 ratio, which in turn leads to vaso-constriction, decreased umbilical–placental blood flow and IUGR. It also results in increased platelet aggregation with consequent TXA_2 release, which further decreases the PGI_2/TXA_2 ratio. This triggers additional platelet aggregation and excess TXA_2 production also on the maternal side with increased coagulation and vasoconstriction. It is possible that the fetoplacental unit produces a humoral compound which goes to the mother and inhibits PGI_2 production; the character of this possible PGI_2-inhibitory factor is not known. It may be possible that not only PGI_2 and TXA_2 but also other vasoactive agents, such as vasoconstrictory endothelin (Lindblom et al, 1991; Mitchell et al, 1990; Mastrogiannis et al, 1991; Myatt et al, 1991) or nitric oxide (a vasodilator) (see Moncada et al, 1991; Myatt et al, 1992), contribute to the development of vascular changes characteristic of pre-eclampsia, perhaps in concert with prostaglandins.

Some attempts have been made to treat pre-eclampsia with PGI_2 infusions (Fidler et al, 1980; Lewis et al, 1981; Jouppila et al, 1985a). Exogenous PGI_2 has led to a fall in blood pressure and to flushing, but it failed to improve the fetoplacental blood flow. Thus, it seems unlikely that PGI_2 infusions could be applicable in the treatment of pre-eclampsia, although the existing data are insufficient for final conclusions. It is also noteworthy that not only PGI_2 but also infusions of PGA_1 have been used to control the blood pressure of pre-eclamptic mothers in early labour (Toppozada et al, 1988, 1991).

IDIOPATHIC FETAL GROWTH RETARDATION

Fetal growth is under genetic and hormonal control; it is also dependent on placental transfer of oxygen and nutrients, all of which require adequate blood circulation in the placenta and fetus. IUGR is often associated with maternal hypertensive pregnancy complications, and therefore it may be a result of occlusive vascular changes in the placenta. However, IUGR may occur also in normotensive pregnancies of healthy women. We may thus ask if the role of vasoactive prostaglandins in the placenta and/or fetus is important in idiopathic IUGR.

It is indeed known that the conversion of exogenous arachidonic acid to PGI_2 is reduced in the umbilical arteries of IUGR fetuses (Stuart et al, 1981). Furthermore, cultured placental cells from pregnancies complicated by IUGR release decreased amounts of PGI_2 (Jogee et al, 1983), and maternal platelet TXA_2 production is enhanced in normotensive pregnancies with IUGR fetuses (Wallenburg and Rotmans, 1982). On the other hand, the concentrations of 6-keto-$PGF_{1\alpha}$ and TXA_2 in amniotic fluid (Ylikorkala et al, 1981a) and the production of PGI_2 by the umbilical artery (Mäkilä et al, 1984b) have been normal in pregnancies complicated by idiopathic IUGR. Thus, PGI_2 deficiency may not be as uniform a finding in pregnancies with IUGR as in pre-eclampsia. The fact that small doses of aspirin accelerate fetal growth, as summarized in Chapter 9, provides further evidence that idiopathic IUGR may be a result of relative PGI_2 deficiency.

Fetal growth retardation often accompanies various fetal chromosomal aberrations like trisomy 21, and, curiously, PGI_2 production by pieces of umbilical artery is lower in Down's syndrome (Mäkilä et al, 1985). In this special case the PGI_2 deficiency might be due to increased peroxide production as a result of over expression of superoxide dismutase, the gene of which is located on chromosome 21 (Antila and Westermarck, 1989).

LUPUS ANTICOAGULANT SYNDROME IN PREGNANCY

Systemic lupus erythematosus (SLE) doubles the risk of such pregnancy complications as spontaneous abortions, thromboembolism, IUGR and stillbirths (see Hadi and Treadwell, 1990; Lubbe and Pattison, 1991). The mechanism of these complications has been poorly understood but seems to be related to the presence of phospholipid antibodies, which can be detected functionally by the lupus anticoagulant test or immunologically (Hadi and Treadwell, 1990). In patients with SLE, the frequency of lupus anticoagulant is 6–10% and that of cardiolipin antibody 20–50% (Love and Santaro, 1990; Orvieto et al, 1991); the large variation in these figures may reflect lack of a proper standardization of tests.

The mechanism by which lupus anticoagulant or phospholipid antibodies threaten the outcome of pregnancy may involve the PGI_2/TXA_2 balance. Lupus anticoagulant decreases the production of PGI_2 by incubated endothelial cells or myometrium in vitro (Carreras and Vermylen, 1982;

Spitz et al, 1984; Lubbe and Pattison, 1991), perhaps by preventing the release of phospholipids from the cell membranes. Lupus anticoagulant may also trigger platelet aggregation by enhancing the synthesis of platelet-activating factor (Silver et al, 1991). These numerous findings imply that pregnancies in women with SLE may be associated with a deficiency of PGI_2, and, therefore, TXA_2 dominance prevails (DeWolf et al, 1982; Orvieto et al, 1991). With the large body of in vitro data as background, it is of interest to note that the imbalance between PGI_2 and TXA_2 is also present in vivo; the excretion of PGI_2 metabolites was only moderately reduced, but that of TXA_2 metabolites increased approximately two-fold in SLE patients with phospholipid antibodies (R. Kaaja et al, personal communication). Therefore, it comes as no surprise that small doses of

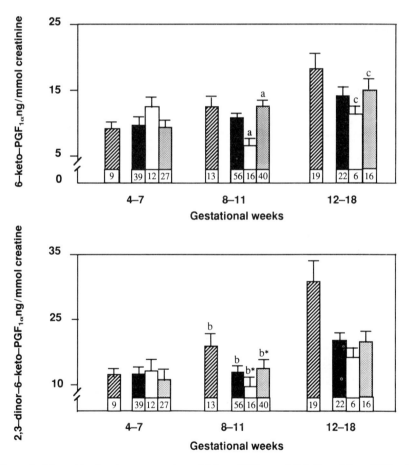

Figure 2. Mean ($\pm$ SE) urinary excretion of 6-keto-$PGF_{1\alpha}$ and 2,3-dinor-6-keto-$PGF_{1\alpha}$ in women with a history of RSA and in healthy control women. The number of samples is given at the bottom of the bars. ▨, control women; ■, RSA women; □, RSA (ending in abortion); ▨, RSA (going to term); a vs a = $p < 0.001$; b vs b and b* vs b* = $p < 0.01$; c vs c = $p < 0.05$. Reproduced with permission from Tulppala et al (1991).

aspirin, which correct this imbalance (see Chapter 9), improve the pregnancy outcome in SLE patients (Elder et al, 1988; Hadi and Treadwell, 1990; Lubbe and Pattison, 1991).

RECURRENT SPONTANEOUS ABORTION

Between 12 and 15% of clinically confirmed pregnancies abort spontaneously. Accordingly, the statistical probability of a woman's experiencing three consecutive miscarriages, namely recurrent spontaneous abortion (RSA), is between 0.2 and 0.3%. The real frequency, however, amounts to 0.4–0.9% of all detected pregnancies, suggesting that RSA is a clinical entity of its

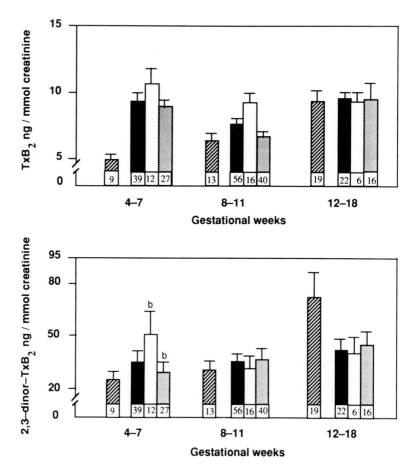

Figure 3. Mean ($\pm$ SE) urinary excretion of TXB_2 and 2,3-dinor-TXB_2 in women with a history of RSA and in healthy control women. The number of samples is given at the bottom of the bars. See Figure 2 for an explanation of the symbols. b vs b = $p < 0.05$. Reproduced with permission from Tulppala et al (1991).

own. The causes of RSA are largely unknown (Stirrat, 1990), but the presence of microthrombosis, vasospastic changes and necrosis in placentas of women with RSA (Rushton, 1988) and the frequent occurrence of endogenous anticoagulants suggest that changes in production of vasoactive and platelet-active prostaglandins may play a part in RSA. Some in vitro evidence suggests the presence of PGI_2 deficiency and/or TXA_2 dominance in doomed pregnancies in women with RSA and phospholipid antibodies or lupus anticoagulant (see Orvieto et al, 1991). Tulppala et al (1991) reported on 22 women with a history of RSA but without circulating anticoagulant who had a lower ratio of PGI_2 to TXA_2 between weeks 4 and 7 of gestation and a lower output of 2,3-dinor-6-keto-$PGF_{1\alpha}$ between weeks 8 and 11 (Figures 2 and 3). That these changes could perhaps be of significance as a cause of RSA is suggested by the finding that alterations to the PGI_2/TXA_2 ratio were more profound in pregnant women whose pregnancies ended in abortion (Tulppala et al, 1991). If these data are confirmed, a placebo-controlled trial is warranted with a low dose of aspirin involving women with a history of RSA but without detectable anticoagulants or phospholipid antibodies.

PRETERM LABOUR

Several maternal factors (for instance poor socioeconomic conditions, young age, short stature) and fetoplacental causes (IUGR, multiple pregnancy, placenta previa, premature rupture of membranes, etc.) predispose women to the occurrence of preterm birth (Keirse et al, 1989). Yet no risk factors are identifiable in 40–50% of preterm births (see Alexander and Keirse, 1989). At least in these cases of idiopathic preterm labour we may assume that the biochemical mechanisms responsible for uterine quiescence have failed or those responsible for initiation of labour have become activated too early. Because prostaglandins, alone or in conjunction with oxytocin, are important in the onset and progress of labour at term (Fuchs et al, 1982a,b; Fuchs and Fuchs, 1984; Casey and MacDonald, 1988; Noort, 1989), their role in preterm labour warrants a closer look.

Increased concentrations of prostaglandins or their metabolites have frequently been reported in maternal plasma (Sellers et al, 1981; Fuchs et al, 1982b; Weitz et al, 1986) or amniotic fluid (Romero et al, 1987a, 1989a) of women judged to be in preterm labour. The rises are, however, smaller than during full-term labour (see Chapter 4). Moreover, in term and preterm labour the lipoxygenase pathway is stimulated, as is evident from elevations of leukotriene levels in amniotic fluid (Romero et al, 1989b) or from elevations in leukotrienes in umbilical plasma during labour (Pasetto et al, 1989). However, the question has remained open of whether the stimulation of arachidonic acid metabolism in labour (either via the cyclooxygenase or the lipoxygenase pathway) is a primary change—and a cause for preterm labour—or a secondary change reflecting stimulation of prostaglandin production by the decidua, placenta and fetal membranes. Interestingly, chorion, which lies between the amnion and the decidua, is the major determinant of the rate of metabolism of PGE_2 in the fetoplacental unit (Sullivan et al, 1991). In any case, suppression of prostaglandin synthesis by cyclooxygenase inhibitors provides one of the most effective tocolytics available in clinical routine (see Chapter 9).

Vasoactive PGI_2 and TXA_2 have also been studied in relation to preterm or full-term birth. In vitro PGI_2 relaxes and TXA_2 contracts the human myometrium (Wilhelmsson et al, 1981). PGI_2 production increases during human full-term parturition, as seen from the rise in 6-keto-$PGF_{1\alpha}$ levels in maternal plasma and urine (Ylikorkala et al, 1981b, 1986b) or amniotic fluid (Mitchell ct al, 1979; Mäkäräinen and Ylikorkala, 1984). During labour TXB_2 levels also rise in amniotic fluid (Mäkäräinen and Ylikorkala, 1984). Abdominal delivery is also followed by rises in PGI_2 and TXA_2 metabolites in maternal plasma (Ylikorkala et al, 1982). Noort (1989) found an increased amount of urinary TXB_2 in all women in imminent preterm labour, these rises being highest in women who progressed to preterm birth. It was thus proposed that urinary TXB_2 assessment could have clinical value in predicting the outcome of tocolysis. In recent work it was found that urinary PGI_2 metabolite output is also elevated in preterm labour, but less than the rise in TXA_2 metabolites. Neither of these elevations predicted the outcome of tocolysis (Kurki et al, 1992).

Besides the baseline production of PGI_2 and TXA_2 in preterm labour, changes in their quantity during and following different tocolytic regimens have also been studied. Maternal indomethacin, which may be a more effective tocolytic than any betamimetic (Besinger and Niebyl, 1990; Kurki et al, 1991), decreases the production of both PGI_2 and TXA_2, but the TXA_2 suppression is more marked and lasts longer (Kurki et al, 1992). No consistent effect of betamimetics on PGI_2 and TXA_2 production were found (Jouppila et al, 1985b; Kurki et al, 1992).

In view of the significant role of PGI_2 in ductal patency (Mitchell, 1986; Walsh, 1990), and of the fact that indomethacin is readily transported through the placenta to the fetus (Moise et al, 1990), suppression of PGI_2 production during maternal indomethacin intake (Kurki et al, 1992) may provide an explanation why maternal indomethacin may cause a transient constriction of ductus arteriosus (Moise et al, 1988). That betamimetic administration did not cause even transient ductal constriction (Eronen et al, 1991) is in harmony with the absence of any effect of betamimetics on PGI_2 production.

Recent interest has focused largely on silent infection in the maternal genital tract as a cause of preterm birth (see Romero and Mazor, 1988; Armer and Duff, 1991). There is indeed evidence that approximately 20% of preterm births occur in women with microbial invasion of the amniotic cavity (see Romero and Mazor, 1988). Bacteria can reach the amniotic cavity from the vagina and cervix, and a two- to three-fold excess of pathological bacteria has been encountered in these sites in women with established preterm labour and/or premature rupture of the membranes (Gravett et al, 1986; Martius et al, 1988; Romero and Mazor, 1988). Infection could trigger uterine contractions through the release of prostaglandins or leukotrienes in the decidua, fetal membranes or adjacent tissues

(Lamont et al, 1985; Bennett et al, 1987a,b; Romero et al, 1987a,b). Cytokines may have an important mediator role: an increasing amount of data suggests that increased production of many of the cytokines is implicated in term and preterm labour (Romero et al, 1991a; Santhanam et al, 1991). Interleukin-1_β (IL-1_β), IL-6 and tumour necrosis factor (TNF) will activate cyclooxygenase in decidual stromal cells and lead to increased prostaglandin production (Khan et al, 1992). Interestingly, the systemic administration of IL-1 induced preterm labour and delivery in all mice so treated (Romero et al, 1991b), and the effect of interleukins may well be prostaglandin mediated. Also of interest are the recent findings that endothelin-1,2 levels are increased in the amniotic fluid of women with preterm labour and microbial invasion of the amniotic cavity (Romero et al, 1992).

POST-TERM PREGNANCY AND LABOUR DYSFUNCTION

The onset of human labour at term or preterm depends on excess availability of prostaglandins in some, or perhaps in all, pregnancy-associated tissues; this change seems to be more a result of increased production than of decreased catabolism (see Fuchs and Fuchs, 1984; Casey and MacDonald, 1988; Noort, 1989). In spite of this, endogenous prostaglandins in post-term pregnancies have not been studied. The fact that women taking large doses of aspirin for rheumatoid arthritis are likely to carry their pregnancies post-term (Lewis and Schulman, 1973) strongly suggests the role of prostaglandin deficiency in post-term pregnancies. The lack of studies on prostaglandins in prolonged pregnancies may have been due in the past to uncertainties about gestational ages (see Bakketeig and Bergsjö, 1989) but, nowadays, the availability of accurate assessment of gestational age by ultrasound has made such studies possible. It is not inconceivable that suppression of production or acceleration of catabolism of prostaglandins could be detected in ultrasonographically verified post-term pregnancies. The fact that post-term pregnancy has a tendency to reoccur (see Bakketeig and Bergsjö, 1989) hints at the possibility that certain women possess a biochemical aberration affecting arachidonic acid metabolism. It is also possible that disturbances in prostaglandins could cause some other labour complications such as prolongation of latent or active phases or too vigorous contractions (see Crowther et al, 1989), although no real data exist to support this view.

POLY- AND OLIGOHYDRAMNIO

Because the amount of amniotic fluid varies greatly in normal pregnancy, diagnosis of poly- and oligohydramnio, even if ultrasound examination is available, is often uncertain. Regulation of the amount of amniotic fluid is poorly understood, but it is evident that fetal urination and swallowing as well as the fetal skin and membranes play important roles (Lind et al, 1972;

Kirshon, 1989; Rabinowiz et al, 1989). Poly- and oligohydramnio may be associated with gross structural and functional abnormalities in the fetus, but may also be present in healthy fetuses. Because prostaglandins may participate in the regulation of renal function, and because they are also present in amniotic fluid, changes in prostaglandins could contribute to the development of poly- and oligohydramnio.

There are no direct measurements of prostaglandins in pregnancies complicated by abnormalities in the volume of amniotic fluid. Yet the fact that maternal indomethacin administration for prevention of preterm births can sometimes be associated with a reduction of amniotic fluid volume (Cantor et al, 1980; Itskovitz et al, 1980; DeWitt et al, 1988; Hendricks et al, 1990) strongly suggests that prostaglandins are involved in the control of the volume of amniotic fluid. Indomethacin-induced reduction of amniotic fluid volume has been utilized clinically for treatment of at least 31 cases with severe symptomatic polyhydramnios (Cabrol et al, 1987; Kirshon et al, 1990; Mamopoulos et al, 1990); in the majority of cases this treatment has decreased the volume of amniotic fluid, or at least prevented further increase in the volume. Because maternal indomethacin readily passes through the placenta (Moise et al, 1990), it is presumed that indomethacin reduces amniotic fluid volume primarily by inhibiting fetal prostaglandins. It probably affects the function of the fetal kidneys and, evidently, the resultant decrease in fetal urine output is one of the most important mechanisms. The coincidental vasoconstrictor effect on the fetal cerebral circulation is a potential cause for concern. However, there is at present no evidence of damage to the fetus.

SMOKING AND ALCOHOL ABUSE

Maternal smoking and alcoholism are among the most common exogenous causes of fetal hazards and mortality today. The mechanism of these risks is not understood, but may involve vasoactive prostaglandins. As regards smoking, this hypothesis is supported by diminished PGI_2 production by the umbilical arteries of the babies of mothers who smoke (Dadak et al, 1981; Busacca et al, 1982) and by the fact that smoking decreases the excretion of PGI_2 metabolite (Nadler et al, 1983). Moreover, smoking increased the ability of platelets to produce TXA_2 (Toivanen et al, 1986). We do not, however, know which constituent of cigarette smoke causes these effects; data on the effect of nicotine on the production of PGI_2 by umbilical arteries are controversial (Stoel et al, 1982; Ylikorkala et al, 1985; Jeremy et al, 1985). Possible TXA_2 stimulation by smoking may not be nicotine-dependent, since the effect was not seen after pipe smoking (Toivanen et al, 1986). By some means, smoking may well shift the balance between PGI_2 and TXA_2 to predominance of the latter and thereby reduce the fetal growth.

Maternal-alcohol-induced fetal damage may result from changes in prostaglandins. This is supported, for example, by the fact that ethanol stimulates PGE synthesis in malformed embryonic hens (Pennington et al, 1985) and that aspirin reduces alcohol-induced damage in mice (Randall and Anton, 1984). Ethanol is known to inhibit production of TXA_2 by platelets from non-pregnant subjects (Kontula et al, 1982; Toivanen et al, 1983), and in fetal tissues ethanol inhibits in vitro production of both TXA_2 and PGI_2 from endogenous substrate but stimulates production from exogenous arachidonic acid (Ylikorkala et al, 1987). Thus, ethanol may inhibit phospholipase A_2, but in the arachidonic acid cascade may stimulate the enzymes distal to it. In pregnant alcohol-drinkers the excretion of metabolites of PGI_2 and TXA_2 increased, the latter more than the former, but these changes were not clearly associated with the development of fetal alcohol effects (Ylikorkala et al, 1988). In their neonates, however, TXA_2 dominance was seen only in those babies who clearly exhibited alcohol effects (Ylikorkala et al, 1988). In conclusion, ethanol certainly affects the prostaglandin system in pregnancy, but a firm cause-and-effect relationship between prostaglandins and alcohol-induced fetal effects in humans has yet to be substantiated.

SUMMARY AND CONCLUSIONS

All pregnancy-associated tissues are capable of producing prostaglandins including PGI_2 and TXA_2. In normal pregnancy there is a dominance of PGI_2 over TXA_2 which may contribute to the maternal circulatory adaptation to pregnancy. Furthermore, both fetoplacental PGI_2 and TXA_2 production are important regulators of the fetal blood supply. It has been clearly established that in pre-eclampsia PGI_2 production decreases in the fetoplacental tissues and quite probably also in the maternal tissues. The effect of this change may be further exaggerated by the simultaneous stimulation in pre-eclampsia of TXA_2 production. The reason for PGI_2 deficiency is not known. Other vasoactive agents, such as endothelin, may act in concert with prostaglandins. Relative PGI_2 deficiency is likely to exist also in IUGR and lupus anti-coagulant syndrome of pregnancy. In the latter, lupus anticoagulant may directly inhibit the synthesis of PGI_2. One study suggests PGI_2 deficiency also in early pregnancies of women with a history of repeated abortions. Prostaglandin production increases during full-term labour, and similar but smaller changes also occur in preterm labour. A silent bacterial infection may trigger the onset of preterm labour through cytokine-stimulated increase of prostaglandin production.

No data were found on prostaglandin production in post-term pregnancies. That oligo-polyhydramnios is possibly prostaglandin mediated is suggested by the control of polyhydramnios by indomethacin treatment. Smoking decreases the production of PGI_2 and possibly increases that of TXA_2, which may lead to decreased blood flow and IUGR. Which constituent of cigarette smoke exerts this effect is not known. Ethanol consumption causes aberrations in prostaglandin metabolism which cannot be directly connected with fetal alcohol effects.

REFERENCES

Alexander S & Keirse MJNC (1989) Formal risk scoring during pregnancy. In Chalmers I, Enkin M & Keirse MJNC (eds) *Effective Care in Pregnancy and Childbirth*, 1st edn, pp 345–365. Oxford: Oxford University Press.

Antila E & Westermarck T (1989) On the etiopathogenesis and therapy of Down syndrome. *International Journal of Developmental Biology* **33:** 183–188.

Armer TL & Duff P (1991) Intra-amniotic infection in patients with intact membranes and preterm labour. *Obstetrical and Gynecological Survey* **46:** 589–593.

Bakketeig L & Bergsjö P (1989) Post-term pregnancy: magnitude of the problem. In Chalmers I, Enkin M & Keirse MJNC (eds) *Effective Care in Pregnancy and Childbirth* 1st Edition, pp 765–775. Oxford: Oxford University Press.

Benedetto C, Massobrio M, Bertini E et al (1989) Reduced serum inhibition of platelet-activating factor in pre-eclampsia. *American Journal of Obstetrics and Gynecology* **160:** 100–104.

Bennett PR, Elder MG & Myatt L (1987a) The effects of lipoxygenase metabolites of arachidonic acid on human myometrial contractility. *Prostaglandins* **33:** 837–844.

Bennett PR, Rose MP, Myatt L & Elder MG (1987b) Preterm labor: stimulation of arachidonic acid metabolism in human amnion cells by bacterial products. *American Journal of Obstetrics and Gynecology* **156:** 649–655.

Besinger RE & Niebyl JR (1990) The safety and efficacy of tocolytic agents for the treatment of preterm labour. *Obstetrical Gynecological Survey* **45:** 415–440.

Bodzenta A, Thompson JM & Poller L (1980) Prostacyclin activity in amniotic fluid in pre-eclampsia. *Lancet* **ii:** 650.

Bønaa KH, Bjerve KS, Straume B et al (1990) Effect of eicosapentaenoic and docosahexanoic acids on blood pressure in hypertension. *New England Journal of Medicine* **322:** 795–801.

Broughton-Pipkin I (1990) Essential fatty acids and pregnancy hypertension. In Horrobin DF (ed.) *Omega-6-essential Fatty Acids. Pathophysiology and Roles in Clinical Medicine*, pp 173–186. New-York: Wiley-Liss.

Busacca M, Dejana E, Balconi G et al (1982) Reduced prostacyclin production by cultured endothelial cells from umbilical arteries of babies born to women who smoke. *Lancet* **ii:** 609–610.

Bussolino E, Benedetto C, Massobrio M et al (1980) Maternal vascular prostacyclin activity in preeclampsia. *Lancet* **ii:** 702.

Cabrol D, Landesman R, Muller J et al (1987) Treatment of polyhydramnios with prosta-glandin synthetase inhibitor (indomethacin). *American Journal of Obstetrics and Gynecology* **157:** 422–426.

Cantor B, Tyler T, Nelson RM & Stein GH (1980) Oligohydramnios and transient neonatal anuria: a possible association with the maternal use of prostaglandin synthetase inhibitors. *Journal of Reproductive Medicine* **24:** 220–223.

Carreras LO & Vermylen JG (1982) 'Lupus' anticoagulant and thrombosis—possible role in inhibition of prostacyclin formation. *Thrombosis and Haemostasis* **48:** 38–40.

Casey ML & MacDonald PL (1988) Biomolecular process in the initiation of parturition decidual activation. *Clinical Obstetrics and Gynecology* **31:** 533–552.

Crowther C, Enkin M, Keirse MJNC & Brow I (1989) Monitoring the progress of labour. In Chalmers I, Enkin, M & Keirse MJNC (eds) *Effective Care in Pregnancy and Childbirth* 1st Edition, pp 833–845. Oxford: Oxford University Press.

Dadak CH, Leithner CH, Sinzinger H & Silberbauer K (1981) Diminished prostacyclin formation in umbilical arteries of babies born to women who smoke. *Lancet* **i:** 94.

DeWitt W, van Mourik I & Wiesenhaan PF (1988) Prolonged maternal indomethacin therapy associated with oligohydramnios. Case reports. *British Journal of Obstetrics and Gynaecology* **95:** 303–305.

DeWolf F, Carreras LO, Moerman P et al (1982) Decidual vasculopathy and extensive placental infarction in a patient with repeated thromboembolic accidents. *American Journal of Obstetrics and Gynecology* **142:** 829–834.

Downing L, Shepherd GL & Lewis PJ (1980) Reduced prostacyclin production in pre-eclampsia. *Lancet* **ii:** 1374.

Dyerberg J & Bang HO (1985) Pre-eclampsia and prostaglandins. *Lancet* **i:** 1267.

Elder MG, de Swiet M, Robertson A et al (1988) Low dose aspirin in pregnancy. *Lancet* i: 410.

Eronen M, Pesonen E, Kurki T, Ylikorkala O & Hallman M (1991) The effects of indomethacin and a β-sympathomimetic agent on the fetal ductus arteriosus during treatment of premature labor. A randomized double blind study. *American Journal of Obstetrics and Gynecology* 164: 141–146.

Erwich JJHM (1991) *Arachidonic acid metabolism in human placenta.* PhD thesis, University of Leiden.

Everett RB, Whorley RJ, MacDonald PC & Gant NF (1978) Effect of prostaglandin synthetase inhibitors on the pressor response to angiotensin II in human pregnancy. *Journal of Clinical Endocrinology and Metabolism* 46: 1007–1010.

Fidler J, Bennet MJ, de Swiet M et al (1980) Treatment of pregnancy hypertension with prostacyclin. *Lancet* ii: 31.

Fitzgerald DJ & FitzGerald GA (1990) Eicosanoids in the pathogenesis of preeclampsia. In Laragh JH & Brenner BM (eds) *Hypertension, Pathophysiology, Diagnosis, and Management,* pp1789–1807. New York: Racon Press.

Fitzgerald DJ, Entman SS, Mulloy K & FitzGerald GA (1987a) Decreased prostacyclin biosynthesis preceding the clinical manifestation of pregnancy-induced hypertension. *Circulation* 75: 956–963.

Fitzgerald DJ, Mayo G, Catella F, Entman SS & FitzGerald GA (1987b) Increased thromboxane in normal pregnancy is mainly derived from platelets. *American Journal of Obstetrics and Gynecology* 157: 325–330.

Fitzgerald DJ, Rocki W, Murray R, Mayo G & FitzGerald GA (1990) Thromboxane A_2 synthesis in pregnancy-induced hypertension. *Lancet* 335: 751–754.

Friedman SA (1988) Preeclampsia: a review of the role of prostaglandins. *Obstetrics and Gynecology* 71: 122–137.

Fuchs A-R & Fuchs F (1984) Endocrinology of human parturition: a review. *British Journal of Obstetrics and Gynaecology* 91: 948–967.

Fuchs A-R, Fuchs F, Husslein P, Soloff MS & Fernström MJ (1982a) Oxytocin receptors and human parturition: a dual role for oxytocin in the irritation of labor. *Science* 251: 1396–1398.

Fuchs A-R, Husslein P, Sumulong L et al (1982b) Plasma levels of oxytocin and 13,14-dihydro-15-keto-prostaglandin F2α in preterm labor and the effect of ethanol and ritodrine. *American Journal of Obstetrics and Gynecology* 144: 753–759.

Gravett MG, Nelson HP, DeRouen T et al (1986) Independent association of bacterial vaginosis and Chlamydia trachomatis infection with adverse pregnancy outcome. *Journal of American Medical Association* 256: 1899–1903.

Griffith FL (1893) A medical papyrus from Egypt. *British Medical Journal* i: 1172–1174.

Hadi HA & Treadwell EL (1990) Lupus anticoagulant and anticardiolipid antibodies in pregnancy. A review. In Immunochemistry and clinical implications. II Diagnosis and management. *Obstetrical and Gynecological Survey* 45: 780–791.

Hendricks SK, Smith JR, Moore DE & Brown EA (1990) Oligohydramnios associated with prostaglandin synthetase inhibitors in preterm labour. *British Journal of Obstetrics and Gynecology* 97: 312–316.

Itskovitz J, Abramovici H & Brandes JM (1980) Oligohydramnios, meconium and perinatal death concurrent with indomethacin treatment in human pregnancy. *Journal of Reproductive Medicine* 24: 137–142.

Jeremy JY, Mikhailidis DP & Dandona P (1985) Cigarette smoke extract, but not nicotine, inhibit prostacyclin (PGI_2) synthesis in human, rabbit and rat vascular tissue. *Prostaglandins, Leukotrienes and Medicine* 19: 261–270.

Jogee M, Myatt L & Elder MG (1983) Decreased prostacyclin production by placental cells in culture from pregnancies complicated by fetal growth retardation. *British Journal of Obstetrics and Gynaecology* 90: 247–250.

Jouppila P, Kirkinen P, Koivula A & Ylikorkala O (1985a) Failure of exogenous prostacyclin to change placental and fetal blood flow in preeclampsia. *American Journal of Obstetrics and Gynecology* 151: 661–665.

Jouppila P, Kirkinen P, Koivula A & Ylikorkala O (1985b) Ritodrine infusion during late pregnancy; effects on fetal and placental blood flow, prostacyclin and thromboxane. *American Journal of Obstetrics and Gynecology* 151: 1028–1032.

Keirse MJNC, Grant A & King JF (1989) Preterm labour. In Chalmers I, Enkin M & Keirse

MJNC (eds) *Effective care in pregnancy and childbirth*, 1st edn, pp 694–745. Oxford: Oxford University Press.

Khan H, Ishihara O, Sullivan MHF et al (1991) A comparison of two decidual cell populations by immunocytochemistry and prostaglandin production. *Histochemistry* **96**: 149–154.

Kirshon B (1989) Fetal urine output in hydramnio. *Obstetrics and Gynecology* **73**: 240–242.

Kirshon B, Mari G & Moise KJ (1990) Indomethacin therapy in the treatment of symptomatic polyhydramnios. *Obstetrics and Gynecology* **75**: 202–205.

Kontula K, Viinikka L, Ylikorkala O & Ylikahri R (1982) Effect of acute ethanol intake on thromboxane and prostacyclin in human. *Life Sciences* **31**: 261–264.

Kurki T, Eronen M, Lumme R & Ylikorkala O (1991) A randomized double-dummy comparison between indomethacin and nylidrin in threatened preterm labor. *Obstetrics and Gynecology* **78**: 1093–1097.

Kurki T, Viinikka L & Ylikorkala O (1992) Urinary excretion of prostacyclin and thromboxane metabolites in threatened preterm labor: effect of indomethacin and nylidrin. *American Journal of Obstetrics and Gynecology* **166**: 150–154.

Lamont RF, Rose M & Elder MG (1985) Effect of bacterial products on prostaglandin E production by amnion cells. *Lancet* **ii**: 1331–1333.

Lewis RB & Schulman JD (1973) Influence of acetylsalicylic acid, an inhibitor of prostaglandin synthesis, on the duration of human gestation and labour. *Lancet* **ii**: 1159–1161.

Lewis PJ, Shepherd GL & Ritter J et al (1981) Prostacyclin and preeclampsia. *Lancet* **i**: 599.

Lind T, Kendall A & Hytten FE (1972) The role of the fetus in the formation of amniotic fluid. *British Journal of Obstetrics and Gynaecology* **79**: 289–298.

Lindblom B, Lindberg JM, Lunell N-O et al (1991) Endothelin—a potent constrictor of small myometrial arteries of term pregnant women. *Acta Obstetrica et Gynecologica Scandinavica* **70**: 267–270.

Lindheimer M & Katz AI (1989) Preeclampsia: pathophysiology, diagnosis and management. *Annual Review of Medicine* **40**: 233–250.

Love PE & Santaro SA (1990) Antiphospholipid antibodies: anticardiolipin and the lupus anticoagulant in systemic lupus erythematosus (SLE) and in non-SLE disorders. *Annals of Internal Medicine* **112**: 682–698.

Lubbe WF & Pattison NS (1991) Antiphospholipid antibody syndrome and recurrent fetal loss. *Current Obstetrics and Gynaecology* **1**: 196–202.

Mäkilä U-M, Jouppila P, Kirkinen P, Viinikka L & Ylikorkala O (1983) Relation between umbilical prostacyclin production and blood-flow in the fetus. *Lancet* **i**: 728–729.

Mäkilä U-M, Viinikka L & Ylikorkala O (1984a) Increased thromboxane A$_2$ production but normal prostacyclin by placenta in hypertensive pregnancies. *Prostaglandins* **27**: 87–95.

Mäkilä U-M, Viinikka L & Ylikorkala O (1984b) Evidence that prostacyclin deficiency is a specific feature in preeclampsia. *American Journal of Obstetrics and Gynecology* **148**: 772–774.

Mäkilä U-M, Viinikka L & Ylikorkala O (1985) Decreased prostacyclin production in Down's syndrome. *Prostaglandins and Leukotrienes in Medicine* **17**: 347–348.

Mäkila U-M, Jouppila P, Kirkinen P, Viinikka L & Ylikorkala O (1986) Placental thromboxane and prostacyclin production in the regulation of placental blood flow. *Obstetrics and Gynecology* **68**: 537–540.

Mäkäräinen L & Ylikorkala O (1984) Amniotic fluid 6-keto-prostaglandin F1α and thromboxane B$_2$ during labour. *American Journal of Obstetrics and Gynecology* **150**: 765–768.

Mamopoulos M, Assimakopoulos E, Reece EA et al (1990) Maternal indomethacin therapy in the treatment of polyhydramnios. *American Journal of Obstetrics and Gynecology* **162**: 1225–1229.

Martius J, Krohn MA, Hillier SL et al (1988) Relationship of vaginal bactobacillus species, cervical chlamydia trachomatis, and bacterial vaginosis to preterm birth. *Obstetrics and Gynecology* **71**: 89–95.

Mastrogiannis DS, O'Brien WF, Krammer J & Benoit R (1991) Potential role of endothelin-I in normal and hypertensive pregnancies. *American Journal of Obstetrics and Gynecology* **165**: 1711–1716.

Mitchell MD (1986) Pathways of arachidonic acid metabolism with specific application to the fetus and mother. *Seminars in Perinatology* **10**: 242–254.

Mitchell MD, Keirse MJNC, Brunt JD, Anderson ABM & Turnbull AC (1979) Concentration of the prostacyclin metabolite 6-keto-prostaglandin F1α in amniotic fluid during late pregnancy and labour. *British Journal of Obstetrics and Gynaecology* **86**: 350–353.

Mitchell MD, Romero RJ, Lepera R, Rittenhouse L & Edwin SS (1990) Actions of endothelin-I on prostaglandin production by gestational tissues. *Prostaglandins* **40:** 627–635.
Moise KJ, Huhta JC, Sharif DS et al (1988) Indomethacin in the treatment of premature labor. *New England Journal of Medicine* **319:** 327–331.
Moise KJ Jr, Ou C-N, Kirshon B et al (1990) Placental transfer of indomethacin in the human pregnancy. *American Journal of Obstetrics and Gynecology* **162:** 549–554.
Moncada S, Palmer RM & Higgs EA (1991) Nitric oxide: physiology, pathophysiology and pharmacology. *Pharmacological Reviews* **48:** 109–142.
Musci TJ, Roberts JM, Rodgers GM & Taylor RN (1988) Mitogenic activity is increased in the sera of preeclamptic women before delivery. *American Journal of Obstetrics and Gynecology* **159:** 1446–1451.
Myatt L, Longdon G, Brewer AS & Brockman DE (1991) Endothelin-I-induced vaso-constriction is not mediated by thromboxane release and action in the human fetal–placental circulation. *American Journal of Obstetrics and Gynecology* **165:** 1717–1722.
Myatt L, Brewer AS, Langdon G & Brockman DE (1992) Attenuation of the vasoconstrictor effects of thromboxane and endothelin by nitric oxide in the human fetal–placental circulation. *American Journal of Obstetrics and Gynecology* **166:** 224–230.
Nadler JL, Velasco JS & Horton R (1983) Cigarette smoking inhibits prostacyclin formation. *Lancet* **i:** 1248–1250.
Noort WA (1989) *Prostanoid excretion in human term and preterm gestation.* PhD thesis, University of Leiden.
Orvieto R, Achiron A, Ben-Rafael Z & Archiron R (1991) Intravenous immunoglobulin treatment for recurrent abortions caused antiphospholipid antibodies. *Fertility and Sterility* **56:** 1013–1020.
Pasetto N, Piccione E, Ticconi C et al (1989) Leukotrienes in human umbilical plasma at birth. *British Journal of Obstetrics and Gynaecology* **96:** 88–91.
Pennington S, Allen Z, Runion J et al (1985) Prostaglandin synthesis inhibitors block alcohol-induced fetal hypoplasia. *Alcoholism: Clinical Experimental Research* **9:** 433–437.
Rabinowiz R, Peters MT, Vyas S, Cambell S & Nicolaides KH (1989) Measurement of fetal urine production in normal pregnancy by real time ultrasonography. *American Journal of Obstetrics and Gynecology* **161:** 1264–1266.
Randall CL & Anton RF (1984) Aspirin reduces alcohol-induced prenatal mortality and malformations in mice. *Alcoholism: Clinical Experimental Research* **8:** 513–515.
Remuzzi G, Marchesi D, Zoja C et al (1980) Reduced umbilical and placental vascular prostacyclin and severe pre-eclampsia. *Prostaglandins* **20:** 105–110.
Roberts JM, Taylor RN, Musci TJ et al (1989) Preeclampsia: an endothelial cell disorder. *American Journal of Obstetrics and Gynecology* **161:** 1200–1204.
Romero R & Mazor M (1988) Infection and preterm labor. *Clinical Obstetrics and Gynecology* **31:** 553–584.
Romero R, Quintero R, Emamian M et al (1987a) Arachidonate lipoxygenase metabolites in amniotic fluid of women with intra-amniotic infection and preterm labor. *American Journal of Obstetrics and Gynecology* **157:** 1454–1460.
Romero R, Emamiam M, Wan M et al (1987b) Prostaglandin concentrations in amniotic fluid of women with intra-amniotic infection and preterm labor. *American Journal of Obstetrics and Gynecology* **157:** 1461–1467.
Romero R, Wu Y, Sirtari M et al (1989a) Amniotic fluid concentrations of prostaglandins F2α, 13,14-dihydro-15-ketoprostaglandin F2α (PGEM) and 11-deoxy-13,14-dihydro-15-keto-11,16-cyclo-prostaglandin E_2 (PGEM-II) in preterm labor. *Prostaglandins* **37:** 149–161.
Romero R, Wu YK, Mazor M et al (1989b) Amniotic fluid arachidonic lipoxygenase metabolites in preterm labor. *Prostaglandins, Leukotrienes, and Essential Fatty Acids* **36:** 69–75.
Romero R, Ceska M, Avila C et al (1991a) Neutrofil attractant/activating peptide-1/interleukin-8 in term and preterm parturition. *American Journal of Obstetrics and Gynecology* **165:** 813–820.
Romero R, Mazor M & Tartakovsky B (1991b) Systemic administration of interleukin-1 induces preterm parturition in mice. *American Journal of Obstetrics and Gynecology* **165:** 969–971.
Romero R, Avila C, Edwin SS & Mitchell MD (1992) Endothelin-1,2 levels are increased in the amniotic fluid of women with preterm labor and microbial invasion of the amniotic cavity. *American Journal of Obstetrics and Gynecology* **166:** 95–99.

Rubin PC & Horn L (1988) Preeclampsia: Platelets and antiplatelet therapy. *Hospital Practice* **23(5A):** 69–73, 76–78.

Rushton DI (1988) Placental pathology in spontaneous miscarriage. In Beard RW & Sharp F (eds) *Early Pregnancy Loss*, pp 149–157. London: Springer-Verlag.

Saeed SA & Mitchell MD (1983) Lipoxygenase activity in human uterine and intrauterine tissues: new prospects for control of prostacyclin production in pre-eclampsia. *Clinical Experimental Hypertension B* **2:** 103–108.

Santhanam U, Avila C, Romero R, Viquet H et al (1991) Cytokines in normal and abnormal parturition: elevated amniotic fluid interleukin-6 levels in women with premature rupture of membranes associated with intrauterine infection. *Cytokine* **3:** 155–163.

Sellers SM, Mitchell MD, Bibby JG, Andersson ABM & Turnbull AC (1981) A comparison of plasma prostaglandin levels in term and preterm labor. *British Journal of Obstetrics and Gynaecology* **88:** 362–366.

Silver RK, Adler L, Hickman AR & Hageman JR (1991) Anticardiolipin antibody-positive serum enhances endothelial cell platelet-activating factor production. *American Journal of Obstetrics and Gynecology* **165:** 1748–1752.

Spitz B, Deckmyn H, van Assche FA & Vermylen J (1984) Prostacyclin in pregnancy. *European Journal of Obstetrics, Gynecology and Reproductive Biology* **18:** 303–308.

Stirrat GM (1990) Recurrent miscarriage II. Clinical associations, causes and management. *Lancet* **336:** 728–733.

Stoel I, Giessen WJ, Wolsman EZ et al (1982) Effect of nicotine on production of prostacyclin in human umbilical artery. *British Heart Journal* **48:** 493–496.

Stuart MJ, Clark DA, Sunderji SG et al (1981) Decreased prostacyclin production: a characteristic of chronic placental insufficiency syndrome. *Lancet* **i:** 1126–1128.

Sullivan MHF, Roseblade CK & Elder MG (1991) Metabolism of prostaglandin E_2 on the fetal and maternal sides of intact fetal membranes. *Acta Obstetrica et Gynecologica Scandinavica* **70:** 425–427.

Toivanen J, Ylikorkala O & Viinikka L (1983) Ethanol inhibits platelet thromboxane A_2 production but has no effect on lung prostacyclin synthesis in humans. *Life Sciences* **33:** 1–8.

Toivanen J, Ylikorkala O & Viinikka L (1986) Effects of smoking and nicotine on human prostacyclin and thromboxane production in vivo and in vitro. *Toxicology Applied and Pharmacology* **82:** 301–306.

Toppozada MK, Ismail AAA, Hegab HM & Kamel MA (1988) Treatment of preeclampsia with prostaglandin A1. *American Journal of Obstetrics and Gynecology* **159:** 160–165.

Toppozada MK, Darwish E & Barakat AAT (1991) Management of severe preeclampsia detected in early labor by prostaglandin A1 or dihydralazine infusions. *American Journal of Obstetrics and Gynecology* **164:** 1229–1232.

Tulppala M, Viinikka L & Ylikorkala O (1991) Thromboxane dominance and prostacyclin deficiency in habitual abortion. *Lancet* **337:** 879–881.

Turk J, Wyche LA & Needleman P (1989) Inactivation of vascular prostacyclin synthetase by platelet lipoxygenase products. *Biochemical and Biophysical Research Communications* **95:** 1628–1632.

Wallenburg HCS & Rotmans N (1982) Enhanced reactivity of the platelet thromboxane pathway in normotensive and hypertensive pregnancies with insufficient fetal growth. *American Journal of Obstetrics and Gynecology* **144:** 523–528.

Walsh SC (1990) Physiology of low-dose aspirin therapy for the prevention of preeclampsia. *Seminars in Perinatology* **14:** 153–170.

Walsh SW & Coulter BS (1989) Increased placental progesterone may cause decreased placental prostacyclin production in preeclampsia. *American Journal of Obstetrics and Gynecology* **161:** 1586–1592.

Weitz CM, Ghodgaonkar RB, Dubin NH & Niebyl JR (1986) Prostaglandin F metabolite concentration as a prognostic factor in preterm labor. *Obstetrics and Gynecology* **67:** 496–499.

Wilhelmsson L, Wikland M & Wiqvist N (1981) PGH_2, TxA_2 and PGI_2 have potent and differential actions on human uterine contractility. *Prostaglandins* **21:** 277–286.

Wisdom SJ, Wilson R, McKillop JH & Walker JJ (1991) Antioxidant systems in normal pregnancy and in pregnancy-induced hypertension. *American Journal of Obstetrics and Gynecology* **165:** 1701–1704.

Ylikorkala O & Mäkilä U-M (1985) Prostacyclin and thromboxane in gynecology and obstetrics. *American Journal of Obstetrics and Gynecology* **152:** 318–329.
Ylikorkala O & Viinikka L (1980) Thromboxane A_2 in pregnancy and puerperium. *British Medical Journal* **281:** 1601–1602.
Ylikorkala O, Mäkilä U-M & Viinikka L (1981a) Amniotic fluid prostacyclin and thromboxane in normal preeclamptic, and some other complicated pregnancies. *American Journal of Obstetrics and Gynecology* **141:** 487–490.
Ylikorkala O, Mäkäräinen L & Viinikka L (1981b) Prostacyclin increases during human parturition. *British Journal of Obstetrics and Gynaecology* **88:** 513–516.
Ylikorkala O, Jouppila R & Viinikka L (1982) Production of prostacyclin and thromboxane during cesarean section. *Obstetrics and Gynecology* **60:** 597–600.
Ylikorkala O, Jouppila P, Kirkinen P & Viinikka L (1983) Maternal prostacyclin, thromboxane, and placental blood flow. *American Journal of Obstetrics and Gynecology* **145:** 730–732.
Ylikorkala O, Jouppila P, Kirkinen P & Viinikka L (1984) Maternal thromboxane, prostacyclin and umbilical blood flow in human. *Obstetrics and Gynecology* **63:** 677–680.
Ylikorkala O, Viinikka L & Lehtovirta P (1985) Effect of nicotine on fetal prostacyclin and thromboxane in humans. *Obstetrics and Gynecology* **102:** 102–105.
Ylikorkala O, Pekonen F & Viinikka L (1986a) Renal prostacyclin and thromboxane in normotensive and preeclamptic pregnant women and their infants. *Journal of Clinical Endocrinology and Metabolism* **63:** 1307–1312.
Ylikorkala O, Paatero H, Suhonen L & Viinikka L (1986b) Vaginal and abdominal delivery increases maternal urinary 6-keto-prostaglandin F1α excretion. *British Journal of Obstetrics and Gynaecology* **93:** 950–954.
Ylikorkala O, Halmesmäki E & Viinikka L (1987) Effect of ethanol on thromboxane and prostacyclin synthesis by fetal platelets and umbilical artery. *Life Sciences* **41:** 371–376.
Ylikorkala O, Halmesmäki E & Viinikka L (1988) Urinary prostacyclin and thromboxane metabolites in drinking women and their infants: relation to the fetal alcohol effects. *Obstetrics and Gynecology* **71:** 61–66.

8

Prostaglandins, prostaglandin inhibitors and their roles in gynaecological disorders

IAN S. FRASER

INTRODUCTION

Prostaglandins in the reproductive tract

Prostaglandins are members of a large family (the eicosanoids) of fatty acid derivatives with related chemical structures, which have important biological actions in the normal female and male genital tracts. These physiological actions have been thoroughly addressed elsewhere in this volume. Disturbances in the synthesis, secretion and action of these various prostaglandin-related substances have been demonstrated to play a role in several gynaecological disorders. The prostaglandins which appear to be of most importance in gynaecological disorders are E_2 and F_{2+} prostaglandins (PGE_2 and $PGF_{2\alpha}$), prostacyclin (PGI_2), possibly thromboxane A_2 (TXA_2), and possibly other eicosanoids such as the leukotrienes (especially leukotriene B_4 (LTB_4)) and the prostaglandin epoxides.

Outline of relevant gynaecological disorders

The gynaecological disorders in which prostaglandins appear most likely to play an important role are those in which symptoms of pain or disturbances of uterine bleeding are prominent.

Pelvic pain

Primary dysmenorrhoea is recognized as a condition associated with elevated production of $PGF_{2\alpha}$ from the endometrium. This is a very common condition and in most cases is very sensitive to treatment with prostaglandin inhibitors.

Secondary dysmenorrhoea is much less common than primary dysmenorrhoea, and prostaglandins appear to play less of a role. However, prostaglandins do appear to have some involvement in the symptomatology, and many patients show some symptomatic response to prostaglandin inhibitors. Conditions which typically cause secondary dysmenorrhoea include endometriosis, adenomyosis, pelvic inflammatory disease and, possibly, 'pelvic congestion syndrome'.

Mid-cycle pain (ovulation pain or 'Mittelschmerz') is a common symptom and, anecdotally, may respond to prostaglandin inhibitors.

Chronic pelvic pain is a relatively common occurrence and, in some cases, may occur in the absence of recognized pathology. It is unclear whether prostaglandins or prostaglandin inhibitors have any role in this condition.

Menstrual disorders

Menorrhagia is excessive menstrual bleeding, and can be associated with local pelvic disease, with certain systemic medical diseases or with dysfunctional uterine bleeding. There is increasing evidence that women with dysfunctional uterine bleeding may have a local abnormality of arachidonic acid metabolism within the endometrium. Prostaglandin inhibitors have a role in the management of some of these conditions.

Intermenstrual bleeding is a common condition in which the involvement of prostaglandins is uncertain. Prostaglandin inhibitors may occasionally have an anecdotal role in management.

Contraceptive-related bleeding disorders are poorly understood, and the mechanisms probably vary depending on the contraceptive method. Subtle abnormalities of endometrial prostaglandins may sometimes occur and prostaglandin inhibitors have a role in some situations.

Other conditions

Premenstrual syndrome is a very poorly understood but common condition in which definite abnormalities of prostaglandin metabolism have not been demonstrated, but in which the use of prostaglandin inhibitors may be of some benefit.

Menstrual migraine is also poorly understood but prostaglandin inhibitors may have a role in management.

Comment on synthetic pathways and prostaglandin inhibitors

The basic pathways have been described in previous chapters but a short summary is relevant in this chapter to set the scene for action of prostaglandin inhibitors. Prostaglandins are derived from phospholipids in the cell membrane where arachidonic acid is predominantly stored at position 2 of the phospholipid molecules. Arachidonic acid is liberated following activation of phospholipase A_2 (Figure 1) or phospholipase C. Stimuli to activation of phospholipase A_2 include thrombin, adrenaline, bradykinin and angiotensin II. The same enzyme can be inhibited by glucocorticoids and some local anaesthetics.

Arachidonic acid is rapidly metabolized through the prostaglandin endoperoxides PGG_2 and then PGH_2 in a manner which depends on the cell type. In general, it appears that each cell type produces predominantly one type of prostaglandin or related prostanoid. The enzyme which acts at this

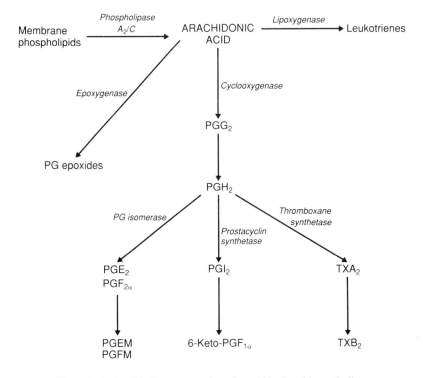

Figure 1. A simplified representation of arachidonic acid metabolism.

point is called cyclooxygenase. Several cell types synthesize PGE_2, $PGF_{2\alpha}$ and PGD_2. Platelets, spleen and lung contain thromboxane synthetase, which is responsible for the synthesis of TXA_2. Blood vessel walls, peritoneum and myometrium are capable of synthesizing prostacyclin via prostacyclin synthetase.

The secondary, and possibly less important, pathway from arachidonic acid in the reproductive tract is through the lipoxygenase enzyme, which is responsible for initiating synthesis of the leukotriene family by hydroxylation of arachidonic acid at carbon 12. These molecules are formed particularly in leukocytes, platelets and macrophages in response to a range of immuno-logical and other stimuli. Leukotrienes are capable of causing muscular contraction and vascular permeability as well as a range of other actions in many tissues. It is possible that these sometimes have important physiological or pathophysiological roles within the genital tract, but their role is largely unknown at present.

The third and probably the least important pathway from arachidonic acid is through the epoxygenase enzyme system to the prostaglandin epoxides. These may occasionally play a role in bleeding disorders but their involve-ment is unclear.

Disturbances of these systems can include:

1. Increased or decreased availability of the arachidonic acid substrate from lipoproteins in the cell membrane. This availability is controlled by the activity of the phospholipase A_2 or C groups of enzymes. All of these appear to be active in the genital tract at certain times and in certain pathological circumstances.
2. Diversion of precursors preferentially through an abnormal route or in increased or decreased amount through a normal synthetic route.
3. Increased precursor which then diffuses into adjacent tissues where other synthetic enzymes are available. This situation appears to occur when prostaglandin endoperoxides diffuse from the endometrium into the myometrium, where large amounts of prostacyclin can be synthesized by myometrial prostacyclin synthetase. Since there is such a large mass of myometrium compared with endometrium, there is potential for secretion of substantial amounts of prostacyclin by this tissue.

There is also great potential for modulation of this synthetic network by drugs. Unfortunately, the realities of drug treatment are still quite limited and the great majority of available agents work solely or predominantly by inhibiting the cyclooxygenase enzyme system. Variable responses and treatment failures suggest a lack of uniformity of underlying pathophysiological mechanisms, perhaps combined with variability of drug absorption, tissue uptake and drug interactions with tissue receptors.

General comment on 'prostaglandin inhibitors' (non-steroidal anti-inflammatory drugs: NSAIDs)

The great majority of 'prostaglandin inhibitors' are inhibitors of the cyclooxygenase enzyme system, although they may also have secondary effects on other prostaglandin synthetase systems. There is also evidence that certain of these agents may have a weak end-organ effect to competitively inhibit the receptor action of prostaglandins which have already been formed. The evidence for this secondary effect is stronger for the fenamates, particularly mefenamic acid and meclofenamic acid, than for prostaglandin inhibitors of different chemical structure (Rees et al, 1988). Meclofenamic acid may also be an inhibitor of the lipoxygenase pathway (Boctor et al, 1986). These agents (Tolman et al, 1985) include derivatives of salicylic acid (aspirin, a complex and weak prostaglandin inhibitor), pyrazolones (phenyl butazone), acetic acids (indomethacin, diclofenac, sulindac), anthranilic and fenamic acids (mefenamic acid, flufenamic acid, tolfenamic acid, meclofenamic acid), oxicams (piroxicam) and arylpropionic acid (ibuprofen, naproxen, ketoprofen, benoxaprofen). The different chemical structures of these drugs affects their absorption and their ability to reach different sites of action.

Although several prostaglandin inhibitors have been available for nearly 30 years, it is only within the last 15 years that their specific antiprostaglandin actions and their gynaecological potential have been widely recognized. Initially, a few isolated cases were reported of treatment of primary dysmenorrhoea with agents like indomethacin and phenylbutazone. The first detailed report of 16 cases of severe primary dysmenorrhoea treated with flufenamic acid (Schwarz et al, 1974) was followed by numerous reports of successful treatment of a variety of gynaecological and obstetric conditions with similar agents (Anderson et al, 1978; Henzl et al, 1980; Kintis and Contifaris, 1980). Aspirin (acetylsalicylic acid) is a moderate prostaglandin synthetase inhibitor, but has little clinical utility in the uterus because it is rapidly de-acetylated in the circulation to the less effective sodium salicylate.

A wide range of minor side-effects and occasional serious complications have been reported with prostaglandin inhibitors (Fraser, 1985a; Tolman et al, 1985). With most of the agents these side-effects are infrequent and of nuisance value only, and in many countries a few of the agents are marketed over the counter without prescription restrictions. This low incidence of side-effects is particularly seen with the repeated short-course regimens widely used for the treatment of menstrual disorders. There do not appear to have been any reports of serious complications with short-term regimens. Mild gastrointestinal disturbances such as nausea, indigestion and diarrhoea have been reported in about 5% of patients using the fenamates or arylpropionic acid derivatives. Occasionally, central nervous system effects such as drowsiness, lethargy and headache have been recorded.

Serious complications such as transient renal failure, major gastro-intestinal bleeding, bone marrow disorders and major central nervous system effects have rarely been recorded, even when these agents are used over long periods of time with repeated daily usage. A few agents, such as phenylbutazone and benoxaprofen, have turned out to have a higher incidence of serious side-effects than the other agents and cannot be recommended for modern use. Indeed, benoxaprofen had to be removed from the market in the UK and the USA after a number of deaths in elderly patients. This saga has led drug regulatory agencies to tighten their pre-marketing requirements for all new prostaglandin inhibitors.

Dosage regimens vary from one drug to another. Absorption is generally fairly rapid, with symptomatic relief beginning within 30–60 minutes and with peak blood levels being reached within 1–2 hours. The sodium salts of some of these agents appear to be absorbed more quickly, e.g. sodium meclofenamate. The duration of effect depends on the particular drug as well as the response of the woman, and the dosage regimen should always be individualized for each patient. A few women may need to take a drug with a relatively short half-life, like mefenamic acid, once every 4–6 hours to provide effective and continuous release. With some of the drugs (e.g. naproxen) it is recommended to start with a double dose to 'load' the system. In a small number of cases, greater relief may be experienced if treatment is started 1–2 days before the menses, although timing of this may be difficult.

An extensive search is continuing for more specific drugs which will inhibit particular parts of the prostaglandin synthetic network. Although some agents have been developed, their use is not yet appropriate in clinical situations either because they are not specific enough, not active enough, or are too toxic.

MENSTRUAL DISORDERS

Dysmenorrhoea

Primary or spasmodic dysmenorrhoea

This extremely common condition typically occurs in adolescence and in the absence of recognizable pelvic disease (Fraser, 1985b). It usually begins within the first few months or years after the menarche, when ovulatory cycles first begin. It has its maximum incidence in the late teens and 20s. Population surveys indicate that well over half of all menstruating women claim to experience dysmenorrhoea at some time in their lives. Around 15% will lose significant time from school or work. The incidence decreases with increasing age and following childbirth. There appears to be a strong association with cigarette smoking and a fairly strong familial trend, with mothers, daughters and sisters often experiencing similar menstrual pain.

The pain of primary dysmenorrhoea usually begins at around the onset of menstrual bleeding and persists through the first 12–48 hours of menstrual flow. In 5–10% of cases pain can be so severe that the patient is confined to bed for some hours or even days. Usually there is a constant background pain upon which is superimposed a succession of severe spasmodic cramping pains. In the more severe cases there may be associated systemic symptoms such as nausea, diarrhoea, headache and extreme lethargy out of proportion to that expected from the pain.

Dysmenorrhoea is often clearly influenced by psychological factors, and it is not surprising that certain personality traits cope with the pain less well than others. Much of the psychological disturbance may be secondary to the experience of severe recurrent pain which has not responded well to previous treatment. This condition has major socioeconomic implications in all Western societies, since it accounts for a substantial proportion of the total number of hours lost from the female workforce.

There is now very strong evidence to link the pain of primary dysmenorrhoea with increased uterine muscular activity resulting in increased uterine tone and excessive spasmodic contractions. Extensive studies of intrauterine pressure waves have been carried out and some sophisticated analyses of pressure velocity changes have been reported (Lumsden and Baird, 1985; Smith, 1989). There are some technical difficulties in measuring absolute pressure inside the small non-pregnant uterine cavity, but it appears that baseline intrauterine pressure in a woman experiencing primary dysmenorrhoea may easily reach 50 mmHg, and pressures up to 100 mmHg have been recorded. Superimposed upon this may be spasmodic pressures commonly up to 200 mmHg and occasionally even up to 400 mmHg during contractions. The non-pregnant uterus appears to be capable of rates of pressure change as high as 120 mmHg/s.

This combination of high resting myometrial tone with superimposed excessive contractions is capable of inhibiting uterine perfusion and causing uterine ischaemia. Simultaneous objective recordings of intrauterine pressure and endometrial blood flow have demonstrated that the flow decreases during contractions, and that pain is at a maximum when the flow is at a minimum (Akerlund et al, 1976). Treatment resulting in decrease in uterine contractions is usually associated with relief of pain. It is proposed that pain results from ischaemia of a type analogous to that seen with myocardial ischaemia and cardiac angina. On the other hand, high-amplitude peak contractions have been observed in the absence of pain, and in some experimental situations pain may be induced without an obvious increase in contractions. This suggests that there may be other mechanisms resulting in pain which are not directly associated with uterine spasm. This is also supported by the fact that dysmenorrhoeic pain can be produced by autologous transfusion of plasma from dysmenorrhoeic women (Irwin et al, 1981).

There is now very strong evidence to implicate excessive synthesis and secretion of $PGF_{2\alpha}$ by the endometrium in the mechanism of primary dysmenorrhoea (Pickles et al, 1965; Lundstrom and Green, 1978; Chan et al, 1981; Lumsden et al, 1983). This appears to be part of a spectrum arising from the modest perimenstrual increase in $PGF_{2\alpha}$ seen in normal cycles. Numerous investigations have reported increased amounts of $PGF_{2\alpha}$ (or its main metabolite) in endometrium, menstrual fluid and peripheral venous blood from women complaining of primary dysmenorrhoea, on the first day of the menstrual flow. There is also evidence that $PGF_{2\alpha}$ concentrations in menstrual fluid correlate with uterine work recorded at the same time. When $PGF_{2\alpha}$ is infused into the uterus it produces an increase in uterine contractility and dysmenorrhoea-like pain (Lundstrom, 1977), and also mimics the associated symptoms of nausea, vomiting, diarrhoea and headache. There is suggestive evidence that LTC_4, LTD_4 and LTE_4 may sometimes have an aetiological role in primary dysmenorrhoea cases (Carraner et al, 1983; Rees et al, 1987). The causal involvement of $PGF_{2\alpha}$ appears to be confirmed by the high rate of therapeutic response of these symptoms to treatment with prostaglandin inhibitors. However, it is not clear what stimulates the excessive endometrial synthesis and secretion of $PGF_{2\alpha}$. It seems likely that this is due to an increase in the availability of arachidonic acid, and this suggests an increase in activity of phospholipase enzymes, although this has not been confirmed. Subtle abnormalities of ovarian secretion of oestradiol or progesterone may be involved. It has been demonstrated in one study (Ylikorkala et al, 1979) that late luteal phase levels of plasma oestradiol are higher in dysmenorrhoea sufferers than in controls (480 pmol/l compared with 260 pmol/l). This relatively elevated oestrogen exposure could lead to increased development of the synthetic apparatus for $PGF_{2\alpha}$ (Abel and Baird, 1980).

It has been known for some years that plasma levels of vasopressin are elevated at the time of menstruation and are significantly higher in women with dysmenorrhoea. Plasma vasopressin levels remain excessively high in women whose dysmenorrhoea is successfully treated with prostaglandin inhibitors, suggesting that vasopressin may have an aetiological role mediated through uterine prostaglandin synthesis or some other pathway (Stromberg et al, 1981). There may also be a role for lipoxygenase products (leukotrienes) in vasopressin-induced uterine contractions. It is not known whether catecholamines and the autonomic nervous system are involved in the mechanism of primary dysmenorrhoea. It has been well demonstrated that the pain of primary dysmenorrhoea can be abolished by presacral neurectomy or laser uterine nerve ablation, and the decrease in dysmenorrhoea following pregnancy could be related to the marked decrease in autonomic innovation in the uterus at that time (Sjoberg, 1979).

In recent years a range of new molecules with biological effects on uterine muscle and vasculature have been identified. It is possible that these may have a role in menstrual symptoms, including dysmenorrhoea. For example, it is now recognized that the endothelins are expressed within the uterus particularly at the time of menstruation. These are the most potent substances known to cause vasoconstriction and they may well have a role in causing uterine ischaemia and initiating menstruation. Their involvement in primary dysmenorrhoea has not been confirmed. Recently discovered inflammatory mediators such as tumour necrosis factor and the interleukins may also be involved in the generation of pain in dysmenorrhoea, but are likely to be mediators rather than primary causal factors.

The exact molecular mechanisms by which prostaglandins cause uterine ischaemia are not clear, but may be mediated partly through the development of gap junctions, which appear with greater frequency in myometrium at the time of menstruation (Garfield and Hayashi, 1980). Gap junctions between adjacent muscle cells facilitate transmission of contractile impulses, and appear to be more frequent in women with dysmenorrhoea. Their appearance is influenced by reproductive steroids and by $PGF_{2\alpha}$.

Secondary or congestive dysmenorrhoea

This is less common than spasmodic dysmenorrhoea and typically occurs in women in their 30s and 40s. It is usually associated with recognizable pelvic pathology such as endometriosis, adenomyosis or pelvic inflammatory disease. It usually has a different symptom pattern from spasmodic dysmenorrhoea, with abdominal bloating, pelvic heaviness and severe dragging pain being prominent. The pain usually builds up during the course of the luteal phase, reaching a maximum around the onset of menstruation and gradually declining during or just after the end of menstruation. Typically, it is also associated with low back pain. The evidence for an involvement of prostaglandins in the mechanism of this pain is limited, and mainly comes from extrapolation from the modest response of symptoms to treatment with prostaglandin inhibitors (Kauppilla et al, 1979). There is some evidence for the involvement of prostaglandins in endometriosis, and this evidence will be discussed later. It should be noted that molecules such as tumour necrosis factor and the interleukins which are released during inflammatory processes may well be important mediators in the generation of symptoms associated with congestive dysmenorrhoea. However, no definite evidence has been produced to support this hypothesis.

Treatment of dysmenorrhoea

Almost every medication used in the management of pain has at some time been proposed for the management of primary dysmenorrhoea. Management is obviously influenced by the severity of pain and individual tolerance of symptoms. A detailed explanation of the physiology and the future implications of the condition (e.g. lack of evidence for any future impairment of fertility), and associated counselling, are an integral part of treatment. A placebo effect has frequently been demonstrated during treatment trials, but this effect usually wears off within 2–3 cycles. The efficacy of any new method of treatment must always be carefully compared on a double-blind and cross-over basis against placebo or an alternative standard mode of therapy. Mild analgesics such as paracetamol and aspirin have often been recommended for mild to moderate dysmenorrhoea, but there is little scientific evidence that they are superior to placebo.

In recent years the prostaglandin-inhibiting agents have been extensively used for primary dysmenorrhoea and in most studies have demonstrated high efficacy. They have become particularly popular because of the simplicity of administration and the relatively low incidence of side-effects. These agents only need to be taken when symptoms are present, but they should be started in appropriate dosage at the very first sign of pain or bleeding in order to obtain an optimum response. On occasion, a better response is obtained by starting the medication 1–2 days before the predicted start of bleeding.

Prostaglandin-inhibiting agents which have shown significantly superior efficacy to placebo include several fenamates, naproxen, naproxen sodium, ibuprofen, ketoprofen, sulindac, diclofenac sodium and indomethacin (Schwarz et al, 1974; Anderson et al, 1978; Henzl et al, 1980; Kintis and Contifaris, 1980; Tolman et al, 1985). Most studies have reported major benefits in 60–90% of subjects when 20% or fewer subjects have responded well to placebo. Following the loading dose, individual response dictates the frequency of subsequent administration. Some women obtain a good response with one agent, but a less satisfactory response with another, indicating the need for individual regimens for all patients.

It must be noted that 10–30% of patients with primary dysmenorrhoea do not respond well to the usual prostaglandin-inhibiting agents. The reason for these treatment failures is unknown and probably reflects our ignorance of all the mechanisms underlying primary dysmenorrhoea. There is preliminary evidence that some cases may be due to an excessive production of LTC_4, LTD_4 or LTE_4 (Rees et al, 1987). In these patients it could be anticipated that a combination of specific lipoxygenase and cyclooxygenase inhibitors would give the best therapeutic response.

Numerous studies have demonstrated that in the majority of primary dysmenorrhoea sufferers prostaglandin inhibitors clearly suppress endometrial prostaglandin secretion, leading to a substantial decrease in uterine tone and contractions. Dramatic differences in the pressure–velocity tocograms of uterine muscle in vivo have been demonstrated before and after mefenamic acid therapy in dysmenorrhoea sufferers (Smith, 1989).

Other agents may also act through a reduction in $PGF_{2\alpha}$ synthesis and release by the endometrium. This includes the combined oral contraceptive pill, which produces almost complete relief of menstrual pain in up to 50% of primary dysmenorrhoea sufferers, with a further 30–40% of women experiencing marked relief (Kremser and Mitchell, 1971). Monophasic preparations with a progestogenic balance appear to be most effective at symptom relief. There is evidence that they reduce the capacity of the endometrium for prostaglandin synthesis. This is probably achieved by suppression of endogenous oestrogen secretion, suppressed secretory changes in endometrial histology and altered uterine contractility patterns. This should usually be the first treatment of choice in the young woman with primary dysmenorrhoea who also wishes contraceptive cover. Alternative approaches to management of primary dysmenorrhoea include β-adrenergic receptor agonists such as terbutaline (5 mg three times daily for the duration of symptoms) (Akerlund et al, 1976). Newer agents include the calcium channel-blocking agents (Andersson and Ulmsten, 1978) and adjuncts to drug therapy such as acupuncture, hypnosis, behavioural modification therapies, relaxation training and osteopathy. Recent evidence suggests that, on their own, these agents are not usually as effective as specific drug therapy, but may be useful adjuncts. An additional degree of benefit may sometimes be achieved by using prostaglandin inhibitors at the time of the withdrawal bleed in women using combined pills. It appears that only about 10% of primary dysmenorrhoea sufferers will not obtain substantial benefit from this regimen. In these women, a useful approach may be continuous use of a monophasic pill in order to prevent menstruation completely. This is highly effective in some women, although a small proportion will experience breakthrough bleeding with associated troublesome cramps.

It is important to recognize that the occasional case of troublesome dysmenorrhoea which occurs in association with use of an intrauterine device may be associated with enhanced prostaglandin synthesis or disturbance of metabolism, and may respond well to treatment with prostaglandin inhibitors. On the other hand, most cases of secondary dysmenorrhoea do not usually respond well to prostaglandin inhibitors. The exception may be seen in some patients with endometriosis or adenomyosis who have been reported to show a partial response to tolfenamic acid (Kauppilla et al, 1979).

Compliance is frequently a problem in the treatment of any chronic condition. Anecdotal evidence suggests that, in most instances where the patient reports that the effect of a prostaglandin inhibitor is wearing off, the attention to compliance was less meticulous than it was initially. In the future it would be valuable to have long-acting delivery systems to provide constant exposure to the drug for the required duration, without the woman having to remember to take repeated pills every 4–8 hours. A device offering such useful flexibility in clinical use would be a vaginal ring loaded with a prostaglandin inhibitor which could be absorbed across the vaginal mucosa. To the author's knowledge, studies on such delivery systems have not yet been carried out.

Menorrhagia

Menorrhagia is a clinical definition indicating that the patient perceives that she is losing excessive amounts of blood at the time of menstruation. In clinical situations the physician's assessment is based on the woman's description of her own perception of her menstrual loss. Her perception is based on visual, tactile and olfactory observations of her total menstrual discharge, which, in most cases, contains a large amount of tissue fluid in addition to blood. Recent evidence suggests that in women with normal menstrual loss 50–60% of the total discharge is probably an endometrial transudate (Fraser et al, 1985). In women with menorrhagia the proportion of endometrial fluid is probably less, at 45–50%. In research studies the objective verification of menorrhagia is usually based solely on measurement of the menstrual haemoglobin content, and the upper limit of the normal range is usually taken as 80 ml per menstrual period (Hallberg et al, 1966). It does appear that in many cases the patient and clinician may be assessing different parameters in determining the complaint. This may partly explain how a majority of studies of women presenting with a complaint of excessively heavy menstrual bleeding have only found 40–60% of the women to have an objectively measured blood loss of greater than 80 ml per menstrual period (Chimbira et al, 1980a; Fraser et al, 1981). Recent attempts have been made to increase the precision of assessment of the volume of menstrual flow by specific questioning (Fraser, 1989) or by use of a pictorial blood loss assessment chart (Higham et al, 1991). It is not yet clear whether these offer a substantial improvement over a general menstrual history when applied in regular clinical practice.

Precise management of menorrhagia depends on precision in diagnosis of the underlying condition, since therapy should usually be aimed at the underlying cause. Aetiologies can be divided into three broad categories, which are to some extent determined by a detailed case history and examination, but require precise imaging or other investigations for optimum management. The major categories are pelvic disease, certain systemic diseases and dysfunctional uterine bleeding. Pelvic disease is the largest category and myomata are the major cause in this category. Objective blood loss measurements indicate that intrauterine, submucous, intramural and subserous myomas are related in decreasing order of severity to the degree of menorrhagia. It is unclear whether disturbances of prostaglandin synthesis or metabolism are significantly involved in the mechanism of bleeding with these tumours. Adenomyosis may be a cause of menorrhagia, but the involvement of prostaglandins is again uncertain. Endometriosis is a controversial cause of menorrhagia. Although many women with this condition do not bleed heavily, others certainly do (Fraser et al, 1986). It is possible that this is mediated through a prostaglandin-related mechanism. This condition will be discussed in more detail below. Menorrhagia may also be caused by endometrial polyps, endometrial carcinoma, and rare causes such as myometrial hypertrophy and uterine vascular malformations. The involvement of prostaglandins and the possible value of prostaglandin inhibitors in these conditions is unknown.

Systemic diseases only account for a very small proportion of all cases of menorrhagia, but they are more commonly detected in the more severe cases, that is, in those who do not respond to initial therapy and in those presenting in early adolescence. The commonest conditions in this category are the coagulation disorders, especially those with a platelet abnormality such as thrombocytopoenia, the thrombocytopathies and von Willebrand's disease. In these cases it is possible that part of the mechanism is mediated through an error in thromboxane metabolism in platelets, although this is probably of minor importance. Other systemic causes of menorrhagia such as hypothyroidism, systemic lupus erythematosus and chronic liver failure are rare in women in these age groups.

Dysfunctional uterine bleeding

Dysfunctional uterine bleeding is a diagnosis of exclusion which should only be made after basic history taking, examination and investigations have excluded disease in the previous two categories. It is, however, a useful clinical working diagnosis even before investigations have been completed (Fraser, 1989). Dysfunctional uterine bleeding is a common diagnosis in association with menorrhagia and it may also include episodes of excessively prolonged or excessively frequent bleeding.

The mechanisms of abnormal bleeding with pelvic disease and systemic disorders are not well understood and there are still large gaps in our understanding of the mechanisms of dysfunctional uterine bleeding. In recent years, increasing evidence has pointed to a role for disturbances of arachidonic acid metabolism as being an important factor in the mechanism of dysfunctional uterine bleeding (Baird et al, 1981).

Aetiology and mechanisms

It is convenient to divide these patients into women who are anovulatory and women who are ovulatory, although it should be remembered that women with a history of anovulation will not infrequently have some ovulatory cycles (Fraser and Baird, 1974).

Anovulatory cycles

Women with dysfunctional bleeding who are anovulatory usually exhibit cyclical ovarian follicular development, sometimes with multiple follicles developing at the same time (particularly in the perimenopausal age range). In some cases, the serum oestradiol levels may be excessive compared with normal cycles, and may be associated with the development of excessive endometrial proliferation and cystic glandular hyperplasia (Brown et al, 1959). It is now clear that the condition of 'metropathia haemorrhagica', with multicystic ovaries, cystic glandular hyperplasia of the endometrium and erratic menorrhagia, is merely the severe end of the spectrum of anovulatory dysfunctional bleeding (Brown et al, 1959). Ovarian synthesis and subsequent metabolism of oestrogens is within normal limits in peri-menopausal women with anovulatory dysfunctional bleeding, but the dynamics of oestrogen secretion are disturbed (Fraser and Baird, 1974). This suggests a disturbance of intraovarian follicular control mechanisms, perhaps as well as subtle abnormalities of pituitary gonadotrophin release (Van Look et al, 1977). By contrast, detailed investigation of adolescent girls with anovulatory dysfunctional bleeding has demonstrated a clear defect in the positive-feedback response to oestrogen (Fraser et al, 1973; Van Look et al, 1978). It is proposed that these girls may be experiencing a delay in the maturation of hypothalamic control.

The erratic, prolonged and excessively heavy bleeding which is typical of anovulatory dysfunctional bleeding is associated with prolonged, unopposed stimulation of the endometrium by fluctuating and sometimes excessively high levels of oestradiol. The exact mechanism of abnormal breakdown of the endometrium with excessive bleeding has not been elucidated. The range of endometrial histological findings has been well documented by Sutherland (1949). Orderly development of the endometrial vasculature does not occur and there is usually poor spiral arterial development with exaggerated venous vascularity and the development of venous sinusoids (Beilby et al, 1971).

There is some evidence to implicate abnormalities of endometrial prosta-glandin metabolism in anovulatory endometrium. The abnormality appears to be an impaired prostaglandin synthetic capacity due to a reduced avail-ability of the precursor arachidonic acid from membrane phospholipids (Smith et al, 1982). It is not clear whether this is due to a reduced activity of phospholipase A_2 or phospholipase C enzymes, or perhaps to an increase in the activity of lipocortin, a natural inhibitor of phospholipase activity. In the study by Smith et al (1982) the PGE_2-to-$PGF_{2\alpha}$ ratio was greater at the time of bleeding than in the normal cycle. There was a highly significant inverse correlation between the ratio of the endogenous concentrations of $PGF_{2\alpha}$ and PGE_2 and the measured menstrual blood loss. This may well be part of the mechanism of menorrhagia in women with anovulation. Unopposed oestrogen may also lead to endometrial vasodilatation and an excessive rate of endometrial blood flow at the time of endometrial breakdown (Fraser et al, 1987). It is uncertain whether abnormalities of fibrinolysis, excessive heparin production or endometrial lysosome function play any role in anovulatory bleeding disturbances.

Ovulatory dysfunctional bleeding

Most of these women appear to have circulating hormone levels indistinguishable from those of normally ovulating women (Haynes et al, 1980). Additionally, there do not appear to be any specific histological abnormalities within the secretory endometrium of these women.

There is increasingly strong evidence to implicate abnormalities of arachidonic acid metabolism in the mechanism of ovulatory dysfunctional bleeding. Elevated endometrial concentrations of PGE_2 and $PGF_{2\alpha}$ have been found throughout the menstrual cycle in women complaining of heavy periods (Willman et al, 1976). In ovulating women with excessively heavy measured menstrual blood loss there appeared to be a shift in the endometrial synthetic capacity in favour of PGE_2 over $PGF_{2\alpha}$ (Smith et al, 1981a). There is also evidence to indicate that the endometrium of patients with ovulatory menorrhagia has an increased capacity to enhance the production of prostacyclin by myometrium from women with normal menstrual blood loss (Smith et al, 1981b). Recent studies have confirmed an increased concentration of PGE in endometrium from women with menorrhagia and have suggested a relationship between the total prostaglandin content of the endometrium and measured menstrual blood loss (Cameron et al, 1987). Recent studies have also demonstrated the finding of increased PGE receptors in the myometrium of women with menorrhagia (Adelantado et al, 1988). Animal models have indicated that local application of $PGF_{2\alpha}$ can induce bleeding from endometrium (Abel et al, 1982), and preliminary experiments in women have suggested that intrauterine $PGF_{2\alpha}$ can do the same in the human uterus.

There is convincing evidence for excessive activity of the endometrial fibrinolytic system in women with menorrhagia (Bonnar et al, 1983; Dockeray et al, 1987). It is clear that the endometrium in the normal uterus already has a high fibrinolytic activity with very limited haemostatic plug formation and the detection of only occasional fragments of mature fibrin strands using electron microscopy of menstrual blood. The menstrual flow contains little fibrinolytically active plasmin but high levels of tissue plasminogen activator, fibrinogen degradation products, and plasmin–inhibitor complexes. The importance of the role of excessive activation of this system in women with menorrhagia is supported by the high efficacy of oral fibrinolytic inhibitors to treat this disorder. It is not clear how important excessive heparin-like activity in endometrium may be in women with menorrhagia (Paton et al, 1980).

Some women with menorrhagia have excessively prolonged bleeding, which suggests an abnormality of surface endometrial healing and perhaps a disturbance of angiogenesis. This could be associated with defective function of a range of endometrial growth factors which remain to be elucidated. Nothing is known about the possible involvement of leukotrienes or prostaglandin epoxides in dysfunctional uterine bleeding.

Management of menorrhagia

Women with menorrhagia due to pelvic or systemic disease should usually be treated with an agent which will specifically deal with the underlying cause. Treatment of dysfunctional uterine bleeding is often more complex, since a high proportion of women (around 50%) with dysfunctional bleeding who present with a complaint of menorrhagia cannot be confirmed to have excessive menstrual bleeding on objective measurements (Fraser et al, 1984). Treatment of menorrhagia is often far from logical and more attention needs to be paid to an individual's history and complaints in order to ensure appropriate precision in management. The major therapeutic approaches are either medical or surgical.

Drug therapy

Numerous pharmacological agents have been used for the treatment of menorrhagia over the past century, and it is probable that the majority were not much more effective than placebos. One of the earliest logical therapies was proposed by Dr H. Beckwith Whitehouse in his historic Hunterian lecture (1915) with the local application of 'thrombokinase in the form of an extract of endometrium or testicle' or, if that did not work, 'fibrin ferment supplied by Messrs Parke, Davis and Co.'. In this chapter the major emphasis on medical therapy will be on the role of prostaglandin inhibitors, although this will be put in context with other established medications.

Prostaglandin inhibitors. Objective studies have been reported of the use of several prostaglandin-inhibiting agents for the treatment of menorrhagia. In practice, any differences in mode of action of individual prostaglandin inhibitors do not seem to make much difference to overall clinical efficacy, although there are individual women who seem to respond well to one agent but less well to another. These clinical differences between preparations have not been explored thoroughly. The majority of reports have studied the use of mefenamic acid (Anderson et al, 1976; Fraser et al, 1981; Muggeridge and Elder, 1983; Hall et al, 1987; Cameron et al, 1990; Grover et al, 1990), but smaller numbers have investigated naproxen (Hall et al, 1987; Fraser and McCarron, 1991), naproxen sodium, meclofenamic acid (Vargyas et al, 1987), ibuprofen (Makarainen and Ylikorkala, 1986a,b), flufenamic acid, diclofenac sodium (Ylikorkala and Viinikka, 1983) or flurbiprofen (Milsom et al, 1991). There is a wide variation in individual patient response, with the overall mean reduction in measured loss during treatment being of the order of 30–40%. There is a suggestion that women with heavier measured loss may experience a greater percentage reduction in loss than those with less heavy bleeding. In women with pretreatment blood loss greater than 60 ml, a mean reduction in menstrual blood loss of 37% was noted with mefenamic acid, whereas no mean reduction was found when pretreatment blood loss was less than 40 ml (Fraser, 1983). This is of major practical importance, because of the high proportion of women who present with a convincing history of menorrhagia when their measured blood loss is not excessive. Meclofenamate sodium is a promising agent because it is somewhat more rapidly absorbed than most other prosta-glandin inhibitors, probably has a more potent clinical effect because of greater end-organ binding (Rees et al, 1988) and may inhibit leukotrienes (Boctor et al, 1986). This promise has been borne out in the one detailed clinical study of its use in menorrhagia which reported reductions in blood loss of the order of 40–50% over four cycles of use (Vargyas et al, 1987).

Dosage regimens are quite variable, depending on the particular agent, and usually need to be individually tailored to the patient's response in order to obtain optimum long-term results. Short-term regimens with initiation of therapy at the onset of bleeding and repeated doses until after the end of excessively heavy bleeding are recommended for most agents. It should be noted that compliance may become a problem after some months because many women find it difficult or distressing to rigidly take regular medication for several days every month, especially when their menorrhagia may be somewhat variable with the occasional 'good' period.

There is a significant incidence of treatment failures with all of these agents (20–30%). A small number of individuals actually experience a consistent increase in measured menstrual loss during treatment with prostaglandin inhibitors (Fraser and McCarron, 1991). The mechanism of this unusual response is unknown, and indicates our lack of understanding of the interactions of prostaglandin-related mechanisms in the causation of dysfunctional uterine bleeding. By contrast, some fortunate women will obtain up to an 80% reduction in measured loss (Fraser, 1983). Overall, it appears that 50–60% of women with objective menorrhagia will gain a sufficient reduction in loss to justify long-term therapy. Most women will also experience a significant reduction in the duration of bleeding during treatment with mefenamic acid (Fraser et al, 1981; Cameron et al, 1990; Grover et al, 1990). These benefits appear to be maintained with long-term therapy. Persistent reductions of the order of 25–35% in measured loss have been reported in 34 women studied over a 16 month period (Fraser et al, 1983). This objective finding is at odds with anecdotal reports from many doctors that the initial reduction in menstrual bleeding is not maintained with long-term therapy. The explanation for this appears to be that patients become less meticulous about dosage as time goes by. It is worth noting that other menstrually related symptoms such as dysmenorrhoea, menstrual headaches and menstrually related diarrhoea, nausea and depression will also improve with mefenamic acid and be maintained for more than 1 year (Fraser et al, 1983).

Menstrual blood loss is significantly increased with use of an intrauterine contraceptive device (IUCD), usually of the order of 50–80% with modern copper IUCDs. Numerous studies confirm the efficacy of a range of prostaglandin inhibitors for the treatment of IUCD-associated menorrhagia (Guillebaud et al, 1978; Ylikorkala et al, 1978; Pizarro et al, 1989). Indeed, the first major report on the use of a prostaglandin inhibitor for menorrhagia was with mefenamic acid and IUCDs (Anderson et al, 1976). There is encouraging evidence that mefenamic acid may be helpful for a substantial number of women with adenomyosis, endometriosis and, occasionally, other conditions causing menorrhagia (Fraser et al, 1981, 1986). There is no good evidence that they are beneficial in menorrhagia due to uterine myomata or coagulation disorders (Fraser et al, 1986; Makarainen and Ylikorkala, 1986a).

A small number of comparative trials have been carried out with different prostaglandin inhibitors or prostaglandin inhibitors and other agents in the same patient. The small number of randomized studies of this type show that mefenamic acid and naproxen are probably similar in effect, provided that appropriate dosages are used (Hall et al, 1987; Fraser and McCarron, 1991). Not all individuals who show a good response to one agent will respond to other agents; hence, there is a place for considering the use of an alternative prostaglandin inhibitor if the first does not work. Mefenamic acid has also been compared with danazol and oral contraception, with remarkably similar results in the first cycle of treatment (Dockeray, 1990; Fraser and McCarron, 1991). Danazol produces a much greater reduction in measured loss with continued use over several cycles compared with other agents. Comparative studies have also been carried out with prostaglandin inhibitors and with the fibrinolytic inhibitor tranexamic acid (Ylikorkala and Viinikka, 1983; Milsom et al, 1991), and with progestogen-releasing IUCDs (Cameron et al, 1990; Milsom et al, 1991), demonstrating that the prostaglandin inhibitors are somewhat less effective than either tranexamic acid or the progestogen-releasing IUCDs. No reports have appeared of combinations of prostaglandin inhibitors with hormonal therapies given at the same time.

Side-effects have been discussed earlier, but it is important to emphasize that, with the simple dosage regimens usually given for menorrhagia treatment, side-effects are uncommon. Mild gastrointestinal and central nervous system side-effects are only slightly more common in active treatment cycles than with placebo and, in long-term studies, treatment withdrawals due to side-effects are less than 10%. The occurrence of minor side-effects, the variability of successive cycles for any one individual and the difficulties of compliance which some women experience point to a need for the development of new systems for delivering prostaglandin inhibitors. It would be ideal if systems could be developed which would deliver constant dosages over several days and could be controlled by the woman herself. The ideal system appears to be a vaginal ring made of a polymer which will deliver adequate dosages of the prostaglandin inhibitors to the vaginal mucosa. Since indomethacin is well absorbed from rectal suppositories, it seems likely that the vaginal surface will also allow adequate and rapid absorption of prostaglandin inhibitors. Research in this area is urgently needed.

Other drug therapies. These therapies have been discussed in detail elsewhere, and will only be briefly addressed in this review (Fraser, 1989).

A variety of hormonal agents are effective for management of ovulatory and anovulatory dysfunctional uterine bleeding. Most of these agents probably act by suppression of endometrial growth, which is probably accompanied by a suppression of prostaglandin synthesis. It is unclear how much the suppression of prostaglandins relates to the efficacy of the hormonal therapy. In the UK the most popular therapy for ovulatory dysfunctional bleeding is luteal phase norethisterone (Bishop and de Almeida, 1960). The original report of this therapy indicated subjective improvement in women with both ovulatory and anovulatory dysfunctional bleeding. However, more recent reports of objective menstrual blood loss measurement have not been able to substantiate this benefit with ovulatory patients (Cameron et al, 1990). On the other hand, luteal phase therapy is probably very useful in women with anovulatory dysfunctional bleeding where objective reductions of more than 50% have been reported (Fraser, 1990). In women with ovulatory dysfunctional bleeding more effective reduction in menstrual blood loss is obtained with progestogen therapy for 3 weeks out of every 4 (Fraser, 1990). Continuous oral progestogen therapy may also be useful in limited cases, and there are anecdotal reports of the beneficial effect of depot medroxyprogesterone acetate (DMPA; Depo-Provera), which will often produce amenorrhoea. Unfortunately, a significant proportion of these women will initially experience erratic and sometimes prolonged breakthrough bleeding. A better approach may be to use oral MPA until amenorrhoea is achieved, and then follow this with DMPA.

The most exciting route for administering progestogens to treat menorrhagia is with an intrauterine device. Dramatic reductions in menstrual blood loss have been reported with use of levonorgestrel-releasing IUCDs (Andersson and Rybo, 1990). These devices can induce reductions in measured menstrual loss of around 85% at 3 months, 90% at 6 months and 95% at 12 months after device insertion. A small proportion of patients experience spotting or somewhat erratic bleeding in the early months after insertion.

The mechanism of action of progestogens is unclear although, histologically, there is initially inhibition of endometrial proliferation followed by suppressed secretory change and, eventually, atrophy. The reduced exposure to unopposed oestrogen and the increased exposure to high-dose local progestogens presumably reduces the capacity of endometrium to mobilize arachidonic acid from membrane phospholipids, and may also affect synthesis of individual prostaglandins from any arachidonic acid or *endo-peroxides* that may be formed. There is also evidence for some inhibition of fibrinolytic activity and a reduction in endometrial vascularity.

Combination oral contraceptives are highly effective and may induce a 40–50% reduction in measured blood loss (Nilsson and Rybo, 1971; Fraser and McCarron, 1991). Danazol is also highly effective, even at dosages as low as 100–200 mg daily over several months (Chimbira et al, 1980b; Fraser and McCarron, 1991), but long-term treatment (beyond 6 months) is generally not advised because of metabolic concerns. Gestrinone is a newer anti-progestogenic and antioestrogenic agent with some minor androgenic activity which has been shown to have beneficial effects for ovulatory menorrhagia when given in a dosage of one capsule twice weekly (Turnbull and Rees, 1990). Gonadotrophin-releasing hormone analogues will produce highly effective reductions in menstrual blood loss in ovulatory menorrhagia (Shaw and Fraser, 1984), but their long-term use is limited by metabolic concerns and cost. These agents may also be useful for shrinking uterine myomata prior to surgery (McLachlan et al, 1986) or for producing endometrial suppression prior to endometrial ablation operations (Petrucco and Fraser, 1992).

Fibrinolytic inhibitors have been extensively evaluated for menorrhagia and are highly effective. Objective reductions in menstrual loss are dose related and reach 50% in most studies (Nilsson and Rybo, 1971; Ylikorkala and Viinikka, 1983; Milsom et al, 1991). Tranexamic acid is the most widely used agent since side-effects are infrequent and complications (such as spontaneous thromboses) are exceedingly rare. Trials of combination therapy with fibrinolytic inhibitors and prostaglandin inhibitors have not been carried out. However, both fibrinolytic and prostaglandin mechanisms appear to be important in the pathogenesis of ovulatory dysfunctional bleeding and a dual approach to therapy could have some merit. Other drugs which may have some utility for ovulatory menorrhagia include ethamsylate, tamoxifen and long-acting injections of vasopressin analogues such as glypressin.

Treatment choices may be difficult and physicians must become familiar with a small range of these agents. Efficacy of these agents depends greatly on the information and encouragement which is given to the patient. Use of medical therapies for dysfunctional bleeding should only be offered as part of a long-term plan which may include cessation of treatment for a trial period, or may involve later use of surgery such as endometrial ablation or hysterectomy. Hysterectomy and the endometrial ablation techniques have been considered elsewhere (Fraser, 1989).

CONTRACEPTIVE-RELATED BLEEDING DISTURBANCES

Troublesome disturbances of bleeding occur with most hormonal agents and with intrauterine devices. Intrauterine devices tend to cause menorrhagia with occasional intermenstrual bleeding, while hormonal agents, particularly the progestogen-only methods, tend to produce erratic and sometimes prolonged spotting or light bleeding. The clinical importance of these has been thoroughly discussed elsewhere (Fraser, 1982; Odlind and Fraser, 1990). Circumstantial evidence strongly suggests abnormalities of endometrial prostaglandin synthesis and secretion in users of intrauterine devices with menstrual disturbances; however, most of the reported studies contain biases or flaws. Perhaps the most important pieces of circumstantial evidence for the involvement of prostaglandins in the genesis of these symptoms is the dramatic reduction in menstrual blood loss that can be demonstrated in many women with IUCD-related menorrhagia using prostaglandin inhibitors (Guillebaud et al, 1978; Ylikorkala et al, 1978; Davis et al, 1981; Makarainen and Ylikorkala, 1986b).

There is some evidence for abnormal endometrial vessel formation, morphology and function, as well as defective endometrial haemostatic response, defective endometrial macrophage and mast cell function and defective endometrial lysozyme function. The importance of each of these mechanisms is unclear. It is probable that abnormalities of spiral arterial function are particularly important in the menorrhagia associated with IUCDs. By contrast, it is probable that the bleeding disturbances with progestogen-only contraceptives are mainly associated with abnormalities of bleeding at a capillary level. These abnormalities are so poorly understood that two major symposia have been organized to identify new leads which may help in the elucidation of their mechanisms and management (Diczfalusy et al, 1980; D'Arcangues et al, 1990).

The possible role of prostaglandins in the mechanisms of progestogen-related bleeding has been studied in some detail (White et al, 1991). There were no significant alterations in the proportion of arachidonic acid which was metabolized by the cyclooxygenase and lipoxygenase enzyme systems in treated cycles compared with controls. However, there was a significant increase in the proportion of arachidonic acid metabolized to an epoxide and to $PGF_{1\alpha}$ after progestogen exposure. The proportions of epoxide metabolite, $PGF_{1\alpha}$ and PGE_2 were positively correlated with serum levonorgestrel levels while PGE_2 and epoxide were correlated with serum oestradiol. The proportion of epoxide formed correlated with the number of bleeding days. An increase in free oxygen radicals in endometrial tissue may be a factor in the disproportionate increase in epoxygenase products compared with the other arachidonic acid metabolites. Some epoxides inhibit platelet aggregation, which could be an important factor relating to abnormalities of bleeding. It has been postulated that persistent exposure of the endometrium to progestogens will diminish overall prostaglandin production as well as increase catabolism by increasing 15-hydroxyprostaglandin dehydrogenase (Smith et al, 1981).

Prostaglandin inhibitors probably have a very limited role in the management of progestogen-related bleeding disturbances, although some reduction in days of breakthrough bleeding with the contraceptive subdermal implant system Norplant may occur with mefenamic acid therapy. The use of prostaglandin inhibitors appears to be much more effective for menorrhagia than for prolonged or erratic bleeding. This is clearly seen in treatments of menorrhagia accompanying IUCD use, as discussed above.

PREMENSTRUAL SYNDROME (PMS)

The aetiology of this poorly defined and highly variable symptom complex is unknown. Symptoms occur in a regular, cyclical fashion during the 1–2 weeks prior to menstruation and usually disappear very soon after the onset of bleeding. Typically they occur in women who are ovulating, and appear to be related to the presence of progesterone after exposure to oestrogen alone. There is suggestive evidence that factors released by the endometrium may contribute to the symptomatology, since great improvements may follow hysterectomy or endometrial ablation, in spite of continued ovarian function.

The predominant symptoms implicate the central nervous system, and current theories of aetiology point to subtle changes in neurotransmitters or neuromodulators. Mood and behavioural symptoms feature prominently and may be accompanied by poor memory, agitation, aggression, indecisiveness, muddled thinking, clumsiness, altered appetite, cravings, headaches and a range of physical symptoms such as breast tenderness and abdominal bloating. However, aetiology is unknown and numerous mechanisms have been implicated.

Several eicosanoids have actions in the central nervous system which could cause symptoms of the type commonly reported with PMS (Craig, 1980). Much of the evidence for the role of prostaglandins in the central nervous system comes from animal studies. Prostaglandins may modify concentrations of biogenic amines and may block dopaminergic receptors in the central nervous system. Prostaglandins of the E series have a profound depressant effect on behaviour, resulting in sedation, reduction in spontaneous motor activity, loss of interest in surroundings, motor incoordination, disturbances of posture, inhibition of conditioned avoidance and escape responses, and decreased skeletal muscle tone. Most prostaglandins also cause anorexia and inhibition of food intake although PGE_1 may produce an increase in food intake through certain hypothalamic centres. PGE_1 is particularly potent in facilitating perception of pain (Juan, 1978). Brush et al (1984) found significantly lower circulating levels of γ-linolenic acid in women with PMS than controls, and felt that this could be a deficiency contributing to symptoms. This could explain why some women respond to evening primrose oil.

Treatment of PMS

Numerous treatments have been reported, but this review will concentrate on the limited evidence for a role of prostaglandin inhibitors in the management of PMS. Double-blind, placebo-controlled studies with luteal phase mefenamic acid have demonstrated a significant reduction in tension, irritability, depression, pain and headaches (Jacubowicz et al, 1982; Mira et al, 1986). This finding suggests that excessive secretion of one or more prostaglandins, probably from the endometrium, constitutes an integral part of PMS, but direct evidence is lacking. A further study utilized evening primrose oil, which contains the dietary prostaglandin precursors linoleic and dihomo-γ-linolenic acids (Brush, 1981). This combination of essential fatty acids should promote the synthesis of some prostaglandins, and may imply an imbalance of certain prostaglandins in PMS rather than an abnormality of absolute levels. All symptoms were found to improve with this treatment in the study by Brush (1981), but a placebo-controlled study was unable to confirm any objective benefit of evening primrose oil (Cerin et al, 1989). It seems probable that anomalies of prostaglandin synthesis and metabolism occur in PMS, but they may only be part of a cascade of factors in both endometrium and the central nervous system.

ENDOMETRIOSIS

Endometriosis is a highly variable and poorly understood condition where tissue histologically similar to endometrium is found in extrauterine sites. Since prostaglandins are synthesized by endometrium, it is to be expected that they will also be synthesized by endometriotic tissue. However, there is considerable controversy about the extent and circumstances of prostaglandin production by this pathological tissue. This may be partly explained by the great variability in symptomatology, site of occurrence, surface morphology and histology, which are likely to be mirrored by variability in biochemical function and responses to cyclical hormone change. The major symptoms of pelvic pain, menstrual disturbance and infertility could all be influenced by disturbances in prostaglandin metabolism.

Peritoneum is the commonest site for endometriosis, and it is now recognized that this tissue probably demonstrates a progressive change in appearance as it develops (Jansen and Russell, 1986; Redwine, 1987). It first appears as a velvety change to the peritoneal surface, followed by the appearance of clear papules, then surrounded by a reddened flare with new vessel formation. These lesions become haemorrhagic and then the centre becomes darkened and brownish, before finally reaching the classical dark 'match head' appearance which may represent a less active old lesion. Sometimes the lesions are associated with fibrosis, and sometimes the peritoneum may be eaten away to form 'windows', with active microscopic endometriosis present in the intact margins. It is unclear why some of the discrete lesions bleed each month at the time of menstruation while others do not: is this a function of tissue mass or of maturation of the implant?

Prostaglandins are present in peritoneal fluid, and some studies have found elevated levels in the presence of endometriosis. However, several other studies have not been able to confirm this finding and the true relationship between endometriosis and the presence of different prostaglandins in peritoneal fluid is unresolved (Syrop and Halme, 1987). These investigations have produced conflicting results because of: difficulties in controlling for stage of the cycle, failure to identify microscopic endometriosis in 'controls'; blood contamination of samples; rapid local release of prostaglandins after minor peritoneal trauma; failure to account for differences in fluid volume; and variations in the extent and 'activity' of lesions. When the day of the cycle was controlled most studies have been unable to show elevated levels of classical prostaglandins in the presence of endometriosis, except perhaps when the tissue is proliferating during the follicular phase. On the other hand, a majority of investigators have reported elevated levels of prostacyclin and TXA_2 (or their metabolites) in the presence of endometriosis. Indeed, Drake et al (1981) reported 6-keto-$PGF_{1\alpha}$ levels of 44.5 ± 13.7 ng/ml in 14 women with endometriosis and only 3.85 ± 2.5 ng/ml in 15 controls with no endometriosis.

The fact that major differences in the prostaglandin content of peritoneal fluid cannot be confirmed in endometriosis sufferers does not mean that prostaglandins are not involved in the function of the lesions or the symptomatology of the disease. In vitro studies have demonstrated that peritoneal endometriotic lesions generally contain and release less $PGF_{2\alpha}$ than uterine endometrium (Vernon et al, 1986). The largest amounts of prostaglandin were released from reddened petechial lesions and the least from dark 'match head' spots, suggesting that there was increased release from the more active lesions. Content and release of prostaglandins appeared to be very low in tissue collected from women with severe or extensive disease. Animal models have also suggested a role for excessive production of prostaglandins at some stages of the disease (Schenken and Asch, 1980; Schenken et al, 1984).

Prostaglandins have a number of biochemical actions which could give them a role in the genesis, function and symptomatology of endometriosis, although this still remains to be proved (Hurst and Rock, 1991; Smith, 1991). Activated peritoneal macrophages are probably present in increased numbers in women with endometriosis, and are capable of secreting prostaglandins. They may influence endometriotic proliferation in this manner. Activated macrophages are capable of secreting a range of regulatory molecules, such as tumour necrosis factor α (TNFα) and interleukins, which in turn have a multitude of actions which interact with prostaglandins. For example, TNFα is capable of increasing the adhesion of endometrial stromal cells to peritoneal mesothelial cells in culture. Preliminary evidence suggests that TNFα, interleukin-1β (IL-1β), IL-6 and IL-8 may all be produced in vitro by experimental endometriosis. Prostaglandins, arachidonic acid and the interleukins may also be involved in stimulating fibroblast proliferation and collagen deposition, probably through the generation of free oxygen radicals. This may contribute to the common finding of peritoneal scarring and adhesion formation in endometriosis. The role of prostaglandins in inflammatory processes indicates that they may contribute to the generation of pain of peritoneal and deeper tissue origin in endometriosis. The possible involvement of leukotrienes is unknown. Undoubtedly, numerous molecular interactions are involved in the pathogenesis of endometriosis, and this may be particularly complex with respect to mechanisms of infertility with endometriosis. At this time, all of these mechanisms are a matter of speculation, and it is likely that the role of prostaglandins is as part of a cascade of interactions, probably as intermediates or modulators rather than primary effectors.

Treatment of endometriosis

Management falls into three categories—expectant, medical and surgical; or may involve a combination. The role of each is gradually being clarified as new therapeutic agents are introduced, and better comparative clinical trials are being reported. The final choice still needs to be individualized, taking into account the extent, duration and site of disease, symptomatology and desire for fertility.

It is not the intention of this review to provide a comprehensive discussion of therapy of endometriosis, but to highlight the possible role of prostaglandin inhibitors and other drugs which may interfere with prostaglandins. The mainstay of medical therapy has been the use of combined oestrogen–progestogen preparations or progestogens alone, but other hormonal preparations such as danazol, gestrinone and the gonadotrophin-releasing hormone analogues may be more effective. It seems probable that these agents will reduce the capability of the endometrium to synthesize and secrete prostaglandins, and this mechanism may make some contribution to the reduction of symptoms.

Studies of the use of prostaglandin inhibitors for the symptoms of endometriosis have been very limited. Tolfenamic acid may produce significant relief of secondary dysmenorrhoea due to endometriosis (Kauppilla et al, 1979), but this relief is not as dramatic as seen with primary dysmenorrhoea, another indicator that prostaglandins only play a subsidiary role in the aetiology of endometriosis. Limited data confirm a small role for prostaglandin inhibitors such as mefenamic acid in the treatment of menorrhagia associated with endometriosis (Fraser et al, 1986). Even more limited data suggest that some women with menorrhagia due to adenomyosis may also respond to mefenamic acid (Fraser et al, 1986).

CONCLUSIONS

Weighty evidence now implicates a role for disturbances of prostaglandin synthesis, secretion and metabolism in several menstrual disorders, of which primary dysmenorrhoea and ovulatory dysfunctional uterine bleeding are the most evident. Prostaglandin inhibitors have an important place in management, but their use needs to be individualized in order to obtain optimal treatment responses. It is not clear which prostaglandin inhibitors are the most effective agents, but the fenamates have been most extensively studied and may have a beneficial end-organ effect. Compliance may be a problem with long-term intermittent therapy, and development of delivery systems would be valuable. Treatment failures occur with all agents, and more research is needed into the reasons for this therapeutic failure. The availability and possible use of more specific synthetic enzyme inhibitors (Poyser, 1985), leukotriene inhibitors or specific prostaglandin receptor blockers would be welcome.

REFERENCES

Abel MH & Baird DT (1980) The effect of 17-β oestradiol and progesterone on prostaglandin production by human endometrium maintained in organ culture. *Endocrinology* **106:** 1599–1605.

Abel MH & Kelly RW (1979) Differential production of prostaglandin within the human uterus. *Prostaglandins* **18:** 821–834.

Abel MH, Zhu C & Baird DT (1982) An animal model to study menstrual bleeding. *Research and Clinical Forums* **4:** 25–34.

Adelantado JM, Rees MCP, Lopez-Bernal A & Turnbull AC (1988) Increased uterine prostaglandin E receptors in menorrhagic women. *British Journal of Obstetrics and Gynaecology* **95:** 162–165.

Akerlund M, Anderssen K-I & Ingermarsson I (1976) Effects of terbutaline on myometrial activity, uterine blood flow and lower abdominal pain in women with primary dysmenorrhoea. *British Journal of Obstetrics and Gynaecology* **83:** 673–681.

Anderson ABM, Haynes PJ, Guillebaud J & Turnbull AC (1976) Reduction of menstrual blood loss by prostaglandin synthetase inhibitors. *Lancet* **i:** 774–776.

Anderson ABM, Fraser IS, Haynes PJ & Turnbull AC (1978) Trial of prostaglandin synthetase inhibitors in primary dysmenorrhoea. *Lancet* **i:** 345–348.

Anderssen K-E & Ulmsten U (1978) Effects of nifedipine on myometrial activity and lower abdominal pain in patients with primary dysmenorrhoea. *British Journal of Obstetrics and Gynaecology* **85:** 142–149.

Andersson K & Rybo G (1990) Levonorgestrel-releasing intrauterine device in the treatment of menorrhagia. *British Journal of Obstetrics and Gynaecology* **97:** 690–694.

Baird DT, Abel MH, Kelly RW & Smith SK (1981) Endocrinology of dysfunctional uterine bleeding: the role of endometrial prostaglandins. In Crosignani PG & Rubin BL (eds) *Endocrinology of Human Infertility; New Aspects*, pp 399–417. New York: Academic Press.

Beilby JOW, Farrer-Brown G & Tarbit MH (1971) The microvasculature of common uterine abnormalities excluding fibroids. *Journal of Obstetrics and Gynaecology of the British Commonwealth* **78:** 361–368.

Bishop PMF & de Almeida JCC (1960) Treatment of functional menstrual disorders with norethisterone. *British Medical Journal* **i:** 1103–1106.

Boctor A, Eickholt M & Pugsley IA (1986) Meclofenamate sodium is an inhibitor of both the 5-lipoxygenase and cyclo-oxygenase pathways of the arachidonic cascade in vitro. *Prostaglandins and Leukotrienes in Medicine* **23:** 229–238.

Bonnar J, Sheppard BL & Dockeray CL (1983) The haemostatic system and dysfunctional uterine bleeding. *Research and Clinical Forums* **5:** 27–36.

Brown JB, Kellar RJ & Matthew GD (1959) Preliminary observations on urinary oestrogen excretion in certain gynaecological disorders. *Journal of Obstetrics and Gynaecology of the British Empire* **66:** 177–211.

Brush MG (1982) Efamol (evening primrose oil) in the treatment of premenstrual syndrome. In Horrobin DF (ed.) *Clinical Uses of Essential Fatty Acids*, pp 156–161. London: Eden Press.

Brush MG, Watson SJ, Horrobin DF & Manker MS (1984) Abnormal essential fatty acid levels in plasma of women with premenstrual syndrome. *American Journal of Obstetrics and Gynecology* **150:** 363–366.

Cameron IT, Leask R, Kelly RW & Baird DT (1987) Endometrial prostaglandins in women with abnormal menstrual bleeding. *Prostaglandins, Leukotrienes and Medicine* **29:** 249–257.

Cameron IT, Haining R, Lumsden MA, Thomas VR & Smith SK (1990) The effects of mefenamic acid and norethisterone on measured menstrual blood loss. *Obstetrics and Gynecology* **76:** 85–88.

Carraher R, Hahn DW, Ritchie DM & McGuire JL (1983) Involvement of lipoxygenase products in myometrial contractions. *Prostaglandins* **26:** 23–34.

Cerin A, Andersson L, Collins A, Landgren B-M & Eneroth P (1989) Effect of Efamol (gammalinolenic acid) treatment in women with premenstrual tension syndrome. *Journal of Psychosomatic Obstetrics and Gynaecology* **10(supplement 1):** 153–154.

Chan WY, Dawood MY & Fuchs F (1981) Prostaglandins in primary dysmenorrhoea: comparison of prophylactic and non-prophylactic treatment with Ibuprofen and use of oral contraceptives. *American Journal of Medicine* **70:** 535–539.

Chimbira T, Anderson ABM & Turnbull AC (1980a) Relation between measured menstrual blood loss and patient's subjective assessment of loss, duration of bleeding, number of sanitary towels used, uterine weight and endometrial surface area. *British Journal of Obstetrics and Gynaecology* **87:** 603–609.

Chimbira T, Anderson ABM & Turnbull AC (1980b) Reduction of menstrual blood loss with danazol in unexplained menorrhagia; lack of effect of placebo. *British Journal of Obstetrics and Gynaecology* **87:** 1152–1157.

Craig G (1980) The premenstrual syndrome and prostaglandin metabolism. *British Journal of Family Planning* **6:** 74–77.

D'Arcangues C, Fraser IS, Newton JR & Odlind V (eds) (1990) *Contraception and Mechanisms of Endometrial Bleeding*. Cambridge: Cambridge University Press.

Davies AJ, Anderson ABM & Turnbull AC (1981) Reduction by naproxen of excessive menstrual bleeding in women using intrauterine devices. *Obstetrics and Gynecology* **57:** 74–78.

Diczfalusy E, Fraser IS & Webb FTG (eds) (1980) *Endometrial Bleeding and Steroidal Contraception*. Bath: Pitman Press.

Dockeray CJ (1990) The use of prostaglandin synthetase inhibitors in dysfunctional uterine bleeding. In Shaw RW (ed.) *Dysfunctional Uterine Bleeding*, pp 117–125. Carnforth: Parthenon Press.

Dockeray CJ, Sheppard BL & Bonnar J (1987) The fibrinolytic enzyme system in normal menstruation and excessive uterine bleeding, and the effect of tranexamic acid. *European Journal of Obstetrics, Gynaecology and Reproductive Biology* **24:** 309–318.

Drake TS, O'Brien WF, Ramwell PW & Metz SA (1981) Peritoneal fluid thromboxane B2 and 6-keto prostaglandin F1a in endometriosis. *American Journal of Obstetrics and Gynecology* **140:** 401–404.

Fraser IS (1982) Abnormal uterine bleeding due to hormonal steroids and intrauterine devices. In Chang CF, Griffin D & Woolman A (eds) *Recent Advances in Fertility Regulation*, pp 265–300. Copenhagen: Atar Press.

Fraser IS (1983) The treatment of menorrhagia with mefenamic acid. *Research and Clinical Forums* **5:** 93–99.

Fraser IS (1985a) Prostaglandin inhibitors in gynaecology. *Australian and New Zealand Journal of Obstetrics and Gynaecology* **25:** 114–116.

Fraser IS (1989) Treatment of menorrhagia. *Baillière's Clinical Obstetrics and Gynaecology* **3:** 391–402.

Fraser IS (1990a) Treatment of ovulatory and anovulatory dysfunctional uterine bleeding with oral progestogens. *Australian and New Zealand Journal of Obstetrics and Gynaecology* **30:** 353–356.

Fraser IS & Baird DT (1974) Blood production and ovarian secretion of estradiol-17β and estrone in women with dysfunctional uterine bleeding. *Journal of Clinical Endocrinology and Metabolism* **39:** 564–570.

Fraser IS & McCarron G (1991) Randomised trial of two hormonal and two prostaglandin inhibiting agents for the treatment of menorrhagia. *Australian and New Zealand Journal of Obstetrics and Gynaecology* **31:** 66–70.

Fraser IS (1990b) Hysteroscopy and laparoscopy in women with menorrhagia. *American Journal of Obstetrics and Gynecology* **162:** 1264–1269.

Fraser IS, Michie EA, Baird DT & Wide L (1973) Pituitary gonadotropins and ovarian function in adolescent dysfunctional uterine bleeding. *Journal of Clinical Endocrinology and Metabolism* **37:** 407–414.

Fraser IS, Pearse C, Shearman RP, Elliott PM, McIlveen J & Markham R (1981) Efficacy of mefenamic acid in patients with a complaint of menorrhagia. *Obstetrics and Gynecology* **58:** 543–551.

Fraser IS, McCarron G & Markham R (1983) Long-term treatment of menorrhagia with mefenamic acid. *Obstetrics and Gynecology* **61:** 109–112.

Fraser IS, McCarron G & Markham R (1984) A preliminary study of factors influencing perception of menstrual blood loss volume. *American Journal of Obstetrics and Gynecology* **149:** 788–793.

Fraser IS, McCarron G & Markham R (1985) Blood and total fluid content of menstrual discharge. *Obstetrics and Gynecology* **65:** 194–198.

Fraser IS, McCarron G & Markham R (1986) Objective measurement of menstrual blood loss in women with a complaint of menorrhagia associated with pelvic disease or coagulation disorder. *Obstetrics and Gynecology* **68:** 630–633.

Fraser IS, McCarron G, Hutton BF & Macey D (1987) Endometrial blood flow measured by xenon-133 clearance in women with normal menstrual cycles and dysfunctional uterine bleeding. *American Journal of Obstetrics and Gynecology* **156:** 158–166.

Garfield RE & Hayashi RH (1980) Presence of gap junctions in the myometrium of women during various stages of menstruation. *American Journal of Obstetrics and Gynecology* **138:** 569–574.

Grover V, Usha R, Gupta U & Kalra S (1990) Management of cyclical menorrhagia with a prostaglandin synthetase inhibitor. *Asia and Oceania Journal of Obstetrics and Gynaecology* **16:** 255–259.

Guillebaud J, Anderson ABM & Turnbull AC (1978) Reduction by mefenamic acid of increased menstrual blood loss associated with intrauterine contraception. *British Journal of Obstetrics and Gynaecology* **85:** 53–60.

Hall P, Maclachlan N, Thorn N, Hudd MWE, Taylor CG & Garrioch DB (1987) Control of menorrhagia by the cyclo-oxygenase inhibitors naproxen sodium and mefenamic acid. *British Journal of Obstetrics and Gynaecology* **94:** 554–558.

Hallberg L, Hogdahl A-M, Nilsson L & Rybo G (1966) Menstrual blood loss—a population study. *Acta Obstetrica et Gynecologica Scandinavica* **45:** 320–351.

Haynes PJ, Flint AP, Hodgson H, Anderson ABM & Turnbull AC (1980) Studies in menorrhagia: a) mefenamic acid; b) endometrial prostaglandin concentration. *International Journal of Gynaecology and Obstetrics* **17:** 567–572.

Henzl MR, Ortega-Herrera E, Rodriguez C & Izu A (1979) Anaprox in dysmenorrhoea; reduction of pain and intrauterine pressure. *American Journal of Obstetrics and Gynecology* **135:** 455–460.

Higham JM, O'Brien PMS & Shaw RW (1990) Assessment of menstrual blood loss using a pictorial chart. *British Journal of Obstetrics and Gynaecology* **97:** 734–739.

Hurst BS & Rock JA (1991) The peritoneal environment in endometriosis. In Thomas E & Rock JA (eds) *Modern Approaches to Endometriosis*, pp 79–96. Dordrecht: Kluwer.

Irwin J, Morse E & Riddick D (1981) Dysmenorrhea induced by autologous transfusion. *Obstetrics and Gynecology* **58:** 286–294.

Jacubowicz D, Goddard E & Dewhurst J (1982) The treatment of premenstrual tension with mefenamic acid; analysis of prostaglandin concentrations. *British Journal of Obstetrics and Gynaecology* **91:** 78–84.

Jansen RPS & Russell P (1986) Non-pigmented endometriosis: clinical, laparoscopic and pathologic definition. *American Journal of Obstetrics and Gynaecology* **155:** 1154–1159.

Juan H (1978) Prostaglandins as modulators of pain. *General Pharmacology* **9:** 403–409.

Kauppila A, Puolakka J & Ylikorkala O (1979) Prostaglandin biosynthesis inhibitors and endometriosis. *Prostaglandins* **18:** 655–661.

Kelly RW & Abel MH (1980) Catechol oestrogens stimulate and direct prostaglandin synthesis. *Prostaglandins* **20:** 613–626.

Kremser E & Mitchell GM (1971) Treatment of primary dysmenorrhoea with combined-type oral contraceptive: a double blind study. *Journal of the American Colleges Health Association* **19:** 195–199.

Lumsden MA & Baird DT (1985) Intrauterine pressure in dysmenorrhoea. *Acta Obstetrica et Gynecologica Scandinavica* **64:** 183–186.

Lumsden MA, Kelly RW & Baird DT (1983) Is prostaglandin $F_{2\alpha}$ involved in the increased myometrial contractility of primary dysmenorrhoea. *Prostaglandins* **25:** 683–691.

Lundstrom V (1977) The myometrial response to intrauterine administration of $PGF_{2\alpha}$ and PGE_2 in dysmenorrhoeic women. *Acta Obstetrica et Gynecologica Scandinavica* **56:** 167–173.

Lundstrom V & Green K (1978) Endogenous levels of $PGF_{2\alpha}$ and its main metabolites in plasma and endometrium of normal and dysmenorrheic women. *American Journal of Obstetrics and Gynecology* **130:** 640–649.

McLachlan RI, Healy DL & Burger HG (1986) Clinical aspects of LHRH analogues in gynaecology: a review. *British Journal of Obstetrics and Gynaecology* **93:** 431–454.

Makarainen L & Ylikorkala O (1986a) Primary and myoma-associated menorrhagia: role of prostaglandins and effect of ibuprofen. *British Journal of Obstetrics and Gynaecology* **93:** 974–983.

Makarainen L & Ylikorkala O (1986b) Ibuprofen prevents IUCD-induced increases in menstrual blood loss. *British Journal of Obstetrics and Gynaecology* **93:** 285–288.

Milsom I, Andersson K, Andersch B & Rybo G (1991) A comparison of flurbiprofen, tranexamic acid and a levonorgestrel-releasing intrauterine contraceptive device in the treatment of idiopathic menorrhagia. *American Journal of Obstetrics and Gynecology* **164:** 879–893.

Mira M, McNeil D, Fraser IS, Vizzard J & Abraham S (1986) The use of mefenamic acid in the treatment of premenstrual tension sufferers. *Obstetrics and Gynecology* **68:** 395–398.

Muggeridge J & Elder MG (1983) Mefenamic acid in the treatment of menorrhagia. *Research and Clinical Forums* **5:** 83–88.

Nilsson L & Rybo G (1971) Treatment of menorrhagia. *American Journal of Obstetrics and Gynecology* **110:** 713–720.

Odlind V & Fraser IS (1990) Contraception and menstrual bleeding disturbances—a clinical overview. In D'Arcangues C, Fraser IS, Newton JR & Odlind V (eds) *Contraception and Mechanisms of Endometrial Bleeding*, pp 5–29. Cambridge: Cambridge University Press.

Paton RC, Tindall H, Zuzel M & McNicol GP (1980) Haemostatic mechanisms in the normal endometrium and endometrium exposed to contraceptive steroids. In Diczfalusy E, Fraser IS & Webb FTG (eds) *Endometrial Bleeding and Steroidal Contraception*, pp 325–341. Bath: Pitman Press.

Petrucco OM & Fraser IS (1992) The potential for use of GnRH agonists for the treatment of dysfunctional uterine bleeding. *British Journal of Obstetrics and Gynecology* **99(supplement 7):** 34–36.

Pickles VR, Hall WJ, Best FA & Smith GN (1965) Prostaglandins in endometrium and menstrual fluid from normal and dysmenorrhoeic women. *Journal of Obstetrics and Gynaecology of the British Commonwealth* **72:** 185–192.

Pizarro E, Schoenstedt G, Mehech G, Hidalgo M, Romero C & Munoz G (1989) Uterine cavity and the location of IUDs following administration of meclofenamic acid to menorrhagic women. *Contraception* **40:** 413–423.

Poyser NL (1985) Prostaglandin pharmacology: five different inhibitors of prostanoid synthesis. *Prostaglandin Perspectives* **2:** 10–11.

Redwine DB (1987) The distribution of endometriosis in the pelvis by age groups and fertility. *Fertility and Sterility* **47:** 173–175.

Rees MCP, Anderson ABM, Demers LM & Turnbull AC (1984) Endometrial and myometrial prostaglandin release during the menstrual cycle in relation to menstrual blood loss. *Journal of Clinical Endocrinology and Metabolism* **58:** 813–818.

Rees MCP, Canete-Soler R, Lopez-Bernal A & Turnbull AC (1988) Effect of fenamates on prostaglandin E receptor binding. *Lancet* **ii:** 541–542.

Schenken RS & Asch RH (1980) Surgical induction of endometriosis in the rabbit: effect on fertility and concentrations of peritoneal fluid prostaglandins. *Fertility and Sterility* **34:** 581–587.

Schenken RS, Asch RH, Williams RF & Hodgen GD (1984) Etiology of infertility in monkeys with endometriosis: measurement of peritoneal fluid prostaglandins. *American Journal of Obstetrics and Gynecology* **150:** 349–355.

Schwarz A, Zor U, Lindner HR & Naor S (1974) Primary dysmenorrhoea: alleviation by an inhibitor of prostaglandin synthesis and action. *Obstetrics and Gynecology* **44:** 709–714.

Shaw RW & Fraser HM (1984) Use of a superactive luteinizing hormone-releasing hormone agonist in the treatment of menorrhagia. *British Journal of Obstetrics and Gynaecology* **91:** 913–919.

Sjoberg N-O (1979) Dysmenorrhoea and uterine neurotransmitters. *Acta Obstetrica et Gynecologica Scandinavica* **87(supplement):** 57–60.

Smith RP (1989) Pressure–velocity analysis of uterine muscle during spontaneous dysmenorrheic contractions in vivo. *American Journal of Obstetrics and Gynecology* **160:** 1400–1405.

Smith SK (1991) The endometrium and endometriosis. In Thomas EJ & Rock JA (eds) *Modern Approaches to Endometriosis*, pp 57–77. Dordrecht: Kluwer.

Smith SK, Abel MH, Kelly RW & Baird DT (1981a) Prostaglandin synthesis in the endometrium of women with ovular dysfunctional uterine bleeding. *British Journal of Obstetrics and Gynaecology* **88:** 434–439.

Smith SK, Abel MH, Kelly RW & Baird DT (1981b) A role for prostacyclin (PGI_2) in excessive menstrual bleeding. *Lancet* **i:** 522–524.

Smith SK, Abel MH, Kelly RW & Baird DT (1982) The synthesis of prostaglandins from persistent proliferative endometrium. *Journal of Clinical Endocrinology and Metabolism* **55:** 284–289.

Stromberg P, Forsling ML & Akerlund M (1981) Effects of prostaglandin inhibition on vasopressin levels in women with primary dysmenorrhoea. *Obstetrics and Gynecology* **58:** 206–208.

Sutherland AM (1949) The histology of the endometrium in functional uterine haemorrhage. *Glasgow Medical Journal* **30:** 1–28.

Syrop CH & Halme J (1987) Peritoneal fluid environment and infertility. *Fertility and Sterility* **48:** 1–9.

Tolman EL, McGuire JL & Rosenthale ME (1985) Pharmacology of non-steroidal anti-inflammatory drugs and their use in dysmenorrhea. In Dawood MY, McGuire JL & Demers LM (eds) *Premenstrual Syndrome and Dysmenorrhea*, pp 159–175. Baltimore: Urban and Schwarzenberg.

Turnbull AC & Rees MCP (1990) Gestrinone in the treatment of menorrhagia. *British Journal of Obstetrics and Gynaecology* **97:** 713–715.

Van Look PFA, Lothian H, Hunter WM, Michie EA & Baird DT (1977) Hypothalamic–pituitary–ovarian function in perimenopausal women. *Clinical Endocrinology* **7:** 13–22.

Van Look PFA, Fraser IS, Hunter WM & Baird DT (1978) Impaired estrogen-induced luteinizing hormone release in young women with anovulatory dysfunctional uterine bleeding. *Journal of Clinical Endocrinology and Metabolism* **46:** 818–823.

Vargyas JM, Campeau JD & Mishell DR Jr (1987) Treatment of menorrhagia with meclofenamate sodium. *American Journal of Obstetrics and Gynecology* **157:** 944–950.

Vernon MW, Beard JS, Graves K & Wilson EA (1986) Classification of endometriotic implants by morphologic appearance and capacity to synthesize prostaglandin F. *Fertility and Sterility* **46:** 801–806.

White JO, Sullivan MHF, Patel L, Croxtall JD, D'Arcangues C, Belsey EM & Elder MG (1991) Prostaglandin production in human endometrium following continuous exposure to low dose levonorgestrel released from a vaginal ring. *Contraception* **43:** 401–412.

Whitehouse HB (1914) The physiology and pathology of uterine haemorrhage. *Lancet* **ii:** 951–957.

Willman EA, Collins WP & Clayton SG (1976) Studies in the involvement of prostaglandins in uterine symptomatology and pathology. *British Journal of Obstetrics and Gynaecology* **83:** 337–345.

Ylikorkala O & Viinikka L (1983) Comparison between antifibrinolytic and antiprosta-glandin treatment in the reduction of increased menstrual blood loss in women with intrauterine contraceptive devices. *British Journal of Obstetrics and Gynaecology* **90:** 78–87.
Ylikorkala O, Kauppila A & Siljander M (1978) Antiprostaglandin therapy in prevention of side-effects of intrauterine contraceptive devices. *Lancet* **ii:** 393–395.

9

Principles and applications of manipulation of prostaglandin synthesis in pregnancy

HENK C. S. WALLENBURG
HENK A. BREMER

The evidence presented in Chapter 7 that important obstetric disorders, including hypertensive disease, fetal growth retardation, and preterm labour, are associated with major changes in prostanoid metabolism has led not only to a better understanding of the key role of members of the eicosanoid family in the physiology of reproduction, but also to attempts to prevent or treat such disorders by manipulation of the eicosanoid system.

Considering manipulation of the eicosanoid system in the pregnant woman, two questions arise: how can it be done, and what are the consequences in terms of benefits and risks for the woman and her fetus. Several approaches are available to manipulate the eicosanoid system and its biological effects. First, exogenous natural prostaglandins or their analogues can be used. This subject is covered in various other chapters of this volume. Second, the endogenous synthesis of eicosanoid products may be selectively stimulated or inhibited, either pharmacologically or by means of dietary manipulation. Third, the effects of eicosanoids on end-organ receptors may be modulated.

The aim of this chapter is to provide the clinician with an assessment of the research-based rationale and the clinical benefits and possible disadvantages of manipulation of the synthesis or biological effects of eicosanoids for prevention or treatment of obstetric disorders.

GENERAL BIOCHEMICAL, PHYSIOLOGICAL AND PATHOPHYSIOLOGICAL BACKGROUND

Prostanoids (prostaglandins) and other derivatives of eicosanoic (20-carbon) polyunsaturated fatty acids (PUFAs) are collectively termed 'eicosanoids' (Corey et al, 1980). They are known to function as autacoids, locally active biochemical mediators released by cells on demand in response to appropriate chemical or physical stimuli.

Biochemistry of eicosanoids

For the purpose of a discussion of the manipulation of eicosanoid synthesis, we may distinguish two main steps in the formation of these autacoids. The initial step consists of the biosynthesis and storage of arachidonic acid, the immediate fatty acid precursor of eicosanoids with two double bonds (dienoic) in their long chains, which constitute the physiologically most important eicosanoids in man. Eicosanoids with one (monoenoic) or three (trienoic) double bonds are derived from different PUFAs and have biological properties that differ from those of products derived from arachidonic acid; they do not seem to be important in man under physiological conditions, but they may modulate the synthesis of dienoic eicosanoids. Arachidonic acid is either ingested as a dietary constituent or synthesized by desaturation and elongation of 18-carbon (linoleic and γ-linolenic acid) or 20-carbon (dihomo-γ-linolenic acid) PUFAs. The enzymes involved in these biochemical processes are not specific and various fatty acids may compete for shared enzymes (Crawford, 1983). Because linoleic acid is an essential fatty acid that cannot be synthesized de novo in human tissues and must be supplied by food, the formation of arachidonic acid and its precursors will depend on the composition of the diet and may be influenced by dietary manipulation (Hoffmann and Mest, 1987).

Much of the arachidonic acid is utilized for energy requirements, but some becomes esterified to the phospholipids of cell membranes and to other lipid pools and may participate in the second step of eicosanoid synthesis, the actual formation of active prostanoids. To that purpose, arachidonic acid must first be liberated from its ester bonds by the hydrolytic action of phospholipases, activated in the presence of calcium and calmodulin (Dennis, 1987). Once released from its cellular stores, the arachidonic acid is either rapidly reincorporated into phospholipids, or metabolized to a series of oxygenated products through the action of a ubiquitous complex of enzymatic oxygenases, including cyclooxygenase, lipoxygenase and epoxygenase (Chapter 1). Cyclooxygenase—also termed 'prostaglandin-endoperoxide synthase' or 'PGH synthase'—catalyses the conversion of arachidonic acid into the very unstable cyclic endoperoxides prostaglandin G_2 (PGG_2) and PGH_2, which are transformed, enzymatically as well as non-enzymatically, into a variety of active compounds, including the classical prostaglandins (PGE_2 and $PGF_{2\alpha}$), prostacyclin (PGI_2) and thromboxane (TXA_2). The cyclooxygenase products are often referred to as 'prostanoids', a terminology that will also be used in this chapter. Through the lipoxygenase pathway arachidonic acid is converted to leukotrienes with four double bonds (4-series), potent mediators in inflammatory and hypersensitivity reactions which also interact at various levels with the cyclooxygenase pathway (Piper, 1984). Also, the eicosanoids of the epoxygenase pathway are biologically active and may interact with cyclooxygenase products (Fitzpatrick et al, 1986). Other PUFAs may undergo the same reactions, resulting in the formation of monoenoic (1-series) or trienoic (3-series) prostanoids, and of leukotrienes of the 3- and 5-series. Because the capacity of the human body for the synthesis of prostanoids is about 1000 times greater than the amount actually produced, activation of the eicosanoid system is countered with negative-feedback reactions of self-catalysed inactivation (Marshall et al, 1987).

An exogenous agent that interferes with the availability or functioning of the various enzymes of the arachidonic acid cascade will necessarily inhibit the formation of prostanoids to some degree. In 1971 Vane discovered that inhibition of the cyclooxygenase enzyme is the mechanism by which acetyl-salicylic acid (aspirin) and nearly all non-steroidal anti-inflammatory agents prevent the formation of the classical prostaglandins, PGI_2 and TXA_2 (Vane, 1971). This finding not only provided a new tool for the investigation of the physiological and pathophysiological effects of endogenous prostanoids in vivo, but it also opened up new pathways for clinical research on prevention and treatment in a variety of diseases, including obstetric disorders, and thus put the clinician in the middle of the field of prostanoid research.

Eicosanoids and maternal adaptation in pregnancy

The data reviewed in Chapter 7 leaves no doubt about the significance of prostanoid metabolism in the control of pregnancy and labour. Prostacyclin and TXA_2 synthesis are closely associated with the adaptational changes of the systemic and uteroplacental circulations in pregnancy, as well as with the initiation of term and preterm labour (Noort and Keirse, 1990). The synthesis of PGE_2 and $PGF_{2\alpha}$ is important in the mechanism of cervical changes and uterine contractions before and during labour. Although a host of data exists as to the potential of local and systemic factors, including steroid hormones, that may modify and modulate prostanoid synthesis and catabolism, the mechanisms that induce and control the changes in eicosanoid metabolism in pregnancy are as yet largely unknown.

In normal pregnancy the synthesis of PGI_2 increases markedly, which leads to a dominance of the biological effects of PGI_2 over those of TXA_2. It is generally accepted that the prostacyclin dominance of pregnancy determines the vasodilatation and the reduced sensitivity of the maternal vascular system to angiotensin II (Wallenburg, 1990) and is involved in the control of myometrial activity (Noort and Keirse, 1990).

Eicosanoids and maternal maladaptation in pregnancy

Some, usually healthy, young women fail to develop or maintain the physiological adaptational responses to pregnancy. In these women the increase in PGI_2 production does not occur or is not sufficiently maintained, resulting in a relative dominance of the opposing effects of TXA_2. Thromboxane dominance appears to be the main mediator of what has been called 'circulatory maladaptation disease', characterized by a relatively increased vascular resistance, increased vascular sensitivity to angiotensin II, and the development of thrombosis in the uteroplacental circulation resulting in placental infarction (Wallenburg, 1988). The clinical expression of circulatory maladaptation disease includes pregnancy-induced hypertensive disorders, uteroplacental circulatory insufficiency with fetal growth retardation and, perhaps, preterm labour. Since the factors that stimulate PGI_2 synthesis in normal pregnancy are not known, the cause of an insufficient formation of prostacyclin remains speculative. However, it seems likely that the relative changes in prostanoid synthesis observed in maladaptation disorders of pregnancy are part of secondary pathophysiological mechanisms rather than the primary cause of the disease (Wallenburg, 1988).

The concept of a prostacyclin–thromboxane imbalance resulting in a dominance of the biological effects of TXA_2 as a key mechanism in the pathophysiology of circulatory maladaptation in pregnancy may well be too simplistic. The complexity of the adaptational vascular processes in pregnancy is only just beginning to emerge and may include various other mediators released from platelets, leukocytes and vascular endothelium (Vane et al, 1990). Nevertheless, the growing understanding of the biochemical pathways of the eicosanoid system and of its involvement in the physiological adaptations to pregnancy has led to attempts to prevent or treat disorders of maladaptation in pregnancy by dietary manipulation of the formation of arachidonic acid and, in particular, by selective pharmacological inhibition of the cyclooxygenase pathway of prostanoid synthesis.

DIETARY MANIPULATION

The dietary manipulation of prostanoid synthesis is in particular associated with the consumption of fish and fish oil. A small number of observational studies suggest a reduced occurrence of pre-eclampsia and eclampsia, longer gestation and higher birthweights in populations with a high consumption of marine fish compared with areas having a lower consumption of fish (Dyerberg and Bang, 1985; Olsen et al, 1986; Andersen et al, 1989). In a questionnaire study of over 6500 pregnant women in Denmark who did not smoke during pregnancy, Olsen et al (1990) showed a significant positive association between fish consumption and placental weight, birthweight and neonatal head circumference, but not gestational age. As Olsen and Secher (1990) have recently pointed out, these observations are supported indirectly by the results of a controlled trial conducted by the People's League of Health (1946) during 1938–1939 in London. In this study of over 5000 pregnant women, allocated alternately to dietary supplements of vitamins, minerals and halibut liver oil, or no treatment, a significant reduction in the occurrence of pre-eclampsia and preterm delivery was observed in women receiving halibut liver oil compared with non-treated women. The usual explanation of the beneficial obstetric effects that are said to be associated with consumption of fish oil is that marine fat has a high content of PUFA precursors of 3-series prostanoids which compete with the formation of arachidonic acid, resulting in a shift in prostanoid synthesis in favour of the biological effects of prostacyclin (Andersen et al, 1989).

Biochemical, physiological and pathophysiological background

Two classes of PUFAs are involved in the processes of desaturation and elongation leading to the formation of direct prostanoid precursors (Figure 1). One class consists of PUFAs with the first of their 3–6 double bonds at the

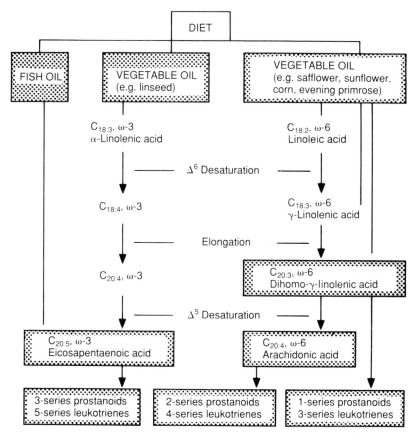

Figure 1. Scheme of the dietary sources and processes of elongation and desaturation of PUFAs resulting in the formation of prostanoids and leukotrienes. PUFAs are indicated by $C_{n:m}$, where n is the number of carbon atoms and m the number of double bonds; $\omega\text{-}n$ indicates the number of carbon atoms counted from the methyl end of the long chain to the first double bond.

third carbon atom from the methyl end of the long chain (ω-3). Members of this class occur in some vegetable oils (linseed oil), but the main source of the precursor of 3-series prostanoids and 5-series leukotrienes, eicosapentaenoic acid (EPA), is marine fish. EPA is reversibly converted to $C_{22:6}$, ω-3 and both PUFAs are synthesized by algae and phytoplankton, and taken up by man in fish and other seafood. In particular, fat marine fish such as the herring, sardine, mackerel, tuna and cod are a rich source of EPA and other ω-3 PUFAs (Bang, 1990). The second class, which contains the 1- and 2-series prostanoids, counts its first double bond at the sixth carbon atom (ω-6) and is derived from linoleic and γ-linolenic acid in various vegetable oils such as corn, sunflower and safflower oil. The immediate precursor of the 2-series prostanoids, arachidonic acid, can also be taken up directly from meat, but since the average diet in developed countries contains less than

0.2% of energy as arachidonic acid, most of the tissue arachidonic acid is derived from linoleate (Manatt et al, 1991). Human metabolism is unable to change ω-3 PUFAs to the ω-6 forms, or vice versa. Although 1- and 3-series prostanoids are not important in man under physiological conditions, both classes of PUFAs are required for many physiological purposes, such as cell membrane structure and transport and oxidation of cholesterol.

The dietary essential PUFAs in both classes compete with one another and with dietary saturated fats for incorporation in cell membranes and lipid pools, and for the shared enzymes which catalyse elongation and desaturation. In addition, EPA and dihomo-γ-linolenic acid may compete with arachidonic acid at the level of cyclooxygenase and lipoxygenase (Crawford, 1983; Hansen, 1983). For that reason, endogenous synthesis of 2-series prostanoids can be modified quantitatively and qualitatively by manipulating the absolute and relative amounts of ω-3 and ω-6 PUFAs in the diet, and such dietary manipulation could affect the function of the many physiological systems in which prostanoids are involved.

A major part of the research on dietary manipulation in non-pregnant individuals concerns attempts to shift the haemostatic balance towards increased vasodilatation and reduced platelet activity with the aim to prevent or treat vascular disease and thrombotic events (Higgs et al, 1986). In the majority of studies the approach has been to manipulate the ω-3 PUFAs, in particular using supplementation of the diet with EPA-rich fish oils or purified EPA. The scientific enthusiasm for this approach is based on the results of epidemiological studies indicating a low incidence of hypertensive, thrombotic and atherosclerotic disorders among Greenland Eskimos (Dyerberg et al, 1978) and certain groups in Japan (Kagawa et al, 1982), who all have a high consumption of fish and sea mammals. Intake of EPA-rich fish meat, fish oil or purified EPA has been shown to lead to a reduced formation of dienoic TXA_2 by collagen-stimulated platelets and an increased synthesis of trienoic thromboxane (TXA_3), which shows only 10% of the biological activity of TXA_2 (Knapp et al, 1986; Hornstra et al, 1990). In addition, consumption of EPA increases the formation in vivo of trienoic Δ^{17}-prostacyclin (PGI_3), biologically equipotent with dienoic PGI_2, whereas synthesis of the latter remains unchanged or may even increase slightly (Knapp and FitzGerald, 1989; Hornstra et al, 1990). These and other experiments indicate that EPA competes with arachidonic acid for incorporation in tissue and plasma phospholipids as well as at the level of the cyclooxygenase enzyme, resulting in inhibition of TXA_2 and its platelet-aggregatory effects while stimulating the synthesis of vasodilator PGI_3. There is evidence that EPA may also affect the arachidonic acid cascade in more complex ways, e.g. by inhibition at the level of Δ^6-desaturation.

The biochemical changes in eicosanoid synthesis associated with manipulation of the ω-3 class of PUFAs explain some, but not all, preventive and therapeutic effects of a diet rich in fish or supplemented with purified EPA with regard to hypertensive, thrombotic and atherosclerotic disease as observed in epidemiological studies and in a large number of clinical trials (Editorial, 1988; Knapp and FitzGerald, 1989). It should be realized that the content of various ω-3 PUFAs is extremely variable in different species of fish, which makes the extrapolation of fish consumption to marine ω-3 fatty acid consumption difficult. For that reason and also because of the marked variations in the design of published studies and the complexity of the mechanisms involved, the putative beneficial effects of dietary supplementation with EPA, although suggestive, remain as yet disputed (Gibson, 1988).

Even more controversial are the effects of dietary manipulation of the ω-6 PUFAs, with supplements of linoleic acid and dihomo-γ-linolenic acid, usually as safflower or sunflower oil. Some studies have used evening primrose oil, which not only has a high content on linoleate (75%), but also contains about 9% of γ-linolenic acid and various substances regarded as cofactors for prostanoid production. Dietary supplementation with linoleic acid has been shown to stimulate synthesis of PGE and PGF, whereas prostacyclin formation remained unaffected (Knapp and FitzGerald, 1989). A diet rich in linoleate appears to reduce platelet TXA_2 formation, a biochemically unexpected effect that seems to be based on incorporation of linoleic acid into platelet lipids without bioconversion into arachidonic acid (Hoffmann and Mest, 1987). A high dietary content of linoleic acid has been linked to reduced blood pressure, an effect that could be mediated by conversion of linoleic acid to arachidonate and subsequent formation of 2-series prostanoids. However, many later studies have failed to confirm such an association (Knapp and FitzGerald, 1989). It has been suggested that evening primrose oil could alleviate the symptoms of the premenstrual syndrome through an increased synthesis of PGE_1, but a recent double-blind placebo-controlled study failed to support such claims (Khoo et al, 1990).

The majority of the studies on dietary manipulation of prostanoid synthesis are not properly controlled and they have applied dietary supplementation in various forms from various sources in variable doses for variable periods of time. For that reason, many doubts and uncertainties remain with regard to the biochemical and biological effects and, in particular, the clinical consequences of the manipulation of dietary PUFAs with the aim to prevent or treat hypertensive, thrombotic and atherosclerotic disorders.

Obstetric applications of dietary manipulation

There is no evidence to suggest that a dietary deficiency of ω-3 or ω-6 PUFAs is involved in the pathophysiology of maladaptation disorders of pregnancy. MacGillivray (1983) in a small-scale study in Aberdeen found no differences in the amount of linoleic, γ-linolenic or arachidonic acid between the diets of 15 pre-eclamptic women and 29 normotensive pregnant controls. The few studies on plasma levels of free and esterified arachidonic acid in women with pre-eclampsia have not revealed any difference with normotensive pregnant women (Ogburn et al, 1984; Wang et al, 1991), but plasma levels of total PUFAs, and of EPA, linoleic, and α-linolenic acid were found to be somewhat reduced in term pre-eclamptic women (Wang et al, 1991). The authors suggest that this could represent altered fatty acid metabolism with altered storage or mobilization from lipid pools.

Experience with dietary manipulation of prostanoid synthesis in pregnancy is extremely limited. Worley (1984) mentions a study by Gant et al, who are said to have found no difference in the incidence of pregnancy-induced hypertension among pregnant women who received a large daily dietary supplement of dihomo-γ-linoleic acid when compared with placebo-treated women; however, no data of this study are presented or could be found in the literature. Moodley and Norman (1989) report a study in which they randomly allocated 47 primigravid patients with mild to moderate pregnancy-induced hypertension (blood pressure of 140/90 mmHg or more) in the third trimester to supplementation with a daily dose of 4 g of evening primrose oil or matched placebo for a minimum period of 2 weeks. No differences were found between the two groups with regard to blood pressure, or course and outcome of pregnancy. This is in fact a therapeutic rather than a prophylactic study. Also using a daily dose of 4 g of evening primrose oil during 7 days, O'Brien et al (1985) investigated the effect of dietary supplementation with ω-6 PUFAs on the pressor response to infusion of angiotensin II in ten normotensive pregnant women accepted for therapeutic termination of pregnancy in the early second trimester, and in five healthy non-pregnant female and five male volunteers. The diastolic pressor response to angiotensin II was significantly blunted in treated pregnant and non-pregnant subjects as compared with non-treated controls, and the effect was greatest in pregnant women. The systolic response was somewhat reduced in treated pregnant women, but not in non-pregnant subjects. Effects on platelet behaviour and prostanoid synthesis were not measured. Accepting that the physiologically reduced sensitivity of the vascular system in pregnancy to the pressor effects of angiotensin II is largely determined by prostacyclin dominance, these results provide indirect evidence that short-term dietary supplementation with ω-6 PUFAs may shift prostanoid synthesis towards an increased prostacyclin dominance, perhaps by reducing platelet TXA_2 formation, as discussed previously.

The effects of supplementation with ω-3 PUFAs on pregnancy duration and on weight and length of the newborn were investigated in 533 healthy women in week 30 of pregnancy who were randomly assigned in a ratio of 2:1:1 to fish oil (about 2.7 g ω-3 fatty acids per day), olive oil, or no supplement (Olsen et al, 1992). Fish oil supplementation was associated with a small but significant increase of, on average, 4 days in the duration of pregnancy compared with women taking olive oil, but no differences were found with regard to neonatal weight and length adjusted for gestational age. These results are in contrast with those of the earlier epidemiological study which showed no association between fish consumption and gestational age at delivery (Olsen et al, 1990). Data on the occurrence of pregnancy-induced hypertension are not presented.

In conclusion, the theoretical basis of dietary manipulation of ω-3 and ω-6 PUFAs to produce physiologically beneficial changes of prostanoid synthesis remains largely speculative, and the results of the studies discussed above are hypothesis-generating rather than providing evidence that such manipulation could reduce the risk of pregnancy-induced hypertensive disorders, preterm labour, or fetal growth retardation. There is a need for more fundamental research as well as for large well-controlled multicentre clinical trials, not only to assess the putative benefits but also the possible side-effects and risks of dietary PUFA manipulation.

Side-effects of dietary manipulation

An important aim of dietary PUFA manipulation is to reduce platelet activity, which could cause problems in pregnancy and delivery due to an increased bleeding tendency. Although to the best of the authors' knowledge no toxic effects of ω-3 or ω-6 PUFAs have been reported in any of the studies in non-pregnant subjects, the highly unsaturated ω-3 fatty acids are easily oxidized, which may produce substances that could be toxic in the mother or the fetus (Secher and Olsen, 1990). The long-term effects of dietary manipulation of fatty acids are not known, but the possibility of deleterious effects due to an increased production of peroxides and radicals has been suggested (Lands, 1986). In 1988 the US Food and Drug Administration banned the import and sale of evening primrose oil as a food or drug (McCollum, 1989). Considering the rapidly growing public interest in the preventive and therapeutic use of PUFAs, in particular of EPA in fish oil, and in view of recent medical publications already proposing EPA as a reasonable alternative to aspirin in the prevention and treatment of pregnancy-induced hypertensive disorders (England et al, 1987; Romero et al, 1988), further research on its maternal and fetal effects should have a high priority.

PHARMACOLOGICAL MANIPULATION

Two decades ago Lewis and Schulman (1973) published the first retrospective observation that gestation was prolonged by an average of 7 days in women who used 3.25 g or more of aspirin daily during the last 6 months of pregnancy as compared with women who took no aspirin. In 42% of these women, gestation lasted 42 weeks or more as compared with only 3% in controls who did not take aspirin. Labour lasted 12 hours in treated women, and 7 hours in untreated controls. These effects were attributed to suppression of endogenous prostanoid synthesis, and 1 year later this principle was applied therapeutically to the inhibition of preterm labour using indomethacin (Zuckerman et al, 1974). The retrospective study by Crandon and Isherwood (1979), indicating that pre-eclampsia occurred less frequently in regular aspirin users than in pregnant women who took no aspirin, forms another landmark in the history of pharmacological manipulation of prostanoid synthesis to prevent and treat maladaptation disorders of pregnancy.

Pharmacological, physiological and pathophysiological background

Three enzyme systems in the eicosanoid cascade can be pharmacologically inhibited: the phospholipases, the cyclooxygenase and the specific isomerases that catalyse the conversion of endoperoxides into the specific prostanoids. Finally, end-organ receptors may be inhibited by specific antagonists

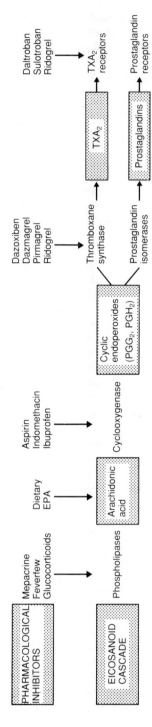

Figure 2. Pharmacological inhibition of the eicosanoid cascade.

(Figure 2). A few agents have been claimed to stimulate prostacyclin synthesis by complex mechanisms.

Inhibition of phospholipases

There are a very large number of drugs and chemical compounds that have been reported to inhibit various phospholipases and thus the availability of arachidonic acid for prostanoid synthesis, including glucocorticoids. The numerous and widespread effects of glucocorticoids and other phospholipase-inhibiting drugs preclude their pharmacological use for specific inhibition of prostanoid synthesis in pregnancy.

Inhibition of cyclooxygenase

A heterogeneous group of pharmacological agents, many of them chemically unrelated, have anti-inflammatory, analgesic and antipyretic effects, and are frequently designated as non-steroidal anti-inflammatory drugs (NSAIDs) or, after their prototype, aspirin-like drugs. Apart from acetylsalicylic acid (aspirin) and sodium salicylate, p-aminophenol derivatives (e.g. paracetamol), acetic acid (e.g. indomethacin) and propionic acid (e.g. ibuprofen, fenoprofen, naproxen) derivatives are well-known representatives. It is generally believed that inhibition of cyclooxygenase, and thus the formation of all prostanoids derived from arachidonic acid, is responsible for many of the beneficial activities and side-effects of NSAIDs, although this concept has been challenged (Abramson and Weissmann, 1989). Individual agents have different mechanisms for inhibition of cyclooxygenase, but their effect is always dependent on reaching the enzyme and, for that reason, the distribution and pharmacokinetic properties of the drugs are important factors determining their activity. For more detailed general pharmacological information on this subject the reader is referred to one of the extensive reviews on this subject (Hart and Huskisson, 1984; Bailey, 1989; Insel, 1990). In the following sections we will briefly discuss some of the pharmacological and pharmacokinetic aspects of aspirin and indomethacin, the two NSAIDs which are most widely applied to manipulate prostanoid synthesis in pregnant women.

Inhibition of isomerases

The evidence implicating platelet TXA_2 as a major factor in the pathophysiology of occlusive vascular events has led to the development of selective inhibitors of thromboxane synthase, the isomerase catalysing the conversion of PGH_2 into TXA_2. Several compounds (e.g. dazoxiben, dazmagrel, pirmagrel, furegrelate) have undergone clinical testing in coronary and peripheral vascular disease, as yet with disappointing results (Fiddler and Lumley, 1990). Only dazoxiben has been used in pregnant patients and will be briefly discussed. On theoretical grounds it was expected that selective inhibition of TXA_2 synthesis would lead to an accumulation of PGH_2 with favourable redirection to formation of PGI_2 ('steal mechanism').

However, PGH_2 itself has biological effects similar to those of TXA_2, and redirection of PGH_2 to prostacyclin is apparently not effective enough to antagonize the functional effects of accumulating PGH_2 (Fiddler and Lumley, 1990).

Inhibition of thromboxane receptor antagonists

Receptor antagonists do not interfere with eicosanoid synthesis but prevent TXA_2 (and PGH_2) from activating platelet and vascular receptors. Some of these agents (daltroban, sulotroban and others) have undergone preliminary clinical testing with variable results (Fiddler and Lumley, 1990). A new and promising approach is the combination of TXA_2 synthase inhibition with TXA_2 receptor antagonism in one drug, such as ridogrel (Patscheke, 1990).

Stimulation of prostacyclin synthesis

In the past decade mainly five pharmacological agents have been reported to stimulate PGI_2 synthesis in experimental conditions in vitro: nitroglycerine, nafazatrom, dipyridamole, magnesium sulphate and the experimental drug proadifen. These findings have not been confirmed in vivo (Boeynaems et al, 1986; FitzGerald, 1987; O'Brien et al, 1990). Of these agents, dipyridamole is the only drug that has been tested in clinical trials, the results of which do not support its use as an antiplatelet agent (FitzGerald, 1987). However in certain patients with bad obstetric histories and in whom there is excessive platelet aggregation that is not inhibited by low dose aspirin, the addition of dipyridamole has produced the desired inhibitory effect on in vitro platelet aggregation.

Acetylsalicylic acid

Acetylsalicylic acid, registered under the name 'aspirin' since 1899, has antipyretic, anti-inflammatory and analgesic effects at high doses of 4–6 g/day. At lower dosages aspirin retains its antipyretic and analgesic effects, but has no anti-inflammatory activity (Abramson and Weissmann, 1989). Most of the effects at lower dosages can be attributed to inhibition of cyclooxygenase by covalent acetylation of a serine residue at the active site of the enzyme (Figure 3). The acetylation is irreversible. Aspirin does not inhibit lipoxygenase; on the contrary, inhibition of cyclooxygenase may lead

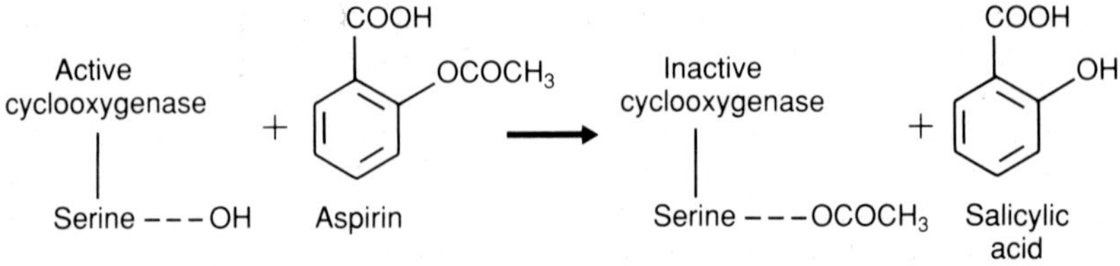

Figure 3. Molecular action of aspirin on cyclooxygenase.

to increased formation of leukotrienes, most likely because of an increase in the amount of free arachidonic acid available to the lipoxygenase enzyme (Piper, 1984). At high doses aspirin and other NSAIDs also inhibit a variety of membrane-associated processes that are not dependent on prostanoid synthesis, including cell-mediated immunological responses and cytokine production (Abramson and Weissmann, 1989).

Low oral doses of aspirin, of the order of 60–80 mg/day, block the formation of TXA_2 in platelets almost completely, resulting in inhibition of thromboxane-dependent platelet aggregation in vitro by arachidonic acid, ADP and a low dose of collagen. Because the reaction between aspirin and the cyclooxygenase enzyme is irreversible, the duration of the inhibitory effect is determined by the rate at which new enzyme is synthesized (Oates et al, 1988). Platelets lack nuclei and are therefore unable to resynthesize cyclooxygenase, so that following administration of aspirin platelet aggregation remains impaired for the duration of platelet life span. Recovery of thromboxane synthesis and platelet aggregation in peripheral blood depends on the formation of new, uninhibited platelets from megakaryocytes (Wallenburg and Van Kessel, 1978). In contrast to platelets, nucleated cells such as endothelium can replace cyclooxygenase, and their capacity to synthesize prostanoids will recover rapidly after aspirin exposure (Oates et al, 1988).

Other factors that determine the systemic effects of aspirin are its absorption and deacetylation by the liver. Aspirin is readily absorbed after oral administration, mainly from the upper small intestine. The rate of absorption is determined by many factors, in particular the disintegration and dissolution rates of tablets or capsules, the pH of the mucosal surfaces, and the gastric emptying time (Insel, 1990). Gastric emptying is known to be slower in pregnant than in non-pregnant women (Hytten, 1991), but the effect of pregnancy on aspirin absorption has not been systematically investigated. Following oral ingestion of a single immediate-release tablet of aspirin peak levels of salicylate in plasma occur after approximately 30 minutes (Kelton, 1983). During the first pass through the liver at least 60% of the aspirin is deacetylated to salicylic acid (salicylate), a weak and reversible inhibitor of cyclooxygenase, which has no measurable effect on platelet aggregation at concentrations achieved in vivo. It acts mainly on the lipoxygenase pathway that leads to formation of leukotrienes (Buchanan et al, 1986). Elimination from plasma after a single therapeutic dose follows a bi-exponential curve; the half-life of the first exponent is 2–5 minutes for aspirin and salicylate, whereas the half-life of the second exponent is 13–19 minutes for aspirin and much longer (3.5–4.5 hours) for salicylate (Insel, 1990). Salicylate is excreted in the urine, mainly as glycine and glucuronic acid conjugate.

Intermittent long-term administration of a conventionally formulated low dose of aspirin of 60–80 mg/day, or even less, inhibits platelet thromboxane synthesis almost completely, with marked inhibitory effects on platelet aggregation in vitro, but has little effect on prostacyclin formation (Oates et al, 1988; Sibai et al, 1989). The selective inhibition of platelet thromboxane synthesis by low oral doses of aspirin is explained by the fact that platelets passing through the gut capillaries are exposed to relatively high concentrations of acetylsalicylic acid, whereas, due to the high first-pass deacetylation by the liver, the concentration in the systemic circulation remains too low to markedly affect the cyclooxygenase enzyme and prostacyclin formation in vascular endothelium (Pedersen and FitzGerald, 1984). If vascular prostacyclin synthesis is slightly reduced after ingestion of a low dose of aspirin, it will recover rapidly because of the formation of new cyclooxygenase enzyme (Ritter et al, 1989). Alternate-day dosing has been proposed to enhance the selectivity of the inhibitory effect of a low dose of aspirin on platelet TXA_2 synthesis (Hanley et al, 1982), but so far the best pharmacological selectivity has been obtained with the use of a controlled-release preparation that 'dribbles' aspirin into the presystemic circulation (Clarke et al, 1991). Based on the concept of dose-dependent selective inhibition of platelet thromboxane synthesis, aspirin has been applied extensively as an antiplatelet, antithrombotic agent in the treatment and prevention of arterial thrombotic disorders, including coronary and cerebral vascular disease (Peto et al, 1988; Steering Committee of the Physicians' Health and Study Research Group, 1989; Dutch TIA Trial Study Group, 1991; SALT Collaborative Group, 1991).

Aspirin in the maternal systemic circulation crosses the placenta rapidly (Jacobson et al, 1991). Fetal plasma concentrations of salicylate reach about 80–90% of maternal levels, 60–90 minutes after administration of an intravenous dose of aspirin to the mother; fetal aspirin levels reach about one-third of maternal concentrations. Maternal–fetal equilibration is slow because approximately 75% of maternal salicylate is bound to plasma protein. Considering the marked first-pass hepatic deacetylation, an extremely low concentration of acetylated salicylic acid may be expected to reach the placenta after a low oral dose of aspirin taken by a pregnant woman. Elimination of salicylate from the fetal circulation is slow because of a low capacity of the glycine and glucuronic acid pathways of conjugation; the half-life of salicylates in the neonate is about 7 hours (Levy and Garrettson, 1974). Determination of thromboxane synthesis by neonatal platelets provides an indirect but sensitive approach to assess placental transfer of aspirin. Ylikorkala et al (1986) found that maternal ingestion of a single dose of 100 mg of aspirin between 30 minutes and 10 hours before birth was associated with a small reduction in neonatal platelet thromboxane synthesis when compared with a control group without aspirin intake, whereas the reduction was significantly greater with 500 mg of aspirin. No inhibition of platelet thromboxane synthesis in cord blood was observed with a maternal intake of 20–80 mg/day of aspirin during approximately 2 weeks before delivery (Ritter et al, 1987; Sibai et al, 1989), but the long-term use of a daily dose of 60 mg of aspirin throughout the second and third trimester was associated with a 63% reduction in platelet thromboxane production (Benigni et al, 1989). Neither a single maternal dose of 100 mg of aspirin during labour (Ylikorkala et al, 1986) nor a daily dose of 80 mg during 2 weeks before delivery (Sibai et al, 1989) had a noticeable effect on fetal prostacyclin synthesis, as judged by measurement of 6-keto-$PGF_{1\alpha}$ levels in cord blood or in neonatal urine.

In conclusion, a low maternal dose of aspirin of the order of 60–80 mg/day causes selective suppression of platelet thromboxane synthesis, which is almost complete in the mother and small in the fetus, with little or no effect on the synthesis of PGI_2 or other prostanoids in the mother or fetus. For that reason, low-dose aspirin may shift prostanoid synthesis in pregnancy towards an increased prostacyclin dominance. The dose-dependent selectivity of the inhibition of cyclooxygenase is a unique feature of aspirin. This concept forms the rationale of clinical attempts of prevention or early treatment of maladaptation disorders of pregnancy, in particular pregnancy-induced hypertensive disorders and fetal growth retardation, with low-dose aspirin.

Indomethacin

Indomethacin was introduced in 1963 for the treatment of rheumatoid arthritis and related disorders (Insel, 1990). It is a potent inhibitor of the cyclooxygenase enzyme but, in contrast with aspirin, it competes with arachidonic acid for utilization and leaves the enzyme intact; it interferes with prostanoid synthesis only as long as its tissue concentration is sufficiently high. In addition, indomethacin inhibits a variety of non-prostanoid-dependent cellular processes (Abramson and Weissmann, 1989). It is rapidly and almost completely absorbed from the gastrointestinal tract after oral or rectal administration. The peak concentration in plasma occurs within about 2 hours, but may be variable. The liver converts most of the indomethacin to glucuronized metabolites eliminated in urine, bile and faeces, but 10–20% is excreted unchanged in the urine. The half-life in plasma is variable, perhaps because of enterohepatic cycling, but averages 3 hours (Insel, 1990).

In contrast to aspirin, dose-dependent biochemical selectivity of cyclooxygenase inhibition does not occur with indomethacin. Administration of indomethacin during labour has been shown to result in a significant reduction in synthesis of $PGF_{2\alpha}$ and PGE_2, (Besinger and Niebyl, 1990), and of PGI_2 and TXA_2 (Kurki et al, 1992). Because of its inhibitory effect on uterine prostanoid synthesis indomethacin has become widely used to suppress unwanted uterine activity. Although a single dose of 50 mg of indomethacin inhibits platelet cyclooxygenase, thromboxane synthesis and aggregation in vitro to the same degree as 500 mg of aspirin (Colli et al, 1988), its effect is reversible and short lived (Rorarius et al, 1989).

Indomethacin crosses the placenta rapidly; it can be demonstrated in the fetal circulation within 15 minutes after maternal ingestion and fetal and maternal concentrations equilibrate after approximately 5 hours (Niebyl, 1981). Moise et al (1990) performed cord blood sampling for diagnostic or therapeutic reasons in 26 pregnant women with a gestational age between 24 and 36 weeks, 6 hours after an oral dose of 50 mg of indomethacin. They found similar levels of indomethacin in maternal and fetal serum, independent of gestational age. Because of relatively deficient processes of hepatic glucuronidation and renal excretion, the neonate eliminates indomethacin rather slowly, in particular if it is preterm; the mean plasma half-life has

H. C. S. WALLENBURG AND H. A. BREMER

Table 1. Characteristics of randomized controlled clinical trials of low-dose aspirin to prevent pregnancy-induced hypertensive disorders.

Reference	Inclusion criteria	Exclusion criteria	Treatment protocol	No. treated	No. controls	Placebo	Clinical end-points	Conclusions
Beaufils et al (1985)	History of complicated pregnancy Vascular risk factors	Secondary hypertension Renal disease	ASA 150 mg/day plus dipyridamole 300 mg/day from 3 months until delivery	48	45	No	PIH, PE BW	Significant reduction in PE and FGR with ASA
Wallenburg et al (1986)	Normotensive primigravidae, positive A-II test at 28 weeks	History of hypertension Cardiovascular disease	ASA 60 mg/day from 28 weeks gestation until delivery	23	23	Yes	PIH, PE BW	Significant reduction of PE and PIH with ASA
Benigni et al (1989)	History of complicated pregnancy Chronic hypertension	Antiphospholipid antibodies	ASA 60 mg/day from 12th week until delivery	17	16	Yes	PIH, BW	Significant increase in duration of pregnancy, and fetal weight with ASA
Schiff et al (1989)	Positive roll-over test in women at risk for pre-eclamptic toxaemia	History of thrombocytopenia History of coagulation disorders History of heart failure Chronic renal/pulmonary disease Hepatic disease	ASA 100 mg/day during the third trimester	34	31	Yes	PIH, PE BW	Significant reduction in PIH and PE with ASA
McParland et al (1990)	Nulliparous women with repeated abnormal wave forms on Doppler ultrasound examination of the uteroplacental circulation	Bleeding disorders Diabetes mellitus Systemic lupus erythematosus	ASA 75 mg/day from 24 weeks until delivery	48	52	Yes	PIH, PE BW	Significant reduction in PE and hypertension <37 weeks with ASA
Uzan et al (1991)	Poor obstetric history	Twin pregnancy Renal disease Cardiovascular disease Diabetes	ASA 150 mg/day or ASA 150 mg/day plus dipyridamole 225 mg/day, from 15–18 weeks until delivery	156	73	Yes	PIH, PE BW	Significant reduction in PE and FGR with ASA

ASA, aspirin; PIH, pregnancy-induced hypertension; PE, pre-eclampsia; BW, birthweight; FGR, fetal growth retardation.

been reported to be 19 hours for infants born before 32 weeks' gestation, and 13 hours for infants born after 32 weeks (Bat et al, 1979).

Obstetric applications of aspirin

Inhibition of preterm labour

Due to the marked first-pass deacetylation by the liver, high doses of aspirin are needed to obtain levels of acetylated salicylic acid that are high enough to inhibit the cyclooxygenase enzyme in uterine tissues. Aspirin has been administered in daily doses of 6 g orally to 10 g intravenously to women in active preterm labour in an attempt to suppress uterine prostanoid synthesis and inhibit uterine contractions (Dornhöfer and Mosler, 1975; Wolff et al, 1981). In one uncontrolled study the investigators claimed successful delay of delivery for more than 7 days in six out of ten cases (Wolff et al, 1981). Considering the availability of other effective tocolytic agents and the potential hazards of high doses of aspirin (see below), there seems to be no indication for the use of aspirin in the treatment of premature labour. If the use of a cyclooxygenase inhibitor is indicated, indomethacin appears to be far more effective with less side-effects.

Prevention and treatment of pregnancy-induced hypertensive disorders and fetal growth retardation

In two early case reports on treatment of established pre-eclampsia, relatively high doses of aspirin (1.5–1.8 g/day) were used (Goodlin et al, 1978; Jespersen, 1980). Although platelet counts showed improvement, one of the two fetuses died after 1 week. In a later study, Goodlin (1983) treated five pre-eclamptic and thrombocytopenic women with 85 mg/day of aspirin in divided doses. Platelet counts improved but no improvement in fetal condition was observed, and two fetuses died.

Following these anecdotal observations, six randomized, controlled clinical trials were conducted and reported until 1992, using low-dose aspirin for the prevention of pregnancy-induced hypertensive disease and/or fetal growth retardation (Table 1). All patients entered were judged to be at high risk, based on obstetric history (Beaufils et al, 1985; Benigni et al, 1989; Uzan et al, 1991) or tests and observations in the present pregnancy (Wallenburg et al, 1986; Schiff et al, 1989; McParland et al, 1990). The dose of aspirin used varied from 60 mg/day (Wallenburg et al, 1986; Benigni et al, 1989) to 150 mg/day (Beaufils et al, 1985; Uzan et al, 1991), and aspirin was combined with dipyridamole in two studies (Beaufils et al, 1985; Uzan et al, 1991). In four trials aspirin was prescribed during the second and the third trimester of pregnancy (Beaufils et al, 1985; Benigni et al, 1989; McParland et al, 1990; Uzan et al, 1991), whereas it was used during the third trimester only in the remaining two trials. All studies, except one (Beaufils et al, 1985), were placebo controlled. Although the findings are in general agreement in that they suggest that low-dose aspirin reduces the risk of pregnancy-induced hypertensive disorders, fetal growth retardation and their sequelae, the numbers in each separate trial are quite small and preclude reliable conclusions. Because the study designs are comparable and criteria and end-points are well defined, systemic pooling of the results across trials by means of meta-analysis provides more precise estimates of the effects of treatment (Chalmers et al, 1989; Imperiale and Petrulis, 1991). Differences in the end-points of hypertension, proteinuria, low birthweight, and perinatal mortality between treated and non-treated groups were accumulated and expressed as 'odds ratios' with 95% confidence intervals. The results, covering 326 treated and 240 untreated patients, are presented graphically in Figure 4. None of the 95% confidence intervals crosses the line

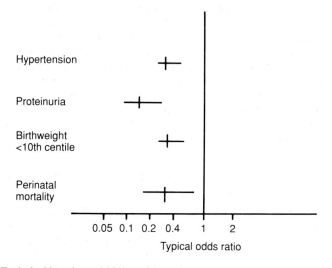

Figure 4. Typical odds ratios and 95% confidence intervals of effects of low-dose aspirin on the occurrence of hypertension, proteinuria and fetal–neonatal sequelae from six randomized controlled clinical trials (see Table 1). All odds ratios are less than 1 in patients at risk receiving low-dose aspirin.

representing a typical odds ratio equal to 1. This means that all variables shown occur significantly less often in aspirin-treated pregnant women than in untreated controls. The widest confidence interval is found for perinatal mortality, which occurred in only nine of the treated and 16 of the untreated patients. The reported data do not allow distinguishment between perinatal deaths related or unrelated to pregnancy-induced hypertensive disorders. Further subgroup analyses show that aspirin-treated women have a significantly reduced risk of preterm birth and caesarean section. However, the specific indications for caesarean section are not stated in most studies, so that it remains to be proven that the higher caesarean section rate in controls is related to the higher incidence of pregnancy-associated hypertensive disorders.

A striking observation in all of these controlled studies is the reduction in the incidence of uteroplacental circulatory insufficiency with fetal growth retardation; this finding reaches significance in the meta-analysis. The positive effect of a low dose of aspirin on birthweight corrected for gestational age was also observed by Trudinger et al (1988) in a randomized placebo-controlled, double-blind study in a small group of patients with a clinical diagnosis of fetal growth retardation and an abnormal Doppler-flow pattern in the umbilical arteries, but not in a small number of uncomplicated twin pregnancies (Trudinger et al, 1989) (Table 2).

The evidence that low-dose aspirin restores a disturbed prostacyclin–thromboxane balance in pregnancy to the dominance of the vascular effects of prostacyclin by means of selective inhibition of platelet TXA_2 synthesis is supported by the results of three studies, showing that a daily dose of 60–80 mg of aspirin during 1–4 weeks significantly increases vascular refractoriness to the vasopressor effects of angiotensin II in pregnant women with an elevated (Spitz et al, 1988; Wallenburg et al, 1991) or physiological (Sanchez-Ramos et al, 1987) angiotensin sensitivity. In contrast, oral ingestion of 650 mg of aspirin twice with an interval of 6 hours between doses has been demonstrated to lead to a marked increase in angiotensin sensitivity (Everett et al, 1978), because in this dose aspirin inhibits the biosynthesis not only of TXA_2 but also of PGI_2.

Also, results of non-randomized controlled studies in patients with a history of recurrent idiopathic severe fetal growth retardation, fetal death, lupus anticoagulant, anticardiolipin antibodies or systemic lupus erythematosus support the concept of a beneficial effect of prophylactic treatment with a low dose of aspirin on uteroplacental blood flow and fetal growth (Wallenburg and Rotmans, 1987, 1988; Elder et al, 1988). Lupus anticoagulant and other antiphospholipid antibodies interfere with vascular and placental synthesis of PGI_2, leading to a relative dominance of platelet thromboxane action with placental thrombosis and infarction (Brown, 1991). Lubbe and Liggins (1988) obtained a successful pregnancy outcome in 80% of 25 patients after prophylactic treatment with 40–60 mg of prednisone and 75 mg of aspirin daily. Also, other centres have reported good results with a similar combination (Farquharson et al, 1984), although some have not (Branch et al, 1985).

In contrast with the prophylactic studies discussed above, the potential benefits of treatment of established circulatory maladaptation in pregnancy with a low dose of aspirin have hardly been investigated. Pregnancy-induced hypertension often occurs early in the third trimester, and if low-dose aspirin treatment would result in even a moderate delay in the progression of the disease, this could have a significant impact on neonatal morbidity and mortality. The results of a recent randomized, double-blind trial in 47 patients with mild pregnancy-induced hypertension using a daily dose of 100 mg of aspirin or placebo did not indicate any improvement in the hypertensive condition or delay in its progression to pre-eclampsia (Schiff et al, 1990).

In conclusion, the results of meta-analysis of published trials indicate that prophylactic treatment with a low dose of aspirin to prevent pregnancy-induced hypertensive disorders, fetal growth retardation and sequelae such as prematurity, caesarean section and low birthweight is effective in women

Table 2. Characteristics of clinical trials of low-dose aspirin to prevent fetal growth retardation.

Reference	Inclusion criteria	Exclusion criteria	Treatment protocol	No. treated	No. controls	Randomized	Placebo	End-points	Conclusions
Wallenburg and Rotmans (1987)	History of at least two previous pregnancies with severe idiopathic FGR		1–1.6 mg/kg/day of ASA and 225 mg of dipyridamole daily from 16 weeks until delivery	24	24	No	No	BW	Reduction in incidence of FGR
Elder et al (1988)	History of severe FGR and/or hypertension SLE		ASA 75 mg/day from the first or second trimester until delivery	42	—	No	No	PE, BW	'Striking' improvement of pregnancy outcome
Trudinger et al (1988)	Abnormal umbilical artery wave forms on Doppler ultrasound gestational age between 28 and 36 weeks	Severe hypertension	ASA 150 mg/day from 28–36 weeks until delivery	22	24	Yes	Yes	BW	Significant increase in BW and head circumference
Trudinger et al (1989)	Uncomplicated twin pregnancy at 28–30 weeks		ASA 100 mg/day until delivery	15	12	Yes	Yes	BW	No effect of ASA on BW

FGR, fetal growth retardation; ASA, aspirin; BW, birthweight; SLE, systemic lupus erythematosus; PIH pregnancy-induced hypertension.

at risk. However, it should be emphasized that the patients in the clinical trials presented above were selected on the basis of high risk and it remains to be determined whether similar effectivity could be obtained in populations at small or moderate risk.

Obstetric applications of indomethacin

Treatment of polyhydramnios

Indomethacin crosses from the mother to the fetus and may suppress fetal renal prostanoid synthesis, resulting in a reversible reduction in urine output (Kirshon et al, 1988). This side-effect has been applied therapeutically to reduce amniotic fluid volume in a few pregnancies complicated by polyhydramnios (Cabrol et al, 1987; Kirshon and Cotton, 1988). The associated inhibition of uterine activity may be considered an advantage of this approach, but experience is too limited to allow assessment of its efficacy and risks.

Inhibition of preterm labour

The first clinical trial on the use of indomethacin as a tocolytic agent was reported in 1974 by Zuckerman et al. This uncontrolled study was followed by many other uncontrolled trials, in which various end-points of tocolytic therapy were used, including short-term and long-term delay in delivery, birthweight, perinatal death rate, and occurrence of the respiratory distress syndrome (Besinger and Niebyl, 1990). These reports all suggest that indomethacin is an effective inhibitor of myometrial contractions, but no conclusions can be drawn as to its clinical benefits or disadvantages.

Only two double-blind, placebo-controlled studies could be found in the literature, together comprising 33 patients in active preterm labour who received indomethacin and the same number treated with placebo (Niebyl et al, 1980; Zuckerman et al, 1984). Treatment failure necessitating the use of an alternative tocolytic agent occurred significantly less frequently in indomethacin-treated patients than in patients receiving placebo. In a comparative trial of 20 patients treated with ethanol combined with indomethacin and 22 patients receiving ethanol alone, the combination with indomethacin delayed delivery for 48 hours in 80% of the cases, as compared with 55% with ethanol alone (Spearing, 1979). The results of two controlled trials with similar design using ritodrine alone or in combination with indomethacin also suggest that the addition of indomethacin may increase the delay in delivery (Gamissans et al, 1978; Katz et al, 1983). On the other hand, two randomized trials comparing short-term (Morales et al, 1989) or long-term (Besinger et al, 1991) indomethacin therapy with ritodrine treatment found no significant differences in the delay of delivery or neonatal outcome.

The marked differences between these studies with regard to the diagnosis of preterm labour, gestational age, cervical effacement and degree of cervical dilatation, as well as with respect to the study design and the end-points used to assess the efficacy of indomethacin treatment, make it hazardous to attempt to draw firm conclusions. In a recent thoughtful overview Keirse et al (1989) present a meta-analysis of the most reliable data that could be extracted from controlled trials published until 1987. The authors conclude that the data suggest that treatment of active preterm labour with indomethacin is more effective than that with ethanol and ritodrine in delaying delivery and, consequently, in increasing birthweight, but that there is no evidence that such treatment is associated with a significant reduction in the incidence of the neonatal respiratory distress syndrome, or of perinatal death. Indomethacin can be a useful drug for tocolysis when betamimetics fail at a gestational age at which even a few days of prolongation of pregnancy may improve neonatal outcome.

Propionic acid-derived cyclooxygenase inhibitors such as naproxen have been shown to reduce myometrial contractions and have been used to inhibit preterm labour (Wiqvist, 1979), but none of these drugs has been subjected to controlled trials.

Obstetric applications of thromboxane synthase and receptor antagonists

There are two reports by the same investigators on the use of dazoxiben in the treatment of nine patients with severe pre-eclampsia in the late second trimester of pregnancy (Van Assche et al, 1984; Van Assche and Spitz, 1988). In two patients dazoxiben reduced the capacity of whole blood to produce TXA_2, whereas the synthesis of PGI_2 increased; the effects on prostanoid synthesis in the other seven patients were not shown. A mean prolongation of pregnancy of 4½ weeks was obtained, but one fetus and three newborns died. Because no further reports could be found in the literature, the putative beneficial effects of dazoxiben in the treatment of pre-eclampsia remain to be proven.

To the best of the authors' knowledge, no reports have been published on the use of thromboxane receptor antagonists in pregnant patients.

Obstetric applications of prostacyclin-stimulating agents

In several trials of prevention of maladaptation disorders in pregnancy, low-dose aspirin was combined with dipyridamole on the premise that the combination would be more effective than aspirin alone (Beaufils et al, 1985; Wallenburg and Rotmans, 1987; Uzan et al, 1991). In the recent EPREDA trial, in which 127 women at risk taking a daily dose of 150 mg of aspirin from 16 weeks gestation until delivery were compared with 119 women taking the same dose of aspirin combined with 225 mg of dipyridamole, no differences were found between the two groups with regard to the incidence of low birthweight or pre-eclampsia (Uzan et al, 1991).

Because large trials in non-pregnant subjects have also not shown an additional effect of dipyridamole on the efficacy of aspirin as an antiplatelet agent, there appears to be no scientific rationale for combining the two drugs. Only one case report was found on the use of nafazatrom in pregnancy (Elder and Myatt, 1984). The drug, combined with dipyridamole, was used successfully in a woman with a history of recurrent abortion and severe placental infarction.

Side-effects of pharmacological manipulation

The general side-effects that can be caused by ingestion of aspirin and other NSAIDs may also occur in pregnant women. Complaints and adverse effects such as gastric irritation, nausea, diarrhoea, constipation, bronchospasm, effects on renal function, skin rashes and angio-oedema are usually—but not always—dose related or associated with hypersensitivity. Since they are not specific for pregnancy, these potential side-effects will not be reviewed.

Pregnancy-specific complications of the use of NSAIDs may be due to unwanted effects of inhibition of prostanoid synthesis in the mother, and to transfer of the drug across the placenta leading to immediate or delayed disturbances in embryonic or fetal development and functions. In particular, the risk of maternal and neonatal haemorrhage, the potential teratogenic effects of aspirin use in pregnancy, and the possible effects of aspirin and indomethacin on the fetal ductus arteriosus and pulmonary circulation, have caused considerable worries among doctors and patients.

Many studies have determined the skin bleeding time in non-pregnant and pregnant aspirin users to assess the risk of haemorrhage, with disparate results. Determination of the bleeding time is most likely not a reliable test to use as a predictor of clinically significant bleeding in individual patients (Rodgers and Levin, 1990); the effects of aspirin on haemostasis must be determined in properly designed clinical trials. Large prophylactic studies in non-pregnant subjects involving long-term use of aspirin in doses between 30 and 500 mg/day have not shown any relevant increase in bleeding tendency (Peto et al, 1988; Steering Committee of the Physicians' Health Study Research Group, 1989; SALT Collaborative Group, 1991; Dutch TIA Trial Study Group, 1991). It is the Australian study by Collins and Turner (1975) that is most often cited to emphasize the maternal bleeding risk associated with the regular consumption of aspirin and salicylate in pregnancy. During the 28 months of the study, 144 pregnant regular users of 'analgesic powders' containing aspirin and salicylate combined with other drugs were identified by testing urine specimens. The rates of anaemia, antepartum and postpartum haemorrhage, and blood transfusion at delivery were increased in the group of aspirin takers compared with controls, not exposed to aspirin, matched for age and parity. This study can be criticized on two main points. First, as part of an abusive habit the women not only used high doses of aspirin and salicylates, but also unknown amounts of 'other drugs', which may have affected pregnancy outcome. Second, aspirin takers were clearly identified to the attendant obstetricians, which introduced an important potential observer bias, in particular because the amount of antepartum and postpartum haemorrhage appears to have been based on estimates rather than on accurate measurements of blood loss. The conclusions of this study have been contradicted by the results of several controlled trials involving pregnant women taking high doses of aspirin in the peripartum period for tocolysis or antithrombotic prophylaxis, and by the recent analysis of a large set of data derived from the prospective Collaborative Perinatal Project, which failed to indicate an increased risk of bleeding problems during labour or after delivery (de Swiet and Fryers, 1990). There has been no report of an increased maternal bleeding tendency in the low-dose aspirin studies in pregnancy carried out so far. The fear of epidural haematoma following epidural analgesia in pregnant women using a low dose of aspirin for prophylaxis of pregnancy-induced hypertensive disorders or fetal growth retardation, expressed in a recent editorial (MacDonald, 1991), seems to be based on theoretical considerations rather than on clinical evidence.

There is no evidence that the use of indomethacin for inhibition of preterm labour is associated with an increased incidence of maternal haemorrhage during or after labour (Besinger and Niebyl, 1990).

As discussed earlier, aspirin and indomethacin transferred to the fetus could have an inhibitory effect on platelet thromboxane synthesis. Based on anecdotal reports and two rather small prospective studies (Rumack et al, 1981; Stuart et al, 1982), this effect has been related to an increased bleeding tendency in the neonate. In contrast, several other studies have not shown an association between maternal use of aspirin or indomethacin and neonatal bleeding (Niebyl et al, 1980; de Swiet and Fryers, 1990). The most powerful study on this issue with regard to aspirin use in pregnancy is based on the prospective Collaborative Perinatal Project and comprises 2269 women who had taken aspirin in the last 10 days of pregnancy, and 7606 unexposed pregnant women. No differences were found between infants of mothers who had taken aspirin and infants not exposed to aspirin, with regard to the incidence of cerebral haemorrhage, and neonatal haemoglobin and haematocrit values (de Swiet and Fryers, 1990). No neonatal bleeding was noted in any of the low-dose aspirin studies in pregnancy reported. In conclusion, the evidence from controlled studies in large numbers of pregnant women taking variable therapeutic doses of aspirin for variable periods of time, and from smaller trials on the use of indomethacin and low-dose aspirin in pregnancy do not support the view that maternal use of aspirin or indomethacin in pregnancy is associated with an increase in maternal or fetal bleeding risk.

The use of aspirin in pregnancy has been associated with teratogenic effects, based on evidence derived from a number of case histories and from four case–control studies designed 'after the fact': data on aspirin exposure were collected after the birth of the (malformed) baby (Richards, 1969; Nelson and Forfar, 1971; Saxen, 1975; Zierler and Rothman, 1985). Such a study design is known to be liable to a great number of potential biases, such as drug recall, which may be more complete in women with abnormal infants than in control women with healthy babies, and observer bias because the interviewers are aware of the outcome of pregnancy. These biases were avoided in the large cohort study by Slone et al (1976) based on data from the prospective Collaborative Perinatal Project. In this study no single malformation was found to occur more frequently in children of over 14 000 mothers who took aspirin regularly in the first 4 months of pregnancy than in those of more than 35 000 mothers who were not exposed to aspirin. The large numbers make this a very powerful study. Results of other large studies support the absence of an association between aspirin use in the first trimester of pregnancy and fetal anatomical malformations in general (Crombie et al, 1970) and cardiac abnormalities in particular (Werler et al, 1989). Although an experimental study in rats had suggested that aspirin could act as a 'behavioural teratogen' by inhibiting learning in the offspring at maternal doses too low to produce anatomical malformations (Butcher et al, 1972), such an effect was not observed in a recent analysis by Klebanoff and Berendes (1988) of the data of a large prospective study on pregnancy and child development as part of the Collaborative Perinatal Project. In conclusion, the evidence that aspirin in therapeutic doses is not teratogenic and does not cause developmental delays in the offspring appears to outweigh data from retrospective case–control studies, case reports and animal studies, suggesting that the use of extremely high doses of aspirin in pregnancy may be associated with a (small) increase in the relative risk of fetal anatomical malformation and developmental retardation.

In the newborn, a physiological decrease in prostanoid synthesis in the wall of the ductus arteriosus is associated with smooth muscle contraction and functional closure of the doctus between 10–96 hours after birth (Coceani and Olley, 1988). Prostanoids are also involved in the vascular dilatation that takes place in the neonatal lung immediately after birth to allow an increase in blood flow to the expanding lungs at a low perfusion pressure. The recognition of the importance of prostanoid action in keeping the ductus open in fetal life has led to the use of indomethacin as an effective pharmacological tool in the treatment of patent ductus arteriosus in the, usually premature, neonate. For the same reason, fetal cyclooxygenase inhibition may be expected to carry a risk of premature constriction or perhaps even closure of the ductus, with diversion of right ventricular outflow into the pulmonary vascular bed. Increased pulmonary blood flow may result in pulmonary arterial hypertrophy (Levin, 1980). In addition, cyclooxygenase inhibition at birth could interfere with pulmonary vasodilatation and lead to pulmonary hypertension and right heart failure. Indeed, such effects have been shown to occur after high doses of aspirin and indomethacin in experimental animals and, although rarely, in pregnant women treated with indomethacin for tocolysis (Levin, 1980; Van Eyck, 1990).

Recent studies using Doppler echocardiography have demonstrated reversible constriction of the fetal ductus in pregnant women treated with indomethacin in a dose of 100–175 mg/day. Ductal constriction was often associated with tricuspid regurgitation, and with changes in the pulsatility index of the middle cerebral artery, suggestive of an increase in blood flow (Moise et al, 1988; Mari et al, 1989; Eronen et al, 1991). Doppler echocardiography has not shown any evidence of constriction of the ductus arteriosus in 30 women receiving a low dose of aspirin in the last 2–3 weeks of pregnancy (Sibai et al, 1989). To the best of the authors' knowledge only two cases of premature closure of the ductus associated with the use of indomethacin (Van Kets et al, 1979; Truter et al, 1986) and another two cases in women using extremely high doses of aspirin (Arcilla et al, 1969; Levin et al, 1978) have been reported in the accessible literature. In an analysis of several clinical trials on the tocolytic effects of indomethacin, Van Eyck (1990) failed to find a single case of premature closure of the ductus in a total of 328 pregnancies. About six case histories describe the occurrence or the suspicion of occurrence of persistent pulmonary hypertension in newborns of women using aspirin or, in particular, long-term indomethacin therapy (Van Eyck, 1990). Clinical experience with short-term indomethacin treatment (less than 48 hours) has failed to document such neonatal complications in a total of 584 exposed fetuses (Besinger et al, 1991). No neonatal vascular or pulmonary complications have been noted in the low-dose aspirin studies reported so far. In conclusion, although results of animal studies indicate that high maternal doses of aspirin and indomethacin can cause closure of the fetal ductus arteriosus, resulting in pulmonary hypertension in the offspring, the available clinical evidence strongly suggests that these complications are exceedingly rare in women receiving tocolytic treatment with indomethacin, in particular when it is of short duration, and even more rare in women using aspirin, even in high doses. Animal data and results of Doppler echocardiography in pregnant women indicate that the constrictor response of the ductus arteriosus to cyclooxygenase inhibition is reduced at lower gestational age (Eronen et al, 1991). This would imply that the smaller risk of fetal cardiovascular effects of indomethacin would be even smaller at gestational ages at which most can be gained from tocolysis and delay of delivery.

The fetal kidney is quite sensitive to indomethacin, and a reduced urinary output is often observed in fetuses of women treated with indomethacin for preterm labour, resulting in a reduction in amniotic fluid volume and even oligohydramnios. The effect seems to be dose-dependent and reversible (Kirshon et al, 1988; Goldenberg et al, 1989). Although oliguria may continue after birth in the neonate, there is no evidence that it leads to permanent impairment of renal function (Gleason, 1987).

IMPLICATIONS FOR CLINICAL PRACTICE

There appears to be a sound scientific rationale for attempts to prevent and treat maladaptation disorders in pregnancy through manipulation of the eicosanoid cascade. The effects of modulation of prostanoid synthesis in pregnancy by dietary supplementation with polyunsaturated fatty acids, in particular fish oil, on prevention of hypertensive disorders and fetal growth retardation are as yet completely speculative, but they deserve further investigation.

The results of a limited number of randomized, controlled trials in women at high risk indicate that selective inhibition of platelet thromboxane synthesis with a low daily dose of aspirin in the second and third trimester of pregnancy may significantly reduce the incidence of pregnancy-induced hypertensive disorders, fetal growth retardation, and sequelae such as prematurity and caesarean section. The potential benefits of the therapeutic use of a low dose of aspirin in pregnant women with established hypertensive disease or fetal growth retardation remain to be investigated. There are no apparent maternal and fetal hazards associated with the use of a low dose of aspirin in pregnancy. The currently available evidence seems strong enough to justify the prophylactic use of low-dose aspirin in women with a high risk of pre-eclampsia, eclampsia, or severe fetal growth retardation as judged from the obstetric history. The final assessment of the benefit–risk ratio of low-dose aspirin in pregnancy awaits the results of large on-going clinical trials that will become available in the course of 1993. The available evidence does not justify widespread clinical use of thromboxane synthase or receptor antagonists in pregnant women. Selective trials of these agents could prove to be of value.

There is no doubt that indomethacin is an effective inhibitor of myometrial contractility and that it may delay delivery. However, there are too few reliable data to support the contention that it reduces neonatal morbidity and mortality and to recommend it as a first-line tocolytic agent. Indomethacin is a useful drug for tocolysis when betamimetics fail at a gestational age at which even a few days of prolongation may improve neonatal outcome, also by referring the patient to a perinatal centre. There is no place for the use of aspirin or other cyclooxygenase inhibitors in the treatment of preterm labour.

REFERENCES

Abramson SB & Weissmann G (1989) The mechanisms of action of nonsteroidal antiinflammatory drugs. *Arthritis and Rheumatism* **32:** 1–9.

Andersen HJ, Andersen LF & Fuchs A-R (1989) Diet, pre-eclampsia, and intrauterine growth retardation. *Lancet* **i:** 1146.

Arcilla RA, Thilenius OG & Ranniger K (1969) Congestive heart failure from suspected ductal closure in utero. *Journal of Pediatrics* **75:** 74–78.

Bailey JM (1989) Biochemistry and pharmacology of cyclooxygenase inhibitors. *Bulletin of the New York Academy of Medicine* **65:** 5–15.

Bang HO (1990) Dietary fish oils in the prevention and management of cardiovascular and other diseases. *Comprehensive Therapy* **16:** 31–35.

Bat R, Vidyasagar D, Vadapalli MD et al (1979) Disposition of indomethacin in preterm infants. *Journal of Pediatrics* **95:** 313–316.

Beaufils M, Uzan S, Donsimoni R & Colau JC (1985) Prevention of pre-eclampsia by early antiplatelet therapy. *Lancet* **i:** 840–842.

Benigni A, Gregorini G, Frusca T et al (1989) Effect of low-dose aspirin on fetal and maternal generation of thromboxane by platelets in women at risk for pregnancy-induced hypertension. *New England Journal of Medicine* **321:** 357–362.

Besinger RE & Niebyl JR (1990) The safety and efficacy of tocolytic agents for the treatment of preterm labor. *Obstetrical and Gynecological Survey* **45:** 415–440.

Besinger RE, Niebyl JR, Keyes WG & Johnson TRB (1991) Randomized comparative trial of indomethacin and ritodrine for the long-term treatment of preterm labor. *American Journal of Obstetrics and Gynecology* **164:** 981–988.

Boeynaems JM, Demolle D & Van Coevorden A (1986) Prostacyclin-stimulating drugs: new prospects. *Prostaglandins* **32:** 145–149.

Branch DW, Scott JR, Kochenour NK & Hershgold E (1985) Obstetric complications associated with the lupus anticoagulant. *New England Journal of Medicine* **313:** 1322–1326.

Brown HL (1991) Antiphospholipid antibodies and recurrent pregnancy loss. *Clinical Obstetrics and Gynecology* **34:** 17–26.

Buchanan MR, Butt RW, Hirsh J, Markham BA & Nazir DJ (1986) Role of lipoxygenase metabolism in platelet function: effect of aspirin and salicylate. *Prostaglandins, Leukotrienes and Medicine* **21:** 157–168.

Butcher RE, Vorhees CV & Kimmel CA (1972) Learning impairment from maternal salicylate treatment in rats. *Nature (New Biology)* **236:** 211–212.

Cabrol D, Landesman R, Muller J et al (1987) Treatment of polyhydramnios with prostaglandin synthetase inhibitor (indomethacin). *American Journal of Obstetrics and Gynecology* **157:** 422–426.

Chalmers I, Hetherington J, Elbourne D, Keirse MJNC & Enkin M (1989) Materials and methods used in synthesizing evidence to evaluate the effects of care during pregnancy and childbirth. In Chalmers I, Enkin M & Keirse MJNC (eds) *Effective Care in Pregnancy and Childbirth*, pp 39–65. Oxford: Oxford University Press.

Clarke RJ, Mayo G, Price P & FitzGerald GA (1991) Suppression of thromboxane A_2 but not of systemic prostacyclin by controlled-release aspirin. *New England Journal of Medicine* **325:** 1137–1141.

Coceani F & Olley PM (1988) The control of cardiovascular shunts in the fetal and perinatal period. *Canadian Journal of Physiology and Pharmacology* **66:** 1129–1134.

Colli S, Caruso D, Tremoli E et al (1988) Effect of single oral administrations of nonsteroidal antiinflammatory drugs to healthy volunteers on arachidonic acid metabolism in peripheral polymorphonuclear and mononuclear leucocytes. *Prostaglandins, Leukotrienes, and Essential Fatty Acids* **34:** 167–174.

Collins E & Turner G (1975) Maternal effects of regular salicylate ingestion in pregnancy. *Lancet* **ii:** 335–338.

Corey EJ, Niwa H, Falck JR et al (1980) Recent studies on the chemical synthesis of eicosanoids. *Advances in Prostaglandins and Thromboxane Research* **6:** 19–25.

Crandon AJ & Isherwood DM (1979) Effect of aspirin on incidence of pre-eclampsia. *Lancet* **i:** 1356.

Crawford MA (1983) Background to essential fatty acids and their prostanoid derivates. *British Medical Bulletin* **39:** 210–213.

Crombie DL, Pinsent RJFH, Slater BC et al (1970) Teratogenic drugs—R.C.G.P. survey. *British Medical Journal* **iv:** 178–179.

Dennis EA (1987) Regulation of eicosanoid production: role of phospholipases and inhibitors. *Biotechnology* **5:** 1294–1300.

De Swiet M & Fryers G (1990) Review: the use of aspirin in pregnancy. *Journal of Obstetrics and Gynaecology* **10:** 467–482.

Dornhöfer W & Mosler KH (1975) Prostaglandine und β-Stimulatoren. In Jung H & Klöck FK (eds) *Th 1165a (Partusisten) bei der Behandlung in der Geburtshilfe und Perinatologie*, pp 196–202. Stuttgart: Georg Thieme.

Dutch TIA Trial Study Group (1991) A comparison of two doses of aspirin (30 mg vs 283 mg a day) in patients after a transient ischemic attack or minor ischemic stroke. *New England Journal of Medicine* **325:** 1261–1266.

Dyerberg J & Bang HO (1985) Pre-eclampsia and prostaglandins. *Lancet* **i:** 1267.

Dyerberg J, Bang HO, Stoffersen E et al (1978) Eicosapentaenoic acid and prevention of thrombosis and atherosclerosis? *Lancet* **ii:** 117–119.

Editorial (1988) Fish oil. *Lancet* **i:** 1081–1083.

Elder MG & Myatt L (1984) First use of nafazatrom, a new antithrombotic drug, in pregnancy. *Lancet* **i:** 1350.

Elder MG, De Swiet M, Robertson A et al (1988) Low-dose aspirin in pregnancy. *Lancet* **i:** 410.

England MJ, Atkinson PM & Sonnendecker EWW (1987) Pregnancy-induced hypertension: will treatment with dietary eicosapentaenoic acid be effective? *Medical Hypotheses* **24:** 179–186.

Eronen M, Pesonen E, Kurki T, Ylikorkala O & Hallman M (1991) The effects of indomethacin and a β-sympathomimetic agent on the fetal ductus arteriosus during treatment of premature labor: a randomized double-blind study. *American Journal of Obstetrics and Gynecology* **164:** 141–146.

Everett RB, Worley RJ, MacDonald PC & Gant NF (1978) Effect of prostaglandin synthetase inhibitors on pressor response to angiotensin II in human pregnancy. *Journal of Clinical Endocrinology and Metabolism* **46:** 1007–1010.

Farquharson RG, Pearson JF & John L (1984) Lupus anticoagulant and pregnancy management. *Lancet* **ii:** 228–229.

Fiddler GI & Lumley P (1990) Preliminary clinical studies with thromboxane synthase inhibitors and thromboxane receptor blockers. A review. *Circulation* **81(supplement 1):** I-69–78.

FitzGerald GA (1987) Dipyridamole. *New England Journal of Medicine* **316:** 1247–1257.

Fitzpatrick FA, Enis MD, Baze ME et al (1986) Inhibition of cyclooxygenase activity and platelet aggregation by epoxyeicosatrienoic acids. *Journal of Biological Chemistry* **261:** 15334–15338.

Gamissans O, Canas E, Cararach V et al (1978) A study of indomethacin combined with ritodrine in threatened preterm labor. *European Journal of Obstetrics, Gynecology and Reproductive Biology* **8:** 123–128.

Gibson RA (1988) The effect of diets containing fish and fish oils on disease risk factors in humans. *Australia and New Zealand Journal of Medicine* **18:** 713–722.

Gleason CA (1987) Prostaglandins and the developing kidney. *Seminars in Perinatology* **11:** 12–21.

Goldenberg RL, Davis RO & Baker RC (1989) Indomethacin-induced oligohydramnios. *American Journal of Obstetrics and Gynecology* **160:** 1196–1197.

Goodlin RC (1983) Correction of pregnancy-related thrombocytopenia with aspirin without inprovement in fetal outcome. *American Journal of Obstetrics and Gynecology* **146:** 862–865.

Goodlin RC, Haesslein HO & Fleming J (1978) Aspirin for the treatment of recurrent toxemia. *Lancet* **ii:** 51.

Hanley SP, Bevan J, Cockbill SR & Heptinstall S (1982) A regimen for low-dose aspirin? *British Medical Journal* **285:** 1299–1302.

Hansen HS (1983) Dietary essential fatty acids and in vivo prostaglandin production in mammals. *World Review of Nutrition and Dietetics* **42:** 102–134.

Hart FD & Huskisson EC (1984) Non-steroidal anti-inflammatory drugs. Current status and rational therapeutic use. *Drugs* **27:** 232–255.

Higgs EA, Moncada S & Vane JR (1986) Prostaglandins and thromboxane from fatty acids. *Progress in Lipid Research* **25:** 5–11.

Hoffmann P & Mest HJ (1987) What about the effects of dietary lipids on endogenous prostanoid synthesis? *Biomedica et Biochimica Acta* **46:** 639–650.

Hornstra G, Van Houwelingen AC, Kivits GAA et al (1990) Influence of dietary fish on eicosanoid metabolism in man. *Prostaglandins* **40:** 311–329.

Hytten FE (1991) The alimentary system. In Hytten F & Chamberlain G (eds) *Clinical Physiology in Obstetrics*, pp 137–149. Oxford: Blackwell Scientific.

Imperiale TF & Petrulis AS (1991) A meta-analysis of low-dose aspirin for the prevention of pregnancy-induced hypertensive disease. *Journal of the American Medical Association* **266:** 261–265.

Insel PA (1990) Analgesic–antipyretics and antiinflammatory agents; drugs employed in the treatment of rheumatoid arthritis and gout. In Goodman Gilman A, Rall TW, Nies AS & Taylor P (eds) *Goodman & Gilman's The Pharmacological Basis of Therapeutics*, pp 638–681. Elmsford, NY: Pergamon Press.

Jacobson RL, Brewer A, Eis A, Siddiqi TA & Myatt L (1991) Transfer of aspirin across the perfused human placental cotyledon. *American Journal of Obstetrics and Gynecology* **165:** 939–944.

Jespersen J (1980) Disseminated intravascular coagulation in toxemia of pregnancy. Correction of the decreased platelet counts and raised levels of serum uric acid and fibrin(ogen) degradation products by aspirin. *Thrombosis Research* **17:** 743–746.

Kagawa Y, Nishizawa M, Suzuki M et al (1982) Eicosapolyenoic acids of serum lipids of Japanese islanders with low incidence of cardiovascular diseases. *Journal of Nutritional Science and Vitaminology* **28:** 441–453.

Katz Z, Lancet M, Yemini M et al (1983) Treatment of premature labor contractions with combined ritodrine and indomethacine. *International Journal of Gynaecology and Obstetrics* **21:** 337–342.

Keirse MJNC, Grant A & King JF (1989) Preterm labour. In Chalmers I, Enkin M & Keirse MJNC (eds) *Effective Care in Pregnancy and Childbirth*, pp 694–745. Oxford: Oxford University Press.

Kelton JG (1983) Antiplatelet agents: rationale and results. *Clinics in Haematology* **12:** 311–354.

Kirshon B & Cotton DB (1988) Polyhydramnios associated with a ring chromosome managed with indomethacin. *American Journal of Obstetrics and Gynecology* **158:** 1063–1064.

Kirshon B, Moise KJ, Wasserstrum N et al (1988) Influence of short-term indomethacin therapy on fetal urine output. *Obstetrics and Gynecology* **72:** 51–53.

Khoo SK, Munro C & Battistutta D (1990) Evening primrose oil and treatment of premenstrual syndrome. *Medical Journal of Australia* **153:** 189–192.

Klebanoff MA & Berendes HW (1988) Aspirin exposure during the first 20 weeks of gestation and IQ at four years of age. *Teratology* **37:** 249–255.

Knapp HR & FitzGerald GA (1989) The antihypertensive effects of fish oil. A controlled study of polyunsaturated fatty acid supplements in essential hypertension. *New England Journal of Medicine* **320:** 1037–1043.

Knapp HR, Reilly IAG, Alessandrini P & FitzGerald GA (1986) In vivo indexes of platelet and vascular function during fish-oil administration in patients with atherosclerosis. *New England Journal of Medicine* **314:** 937–942.

Kurki T, Viinikka L & Ylikorkala O (1992) Urinary excretion of prostacyclin and thromboxane metabolites in threatened preterm labor: effect of indomethacin and nylidrin. *American Journal of Obstetrics and Gynecology* **166:** 150–154.

Lands WE (1986) Renewed questions about polyunsaturated fatty acids. *Nutrition Reviews* **44:** 189–195.

Levin DL (1980) Effect of inhibition of prostaglandin synthesis on fetal development, oxygenation, and the fetal circulation. *Seminars in Perinatology* **4:** 35–44.

Levin DL, Fixler DE, Morriss FC & Tyson J (1978) Morphologic analysis of the pulmonary vascular bed in infants exposed in utero to prostaglandin synthetase inhibitors. *Journal of Pediatrics* **92:** 478–483.

Levy G & Garrettson LK (1974) Kinetics of salicylate elimination by newborn infants of mothers who ingested aspirin before delivery. *Pediatrics* **53:** 201–210.

Lewis RB & Schulman JD (1973) Influence of acetylsalicylic acid, an inhibitor of prostaglandin synthesis, on the duration of human gestation and labour. *Lancet* **ii:** 1159–1161.

Lubbe WF & Liggins GC (1988) Role of lupus anticoagulant and autoimmunity in recurrent pregnancy loss. *Seminars in Reproductive Endocrinology* **6:** 181–190.

McCollum JR (1989) FDA alert on evening primrose oil. *Journal of the American Dietetic Association* **89:** 622.

MacDonald R (1991) Editorial: aspirin and extradural blocks. *British Journal of Anaesthesia* **66:** 1–3.

MacGillivray I (1983) *Pre-eclampsia: The Hypertensive Disease of Pregnancy*, p 229. London: WB Saunders.

McParland P, Pearce JM & Chamberlain GVP (1990) Doppler ultrasound and aspirin in recognition and prevention of pregnancy-induced hypertension. *Lancet* **i:** 1552–1555.

Manatt MW, Garcia PA, Kies C & Dupont J (1991) Studies of women eating diets with different fatty acid composition. II Urinary eicosanoids and sodium, and blood pressure. *Journal of the American College of Nutrition* **10:** 322–326.

Mari G, Moise KJ, Deter RL et al (1989) Doppler assessment of the pulsatility index of the middle cerebral artery during constriction of the fetal ductus arteriosus after indomethacin therapy. *American Journal of Obstetrics and Gynecology* **161:** 1528–1531.

Marshall PJ, Kilmacz RJ & Lands WEM (1987) Constraints on prostaglandin biosynthesis in tissues. *Journal of Biological Chemistry* **262:** 3510–3517.

Moise KJ, Huhta JC, Sharif DS et al (1988) Indomethacin in the treatment of premature labor. Effects on the fetal ductus arteriosus. *New England Journal of Medicine* **319:** 327–331.

Moise KJ, Ou C-N, Kirshon B et al (1990) Placental transfer of indomethacin in the human pregnancy. *American Journal of Obstetrics and Gynecology* **162:** 549–554.

Moodley J & Norman RJ (1989) Attempts at dietary alteration of prostaglandin pathways in the management of pre-eclampsia. *Prostaglandins, Leukotrienes, and Essential Fatty Acids* **37:** 145–147.

Morales WJ, Smith SG, Angel JL et al (1989) Efficacy and safety of indomethacin versus ritodrine in the management of preterm labor: a randomized study. *Obstetrics and Gynecology* **74:** 567–572.

Nelson MM & Forfar JO (1971) Associations between drugs administered during pregnancy and congenital abnormalities of the fetus. *British Medical Journal* **i:** 523–527.

Niebyl JR (1981) Prostaglandin synthetase inhibitors. *Seminars in Perinatology* **5:** 274–287.

Niebyl JR, Blake DA, White RD et al (1980) The inhibition of premature labor with indomethacin. *American Journal of Obstetrics and Gynecology* **136:** 1014–1019.

Noort WA & Keirse MJNC (1990) Prostacyclin versus thromboxane metabolite excretion: changes in pregnancy and labor. *European Journal of Obstetrics, Gynecology and Reproductive Biology* **35:** 15–21.

Oates JA, FitzGerald GA, Brand RA et al (1988) Clinical implications of prostaglandin and thromboxane A_2 formation. *New England Journal of Medicine* **319:** 689–698.

O'Brien PMS, Morrison R & Broughton Pipkin F (1985) The effect of dietary supplementation with linoleic and gammalinolenic acids on the pressor response to angiotensin II—a possible role in pregnancy-induced hypertension? *British Journal of Clinical Pharmacology* **19:** 335–342.

O'Brien WF, Williams MC, Benoit R, Sawai SK & Knuppel RA (1990) The effects of magnesium sulfate infusion on systemic and renal prostacyclin production. *Prostaglandins* **40:** 529–538.

Ogburn PL, Williams PP, Johnson SB & Holman RT (1984) Serum arachidonic acid levels in normal and preeclamptic pregnancies. *American Journal of Obstetrics and Gynecology* **148:** 5–9.

Olsen SF & Secher NJ (1990) A possible preventive effect of low-dose fish oil on early delivery and pre-eclampsia: indications from a 50-year-old controlled trial. *British Journal of Nutrition* **64:** 599–609.

Olsen SF, Hansen HS, Sorensen TIA et al (1986) Intake of marine fat, rich in (*n*-3)-polyunsaturated fatty acids, may increase birthweight by prolonging gestation. *Lancet* **ii:** 367–369.

Olsen SF, Olsen J & Frische G (1990) Does fish consumption during pregnancy increase fetal growth? A study of the size of the newborn, placental weight and gestational age in relation to fish consumption during pregnancy. *International Journal of Epidemiology* **19:** 971–977.

Olsen SF, Sørensen JD, Secher NJ et al (1992) Randomised controlled trial of effect of fish-oil supplementation on pregnancy duration. *Lancet* **339:** 1003–1007.

Patscheke H (1990) Thromboxane A_2/prostaglandin H_2 receptor antagonists. A new therapeutic principle. *Stroke* **21(supplement IV):** IV-139–142.

Pedersen AK & FitzGerald GA (1984) Dose-related kinetics of aspirin. Presystemic acetylation of platelet cyclooxygenase. *New England Journal of Medicine* **311:** 1206–1211.

People's League of Health (1946) The nutrition of expectant and nursing mothers in relation to maternal and infant mortality and morbidity. *Journal of Obstetrics and Gynaecology of the British Empire* **53:** 498–509.

Peto R, Gray R, Collins R et al (1988) Randomised trial of prophylactic daily aspirin in British male doctors. *British Medical Journal* **196:** 313–316.

Piper PJ (1984) Formation and actions of leukotrienes. *Physiological Reviews* **64:** 744–761.

Richards IDG (1969) Congenital malformations and environmental influences in pregnancy. *British Journal of Preventive and Social Medicine* **23:** 218–225.

Ritter JM, Farquhar C, Rodin A & Thom MH (1987) Low-dose aspirin treatment in late pregnancy differentially inhibits cyclooxygenase in maternal platelets. *Prostaglandins* **34:** 717–722.

Ritter JM, Cockcraft JR, Doktor HS et al (1989) Differential effect of aspirin on thromboxane and prostaglandin biosynthesis in man. *British Journal of Clinical Pharmacology* **28:** 573–579.

Rodgers RPC & Levin J (1990) A critical review of the bleeding time. *Seminars in Thrombosis and Hemostasis* **16:** 1–20.

Romero R, Lockwood C, Oyarzun E & Hobbins JC (1988) Toxemia: new concepts in an old disease. *Seminars in Perinatology* **12:** 302–323.

Rorarius MGF, Baer GA, Metsä-Ketelä T et al (1989) Effects on peri-operatively administered diclofenac and indomethacin on blood loss, bleeding time, and plasma prostanoids in man. *European Journal of Anaesthesiology* **6:** 335–342.

Rumack CM, Guggenheim MA, Rumack BH et al (1981) Neonatal intracranial hemorrhage and maternal use of aspirin. *Obstetrics and Gynecology* **58:** 52S–56S.

SALT Collaborative Group (1991) Swedish Aspirin Low-Dose Trial (SALT) of 75 mg aspirin as secondary prophylaxis after cerebrovascular ischaemic events. *Lancet* **338:** 1345–1349.

Sanchez-Ramos L, O'Sullivan MJ & Garrido-Calderson J (1987) Effect of low-dose aspirin on angiotensin II pressor response in human pregnancy. *American Journal of Obstetrics and Gynecology* **156:** 193–194.

Saxen I (1975) Associations between oral clefts and drugs taken during pregnancy. *International Journal of Epidemiology* **4:** 37–44.

Schiff E, Peleg E, Goldenberg M et al (1989) The use of aspirin to prevent pregnancy-induced hypertension and lower the ratio of thromboxane A_2 to prostacyclin in relatively high risk pregnancies. *New England Journal of Medicine* **321**: 351–356.

Schiff E, Barkai G, Ben-Baruch G & Mashiach S (1990) Low-dose aspirin does not influence the clinical course of women with mild pregnancy-induced hypertension. *Obstetrics and Gynecology* **76**: 742–744.

Secher NJ & Olsen SF (1990) Fish-oil and pre-eclampsia. *British Journal of Obstetrics and Gynaecology* **97**: 1077–1079.

Sibai BM, Mirro R, Chesney CM & Leffler C (1989) Low-dose aspirin in pregnancy. *Obstetrics and Gynecology* **74**: 551–557.

Slone D, Sikind V, Heinonen OP et al (1976) Aspirin and congenital malformations. *Lancet* **i**: 1373–1375.

Spearing G (1979) Alcohol, indomethacin and salbutamol. A comparative trial of their use in preterm labor. *Obstetrics and Gynecology* **53**: 171–174.

Spitz B, Magness RR, Cox SM et al (1988) Low-dose aspirin. I. Effect on angiotensin-II pressor responses and blood prostaglandin concentrations in pregnant women sensitive to angiotensin-II. *American Journal of Obstetrics and Gynecology* **159**: 1035–1043.

Steering Committee of the Physicians' Health Study Research Group (1989) Final report on the aspirin component of the ongoing physicians' health study. *New England Journal of Medicine* **321**: 129–135.

Stuart MJ, Gross SJ, Elrad H & Graeber JE (1982) Effects of acetylsalicylic-acid ingestion on maternal and neonatal hemostasis. *New England Journal of Medicine* **307**: 909–912.

Trudinger BJ, Cook CM, Thompson RS, Giles WB & Connelly A (1988) Low-dose aspirin therapy improves fetal weight in umbilical placental insufficiency. *American Journal of Obstetrics and Gynecology* **159**: 681–685.

Trudinger BJ, Cook CM, Giles WB, Connelly AJ & Thompson RS (1989) Low-dose aspirin and twin pregnancy. *Lancet* **ii**: 1214.

Truter PJ, Franszen S, Van der Merwe JV & Coetzee MJ (1986) Premature closure of the ductus arteriosus causing intra-uterine death. *South African Medical Journal* **70**: 557–558.

Uzan S, Beaufils M, Breart G et al (1991) Prevention of fetal growth retardation with low-dose aspirin: findings of the EPREDA trial. *Lancet* **i**: 1427–1431.

Vane JR (1971) Inhibition of prostaglandin synthesis as a mechanism of action for aspirin-like drugs. *Nature* **231**: 232–235.

Vane JR, Änggård EE & Botting RM (1990) Regulatory functions of the vascular endothelium. *New England Journal of Medicine* **323**: 27–36.

Van Assche FA & Spitz B (1988) Thromboxane synthetase inhibition in pregnancy-induced hypertension. *American Journal of Obstetrics and Gynecology* **159**: 1015–1016.

Van Assche FA, Spitz B, Vermylen J & Deckmijn H (1984) Preliminary observations on treatment of pregnancy-induced hypertension with a thromboxane synthetase inhibitor. *American Journal of Obstetrics and Gynecology* **148**: 216–218.

Van Eyck J (1990) The ductus arteriosus. *Fetal Medicine Review* **2**: 207–223.

Van Kets H, Thiery M, Derom R et al (1979) Perinatal hazards of chronic antenatal tocolysis with indomethacin. *Prostaglandins* **18**: 893–907.

Wallenburg HCS (1988) Prevention of hypertensive disorders in pregnancy. *Clinical and Experimental Hypertension* **B7**: 121–137.

Wallenburg HCS (1990) Maternal haemodynamics in pregnancy. *Fetal Medicine Review* **2**: 45–66.

Wallenburg HCS & Rotmans N (1987) Prevention of recurrent idiopathic fetal growth retardation by low-dose aspirin and dipyridamole. *American Journal of Obstetrics and Gynecology* **157**: 1230–1235.

Wallenburg HCS & Rotmans N (1988) Prophylactic low-dose aspirin and dipyridamole in pregnancy. *Lancet* **i**: 939.

Wallenburg HCS & Van Kessel PH (1978) Platelet lifespan in normal pregnancy as determined by a nonradioisotopic technique. *British Journal of Obstetrics and Gynaecology* **85**: 33–36.

Wallenburg HCS, Dekker GA, Makovitz JW & Rotmans P (1986) Low-dose aspirin prevents pregnancy-induced hypertension and pre-eclampsia in angiotensin-sensitive primigravidae. *Lancet* **i**: 1–3.

Wallenburg HCS, Dekker GA, Makovitz JW & Rotmans N (1991) Effect of low-dose aspirin on vascular refractoriness in angiotensin-sensitive primigravid women. *American Journal of Obstetrics and Gynecology* **164**: 1169–1173.

Wang Y, Kay HH & Killam AP (1991) Decreased levels of polyunsaturated fatty acids in preeclampsia. *American Journal of Obstetrics and Gynecology* **164**: 812–818.

Werler MM, Mitchell AA & Shapiro S (1989) The relation of aspirin use during the first trimester of pregnancy to congenital cardiac defects. *New England Journal of Medicine* **321**: 1639–1642.

Wiqvist N (1979) The use of inhibitors of prostaglandin synthesis in obstetrics. In Keirse MJNC, Anderson ABM & Bennebroek Gravenhorst J (eds) *Human Parturition*, pp 189–200. The Hague: Leiden University Press.

Wolff F, Berg R & Bolte A (1981) Klinische Untersuchungen zur wehenhemmenden Wirkung der Azetylsalizylsäure (ASS) und ihrer Nebenwirkungen. *Geburtshilfe und Frauenheilkunde* **41**: 96–100.

Worley RJ (1984) Pathophysiology of pregnancy-induced hypertension. *Clinical Obstetrics and Gynecology* **27**: 821–835.

Ylikorkala O, Mäkilä U-M, Kääpä P & Viinikka L (1986) Maternal ingestion of acetylsalicylic acid inhibits fetal and neonatal prostacyclin and thromboxane in humans. *American Journal of Obstetrics and Gynecology* **155**: 345–349.

Zierler S & Rothman KJ (1985) Congenital heart disease in relation to maternal use of bendectin and other drugs in early pregnancy. *New England Journal of Medicine* **313**: 347–352.

Zuckerman H, Reiss U & Rubinstein I (1974) Inhibition of human premature labor by indomethacin. *Obstetrics and Gynecology* **44**: 787–792.

Zuckerman H, Shalev E, Gilad G & Katzuni E (1984) Further study of the inhibition of premature labor by indomethacin. Part II. Double-blind study. *Journal of Perinatal Medicine* **12**: 25–29.

10

Prostaglandin analogues and their uses

MARC BYGDEMAN

INTRODUCTION

The prostaglandins of both the E and F groups are potent stimulants of the human uterus in vivo at any stage of pregnancy. They are extensively used clinically for termination of pregnancy and induction of labour. The main disadvantages of these compounds are a short half-life and the occurrence of gastrointestinal side-effects. The primary prostaglandins (prostaglandin $F_{2\alpha}$ ($PGF_{2\alpha}$) and PGE_2) are rapidly metabolized in the body. The initial steps in the enzymatic degradation are the oxidation of the 15-hydroxy group to a keto group and the reduction of the 13,14 double bond. The resulting 15-keto-13,14-dihydro compounds are essentially biologically inactive. When it comes to termination of pregnancy, these drawbacks are partly overcome by using intrauterine administration. Another alternative has been the development of prostaglandin analogues which are not substrates for the initial steps of enzymatic degradation by 15-dehydrogenase and have a more specific effect towards uterine rather than gastrointestinal muscle. A number of such analogues have been developed, some of which are in routine clinical use. These are $15(S)$-15-methyl-$PGF_{2\alpha}$ (carboprost, Upjohn Company), 16-phenoxy-17,18,19,20-tetranor-PGE_2 methyl sulphonylamide (sulprostone, Schering AG) and 16,16-dimethyl-*trans*-Δ^2-PGE_1 methyl ester (gemeprost, Rhône-Poulenc Rover). In contrast to the primary prostaglandins, these compounds can be administered by non-invasive routes, gemeprost vaginally and sulprostone and carboprost intramuscularly. Carboprost is also available for intravenous and intrauterine administration.

The fact that the analogues are administered vaginally or intramuscularly has allowed an extended clinical use for pregnancy termination. In contrast to primary prostaglandins, which are mainly used for termination of second trimester pregnancy, the analogues are useful for termination of early pregnancy, for preoperative dilatation of the cervical canal and for termination of second trimester pregnancy. Prostaglandin analogues have so far not been tried for induction of labour at or near term. In this situation, the longer duration of action is a drawback.

Baillière's Clinical Obstetrics and Gynaecology—
Vol. 6, No. 4, December 1992
ISBN 0–7020–1694–2

TERMINATION OF EARLY PREGNANCY

The possibility of using prostaglandins for termination of very early pregnancy has been evaluated since the beginning of the 1970s. The initial trials using $PGF_{2\alpha}$ or PGE_2 were mainly discouraging. The only effective route was intrauterine administration and premedication was necessary to reduce the frequency of side-effects. If analogues are used the situation is somewhat different. Repeated or single vaginal administration of the methyl ester of carboprost has been shown to be highly effective. This is also true for vaginal administration of gemeprost and meteneprost (9-deoxo-16,16-dimethyl-9-methylene PGE_2, Upjohn Company) or intramuscular injection of sulprostone. In a comparative study, gemeprost and meteneprost administered vaginally, and sulprostone given as intramuscular injections were found to be equally effective. The frequency of complete abortion was between 92 and 94% if the treatment was limited to the first 3 weeks following the first missed menstrual period. With the PGE analogues the side-effects were limited to occasional vomiting and diarrhoea in approximately 50% of the patients (Bygdeman et al, 1983). Even self-administration at home was shown to be possible (Bygdeman et al, 1984). The treatment results in an increase in uterine contractility followed by bleeding, which generally starts 3–6 hours after the initiation of therapy and lasts for 1–2 weeks. Most patients abort during the first 24 hours but minor residues of the conceptus without clinical importance may remain in the cavity for several weeks (Mandelin, 1978). The bleeding is described by most patients as heavier than a menstrual period but it does not generally affect the haemoglobin values. Heavy blood loss and pelvic infection occur in less than 2% of the patients (WHO Prostaglandin Task Force, 1982a). In a recent randomized study including 473 women, in whom repeated intramuscular injections of 0.5 mg of sulprostone were administered, this administration was shown to be equally effective as vacuum aspiration in terminating early pregnancy (WHO Prostaglandin Task Force, 1987).

In spite of the fact that in an acceptability study both prostaglandin and vacuum aspiration was equally appreciated (Rosén et al, 1984), no pharmaceutical company has introduced a prostaglandin analogue for termination of early pregnancy. It was not until the introduction of anti-progestin and its use in combination with prostaglandin analogues that a medical method to terminate pregnancy started to be accepted. The only antiprogestin in clinical use is RU 486 (mifepristone, Roussel Uclaf). Mifepristone is a progesterone receptor blocker which interferes with the action of progesterone at the target organ level (Baulieu, 1985). Treatment with mifepristone during early pregnancy will, after a latency period of 24–36 hours, result in increased uterine contractility due to withdrawal of progesterone inhibition of myometrial activity (Swahn and Bygdeman, 1988). It is possible that this treatment also to some extent stimulates endogenous $PGF_{2\alpha}$ production (Smith and Kelly, 1987), and the sensitivity of the myometrium to prostaglandin will be significantly increased (Swahn and Bygdeman, 1988). Although progesterone is regarded as essential for the maintenance of early pregnancy, treatment with mifepristone alone will not be sufficiently effective in terminating early pregnancy to compete with vacuum aspiration. However, if a small dose of prostaglandin analogue is added, the efficacy of treatment increases to almost 100% (Bygdeman and Swahn, 1985). The difference in efficacy of the different procedures to terminate early pregnancy is illustrated in a comparative study by Cameron and Baird (1988). Complete abortion occurred more often in women treated with vacuum aspiration (96%), gemeprost alone (97%) and mifepristone plus gemeprost (95%) than in those treated with mifepristone alone (60%). The treatments used were 1.0 mg of gemeprost every third hour five times; 150 mg of mifepristone daily for 4 days plus 1.0 mg gemeprost on day 3; and 150 mg mifepristone alone given daily for 4 days, respectively. While the combined treatment was equally effective as gemeprost alone, side-effects and analgesic requirements were much reduced in the women who received mifepristone alone or in combination with a single gemeprost pessary.

Mifepristone is at present registered for clinical use in France and the UK. Registration is expected in the Scandinavian countries by late 1992. Approximately 30% of all early abortions in France are treated with a combination of mifepristone and a prostaglandin analogue. A common treatment is a single dose of 600 mg of mifepristone followed 48 hours later by either 1.0 mg of gemeprost or an intramuscular injection of 0.25–0.50 mg of sulprostone. Silvestre et al (1990) have recently summarized the French experience of routine clinical use of the procedure, including 2115 early pregnant women (Table 1). The overall frequency of complete abortion was 96% with very little difference between the different dose schedules.

Table 1. Termination of early pregnancy with 600 mg of mifepristone followed 48 hours later by either 1.0 mg of cervagem or 0.25–0.5 mg of sulprostone (Silvestre et al, 1990).

Outcome of therapy	Patients (%)
Complete abortion	96.0
Incomplete abortion	2.1
Pregnancy continuation	1.0
Haemostatic procedure	0.9
Fever (infection)	0.3

However, the frequency of uterine pain was significantly lower with 0.25 mg of sulprostone and 1.0 mg of cervagem (14.9 and 21.3%, respectively) than with 0.375 and 0.5 mg of sulprostone (33.3 and 51.2%, respectively). Almost all patients started to bleed on the second day following mifepristone treatment and the mean duration of bleeding was between 7 and 12 days. The frequency of heavy bleeding needing curettage was, however, low (0.9%). Fever as a sign of infection was also very uncommon (0.3%) in the French study. The frequency of heavy bleeding and fever compares favourably with that often reported after vacuum aspiration performed during the first trimester of pregnancy. Serious complications associated with the therapy are very rare. However, one death has been reported. It occurred in association with the administration of sulprostone and the cause was a spasm in the coronary artery resulting in a massive infarction. The reason for this was unclear, but, since the woman was a heavy smoker, the pharmaceutical company has recommended that heavy smokers should not be treated with this therapy.

The best dose schedule of mifepristone and a prostaglandin analogue remains to be established. It is very likely, however, that the dose of mifepristone may be significantly reduced to 200 or even 50 mg. It is also likely that 0.5 mg of gemeprost would be sufficient.

Very recently, the combination of mifepristone and the orally active prostaglandin analogue misoprostol (15(S)-15-methyl-PGE$_2$ methyl ester, Searle AG) has been evaluated. Misoprostol is used in many countries for the treatment of gastric ulcers. It is considerably cheaper and more stable than cervagem and sulprostone. Preliminary studies indicate that a combination of 200 mg of mifepristone and 600 μg of misoprostol may be equally effective as previously described combinations (Aubernu and Baulieu, 1991; Norman et al, 1991). A potential problem with misoprostol is the risk of fetal malformations if the pregnancy continues in spite of treatment (Schönhöfer, 1991).

PREOPERATIVE CERVICAL DILATATION

Vacuum aspiration is the preferred method for termination of first and early second trimester pregnancy in many countries. If the procedure is performed after the seventh week of gestation, dilatation of the cervical canal is necessary. The need for greater mechanical dilatation of the cervix causes an increased risk of cervical laceration and uterine perforation and may have an adverse long-term effect on subsequent fertility. In addition, complications such as haemorrhage and incomplete evacuation of the products of conception may arise as a result of insufficient or difficult dilatation. For these reasons a variety of procedures has been investigated with the aim of developing a simple and safe method for preparing the cervix before dilatation and suction or mechanical curettage. Two alternatives are mainly used, either administration of prostaglandins or a cervical dilator such as a laminaria tent or lamicel, a synthetic hydrophilic polymer impregnated with magnesium sulphate. That prostaglandins can be used for this purpose was suggested at the start of the 1970s. A large number of studies have been published illustrating the advantages and disadvantages of prostaglandin treatment. In this review, reference will mainly be made to two large World Health Organization (WHO) studies. For more detailed references, the reader is referred to Lauersen (1986) and Herczeg (1990).

The first large clinical study was published some 10 years ago by the WHO Prostaglandin Task Force (1981). In this multicentre study with over 1000 patients, pretreatment with a vaginal suppository containing 1.0 mg of 15-methyl-PGF$_{2\alpha}$ methyl ester was randomly compared with placebo. The pretreatment time was either 3 or 12 hours. The study showed that a 3 hour pretreatment period resulted in a significant degree of cervical dilatation, fewer operative complications, shorter duration of postoperative bleeding and a lower frequency of recurettage and treatment of infection in comparison with pretreatment with placebo. The drawback of the treatment was a higher frequency of uterine pain and gastrointestinal side-effects with the active suppositories. These problems seem to be substantially reduced if PGE analogues are used instead. Both 1.0 mg of gemeprost administered vaginally and 0.5 mg of sulprostone given as an intramuscular injection are extensively used for cervical dilatation at present. Both compounds have been randomly compared in another WHO study (WHO Prostaglandin Task Force, 1986). Included in that study were also vaginal administration of meteneprost, the methyl ester of carboprost, and one laminaria tent (Table 2). The study showed that all three PGE analogues were equally effective as

Table 2. Randomized comparison between the laminaria tent, 1.0 mg of gemeprost and 0.5 mg of sulprostone for preoperative dilatation of the cervical canal. Outcome after 3 hours. Mean values ± SD.

| Method | Degree of cervical dilatation (mm) | Percentage of patients with | | | Blood loss (ml) |
		Vomiting	Diarrhoea	Analgesic injection	
Laminaria tent	6.9 ± 1.5*	0*	0.8	0*	67.9 ± 45.8
Gemeprost	7.4 ± 2.1	6.4*	0.8	10.3*	57.5 ± 56.3
Sulprostone	7.7 ± 2.2*	14.3*	4.8	4.0	57.3 ± 43.2

From WHO Prostaglandin Task Force (1986).
* Significant difference, $p < 0.05$.

one medium-sized laminaria tent and more effective than the PGF analogue after 3 hours. Both types of treatment are associated with a low frequency of side-effects. With the three PGE analogues the percentage of patients experiencing occasional episodes of vomiting varied from 6.4 to 14.3% and of diarrhoea from 0.8 to 4.8%. The frequency of vomiting was significantly higher than for a laminaria tent, but not statistically different for diarrhoea. Prostaglandin therapy has a practical advantage over the laminaria tent. The introduction of the tent, which is not always easy, has to be performed by medical staff, whereas prostaglandin treatment can be overseen by paramedical personnel.

Based on these and other studies, The Medical Advisory Committee of the International Planned Parenthood Federation has recommended either prostaglandin therapy or a laminaria tent to be used prior to vacuum aspiration in first trimester abortion (Editorial, 1984). Pretreatment with, for instance, gemeprost followed by vacuum aspiration may also be used during the first 2 weeks of the second trimester instead of conventional two-stage procedures. In a recent study comprising 1000 patients, the outcome of vacuum aspiration up to the 15th week of gestation was evaluated. All late first trimester primipara patients were pretreated with prostaglandin for 3 hours and the patients in early second trimester for 12 hours (Fried et al, 1989). Normally, the frequency of complications increases with gestational age. In this study, the overall complication rate was around 5% and the same in all stages of pregnancy, indicating that, if pretreatment with prostaglandin is used, vacuum aspiration can be safely carried out even in early second trimester abortion.

SECOND TRIMESTER PREGNANCY

Intra-amniotic and extra-amniotic administration of $PGF_{2\alpha}$ and extra-amniotic administration of PGE_2 is widely used for termination of second trimester pregnancy. An alternative is intra-amniotic injection of carboprost. This $PGF_{2\alpha}$ analogue is more potent and has a longer duration of action. The half-life of the analogue in amniotic fluid is approximately double that of $PGF_{2\alpha}$ itself (Gréen et al, 1976). Intra-amniotic administration of this analogue has been evaluated on a large scale in two multicentre studies involving 2506 subjects. A single dose of 2.5 mg of carboprost was compared randomly with either 40 or 50 mg of $PGF_{2\alpha}$ (WHO Prostaglandin Task Force, 1977a; Tejuja et al, 1978). With a success rate of almost 95%, the analogue was significantly more effective than $PGF_{2\alpha}$ (81–88%). The mean induction-to-abortion interval (18–20 hours) and the frequency of complete abortion (about 50%) were similar with both compounds, and gastrointestinal side-effects were within clinically acceptable limits. Injuries to the cervix were observed in 2.9% of the patients with both compounds in the WHO study, but were more common following treatment with 50 mg of $PGF_{2\alpha}$ in the Indian study. If a single-injection method is aimed at, carboprost seems to be a better alternative than the parent compound.

The most important advantage of the analogues carboprost, sulprostone and gemeprost is that these compounds can be administered by non-invasive routes. Some of the major complications associated with second trimester abortion are due to an inadvertent intravenous injection of the compound when it is administered intra-amniotically. If the vaginal or intramuscular route is used, such complications are avoided. These routes offer the additional advantage that the treatment is equally useful during both the early and late parts of the second trimester.

All three analogues have been used for termination of second trimester pregnancy. The results of a multicentre study performed by the WHO Prostaglandin Task Force (1977b) showed that repeated intramuscular injections of carboprost (initial dose 0.2 mg followed by 0.3 mg every 3 hours) was an effective method. About 85% of the patients aborted within 30 hours. The treatment was, however, associated with a high frequency of gastrointestinal side-effects. It was therefore concluded that this method has limited value as a primary abortion method but can be useful in order to complete the abortion process when another method has failed. If sul-prostone is used instead, the efficacy seems equally good, but the frequency of gastrointestinal side-effects are lower (WHO Prostaglandin Task Force, 1982). The efficacy of the treatment can be increased if the patients are pretreated with one laminaria tent. In a multicentre study performed by the WHO Prostaglandin Task Force (1988) 529 patients in the 13th to 22nd week of pregnancy who received this pretreatment were then randomly allocated either 0.25 mg of carboprost every second hour or 0.5 mg of sulprostone every fourth hour. Both treatment schedules were equally effective. The success rate was 95.6 and 94.5% for the PGE and PGF analogues, respectively, within 24 hours from start of prostaglandin therapy. The mean duration of prostaglandin administration was 10.8 hours and 11.3 hours, respectively. The study also showed that the treatment with sulprostone was associated with a significantly lower frequency of gastrointestinal side-effects than carboprost. With the former compound, 16.8% of the patients experienced occasional episodes of diarrhoea. The corresponding figure for vomiting was 41.1%. These figures are only slightly higher than those normally reported for intra-amniotic administration of hypertonic saline and comparable to those following intrauterine administration of PGE_2 or $PGF_{2\alpha}$.

Although studies randomly comparing vaginal administration of geme-prost and intramuscular injection of sulprostone have not been performed, available data indicate that the vaginal approach is an equally good alternative. The dose of gemeprost mainly used is 1.0 mg every 3 hours five times. If the abortion has not occurred within 24 hours, a further course of five pessaries is prescribed. When this treatment was given to 113 women in the 12th to 16th week of pregnancy, 82% of the patients aborted within 24 hours and an additional 14% during the second 24 hour period, giving an overall success rate of 96%. Vomiting and diarrhoea occurred in 14 and 20%, respectively (Cameron et al, 1987). In a more recent study, pregnancies up to the 18th week were included with equally good results (Rodger and Baird, 1990). Vaginal administration of gemeprost has also been shown to be equally effective as extra-amniotic administration of PGE_2. The treatment with gemeprost was less painful, and the simplicity of the treatment was another advantage appreciated by both patients and staff (Cameron and Baird, 1984) (Table 3).

Some recent studies indicate that pretreatment with an antiprogestin will increase the efficacy of prostaglandin treatment during the second trimester. If 200 mg of mifepristone was administered 24 hours prior to extra-amniotic administration of PGE_2 both the induction-to-abortion interval and total dose of PGE_2 were significantly reduced in comparison to pretreatment with placebo (Urquhart and Templeton, 1987). In another study patients were randomly allocated to receive either 600 mg of mifepristone or placebo prior to vaginal administration of 1.0 mg of cervagem every third hour. In the mifepristone pretreated group, 94% of the patients aborted within 24 hours compared with 80% of the placebo group. The median interval between administration of prostaglandin and abortion was significantly shorter in the mifepristone group (6.8 hours) compared with the placebo group (15.8 hours). The women pretreated with mifepristone also reported significantly less pain than the women who received placebo (Rodger and Baird, 1990). The outcome of a third study indicates that a combination of mifepristone and vaginal prostaglandin therapy may be highly effective even in late second trimester pregnancy (up to the 23rd week of gestation). In this study the patients were treated with either 200 mg of mifepristone orally or 0.5 mg of PGE_2 administered into the cervical canal. Twenty-four hours later the

Table 3. Termination of second trimester pregnancy by different prostaglandin analogues. Selected studies.

Compound	Dose	Route of administration	Success rate (%)		Reference
			24 hours	48 hours	
Carboprost	2.5 mg	Intra-amniotic		94.4	WHO Prostaglandin Task Force (1977a)
Laminaria + sulprostone	0.5 mg every 4th hour	Intracervical Intramuscular	95.6		WHO Prostaglandin Task Force (1988)
Cervagem	1.0 mg every 3rd hour	Vaginal	82		Cameron et al (1987)
Mifepristone + cervagem	600 mg 1.0 mg every 3rd hour	Oral Vaginal	94	96	Rodger and Baird (1990)
Mifepristone + metheneprost	200 mg 5.0 mg every 4th hour	Oral Vaginal	100		Gottlieb and Bygdeman (1991)

patients received 5 mg of meteneprost every fourth hour for up to 24 hours. All patients pretreated with mifepristone aborted within 24 hours while, following pretreatment with intracervical PGE_2, three patients out of 21 needed additional treatment. Pretreatment with mifepristone resulted in a shorter induction-to-abortion interval, a reduction in the total dose of meteneprost and less pain in comparison with pretreatment with intracervical PGE_2 gel (Gottlieb and Bygdeman, 1991).

CONCLUSIONS

The development of prostaglandin analogues represents a major breakthrough in abortion technology. In combination with the antiprogestin mifepristone, both vaginal administration of gemeprost and intramuscular injection of sulprostone have been demonstrated to be highly effective in terminating early pregnancy. This non-surgical method is increasingly used as an alternative to vacuum aspiration.

In late first and early second trimester abortion, pretreatment with these analogues will significantly facilitate vacuum aspiration and reduce the frequency of both operative and postoperative complications.

Both vaginal administration of gemeprost and intramuscular injections of sulprostone are highly effective methods of terminating mid- and late second trimester pregnancy. The simplicity of the therapy is an important advantage in comparison with intrauterine administration of abortifacient drugs. Preliminary data indicate that if the patients are pretreated with mifepristone the efficacy of the analogues will be further enhanced and both duration of labour and frequency of side-effects reduced.

REFERENCES

Auberny B & Baulieu EE (1991) Contragestion with RU 486 and an orally active prostaglandin. *Comptes Rendus Hebdomadaires des Séances de l'Académie des Sciences* **312:** 539–564.

Baulieu EE (1985) RU 486: an antiprogestin steroid with contragestive activity in women. In Baulieu EE & Segal SJ (eds) *The Antiprogestin Steroid RU 486 and Human Fertility Control*, pp 1–25. New York: Plenum Press.

Bygdeman M & Swahn ML (1985) Progesterone receptor blockage. Effect on uterine contractility in early pregnancy. *Contraception* **32:** 45–51.

Bygdeman M, Christensen NJ & Gréen K (1983) Termination of early pregnancy—future development. *Acta Obstetrica et Gynecologica Scandinavica* **supplement 113:** 125–129.

Bygdeman M, Christensen NJ, Gréen K & Vesterqvist O (1984) Self-administration at home of prostaglandin for termination of early pregnancy. In Toppozada M, Bygdeman M & Hafez ESE (eds) *Advances in Reproductive Health Care*, pp 83–90. Lancaster: MTP Press.

Cameron IT & Baird DT (1984) The use of 16,16-dimethyl-*trans*-Δ^2 prostaglandin E_1 methyl ester (gemeprost) vaginal pessaries for the termination of pregnancy in the early second trimester. A comparison with extra-amniotic prostaglandin E_2. *British Journal of Obstetrics and Gynaecology* **91:** 1136–1140.

Cameron IT & Baird DT (1988) Early pregnancy termination—a comparison between vacuum aspiration and medical abortion using prostaglandin (16,16-dimethyl-*trans*-Δ^2 PGE_1 methyl ester) or the antiprogestogen RU-486. *British Journal of Obstetrics and Gynaecology* **95:** 271–276.

Cameron IT, Michie AF & Baird DT (1987) Prostaglandin-induced pregnancy termination: further studies using gemeprost (16,16-dimethyl-*trans*-Δ^2 PGE$_1$ methyl ester) vaginal pessaries in the early second trimester. *Prostaglandins* **34:** 111–117.

Editorial (1984) *IPPF Medical Bulletin* **18:** 2–4.

Fried G, Östlund E, Ullberg C & Bygdeman M (1989) Somatic complications and contraceptive techniques following legal abortion. *Acta Obstetrica et Gynecologica Scandinavica* **68:** 515–521.

Gottlieb C & Bygdeman M (1991) The use of antiprogestin (RU 486) for termination of second trimester pregnancy. *Acta Obstetrica et Gynecologica Scandinavica* **70:** 199–203.

Gréen K, Granström E, Bygdeman M & Wiqvist N (1976) Kinetic and metabolic studies of 15-methyl PGF$_{2\alpha}$ administered intraamniotically for induction of abortion. *Prostaglandins* **11:** 699–711.

Herczeg J (1990) Pretreatment of the cervix prior to surgical evacuation of the uterus in the late first and early second trimester of pregnancy. *Baillière's Clinical Obstetrics and Gynaecology* **4(2):** 307–326.

Lauersen NH (1986) Induced abortion. In Bygdeman M, Berger GS & Keith L (eds) *Prostaglandins and their Inhibitors in Clinical Obstetrics and Gynaecology*, pp 271–314. Lancaster: MTP Press.

Mandelin M (1978) Termination of early pregnancy by a single-dose of 3.0 mg 15-methyl PGF$_{2\alpha}$ methyl ester vaginal suppository. *Prostaglandins* **16:** 143–152.

Norman JE, Thong KJ & Baird DT (1991) Uterine contractility and induction of abortion in early pregnancy by mesoprostol and mifepristone. *Lancet* **338:** 1231–1236.

Rodger MW & Baird DT (1990) Pretreatment with mifepristone (RU 486) reduces interval between prostaglandin administration and expulsion in second trimester abortion. *British Journal of Obstetrics and Gynaecology* **97:** 41–45.

Rosén A-S, von Knorring K, Bygdeman M & Christensen NJ (1984) Randomized comparison of prostaglandin treatment in hospital or at home with vacuum aspiration for termination of early pregnancy. *Contraception* **29:** 423–435.

Schönhöfer PS (1991) Misuse of misoprostol as an abortifacient may induce malformations. *Lancet* **337:** 1534–1535.

Silvestre L, Dubois C, Renault M, Rezvani Y, Baulieu EE & Ulmann A (1990) Voluntary interruption of pregnancy with mifepristone (RU 486) and a prostaglandin analogue. *New England Journal of Medicine* **322:** 645–648.

Smith SK & Kelly RW (1987) The effect of the antiprogestins RU-486 and ZK 98.734 on the synthesis and metabolism of prostaglandins F$_{2\alpha}$ and E$_2$ in separated cells from early human decidua. *Journal of Clinical Endocrinology and Metabolism* **65:** 527–534.

Swahn ML & Bygdeman M (1988) The effect of the antiprogestin RU 486 on uterine contractility and sensitivity to prostaglandin and oxytocin. *British Journal of Obstetrics and Gynaecology* **95:** 126–134.

Tejuja S, Choudhury SD & Manchanda PK (1978) Use of intra- and extra-amniotic prostaglandin for the termination of pregnancies. Report of multicentric trial in India. *Contraception* **18:** 641–652.

Urquhart DR & Templeton AA (1987) Mifepristone (RU 486) and second trimester pregnancy. *Lancet* **ii:** 1405.

WHO Prostaglandin Task Force (1977a) Comparison of single intra-amniotic injection of 15-methyl prostaglandin F$_{2\alpha}$ and prostaglandin F$_{2\alpha}$ for termination of second trimester pregnancy. An international multicentre study. *American Journal of Obstetrics and Gynecology* **129:** 597–600.

WHO Prostaglandin Task Force (1977b) Intramuscular administration of 15-methyl prostaglandin F$_{2\alpha}$ for induction of abortion in weeks 10 to 20 of pregnancy. *American Journal of Obstetrics and Gynecology* **129:** 593–600.

WHO Prostaglandin Task Force (1981) Vaginal administration of 15-methyl PGF$_{2\alpha}$ methyl ester for preoperative cervical dilatation. *Contraception* **23:** 251–259.

WHO Prostaglandin Task Force (1982a) Termination of early first trimester pregnancy by vaginal administration of 16,16-dimethyl-*trans*-Δ^2 PGE$_1$ methyl ester. *Asia Oceania Journal of Obstetrics and Gynaecology* **8:** 263–268.

WHO Prostaglandin Task Force (1982b) Termination of second trimester pregnancy by intramuscular injection of 16-phenoxy-ω-17,18,19,20-tetranor PGE$_2$ methyl sulfonylamide. *International Journal of Obstetrics and Gynecology* **20:** 383–386.

WHO Prostaglandin Task Force (1986) Randomized comparison of different prostaglandin analogues and laminaria tent for preoperative cervical dilatation. *Contraception* **34:** 237–251.

WHO Task Force on Postovulatory Methods for Fertility Regulation (1987) Menstrual regulation by intramuscular injections of 16-phenoxy-tetranor PGE$_2$ methyl sulfonylamide or vacuum aspiration. A randomized, multicenter study. *British Journal of Obstetrics and Gynaecology* **94:** 949–956.

WHO Prostaglandin Task Force (1988) Termination of second trimester pregnancy with laminaria and intramuscular 15-methyl PGF$_{2\alpha}$ or 16-phenoxy-ω-17,18,19,20-tetranor PGE$_2$ methyl sulfonylamide. A randomized multicentre study. *International Journal of Obstetrics and Gynecology* **26:** 129–135.

Index